PROBE MICROPHONE MEASUREMENTS

HEARING AID SELECTION AND ASSESSMENT

- H. GUSTAVE MUELLER, Ph.D. -
- JERRY L. NORTHERN, Ph.D. -
- DAVID B. HAWKINS, Ph.D. -

SINGULAR PUBLISHING GROUP, INC.
SAN DIEGO · LONDON

Singular Publishing Group, Inc.
4284 41st Street
San Diego, California 92105-1197

19 Compton Terrace
London N1 2UN, U.K.

Typeset in 10/12 Palatino by CFW Graphics
Printed in the United States of America by McNaughton & Gunn

Library of Congress Cataloging-in-Publication Data

Mueller, H. Gustav.
   Probe microphone measurements : hearing aid selection and
assessment / H. Gustav Mueller, David B. Hawkins, Jerry L. Northern.
     p.   cm.
   Includes bibliographical references and index.
   ISBN 1-879105-68-3
   1. Hearing aids — fitting. 2. Probe microphone measurment
(Audiology)   I. Hawkins, David B. II. Northern, Jerry L.
III. Title
   [DNLM: 1. Audiometry — instrumentation. 2. Hearing Aids.   WV 247
M946p]
RF300.M84 1992
617.8'9 — dc20
DNLM/DLC
for Library of Congress   92-9618
                                                 CIP

■ CONTENTS ■

▪ PREFACE ▪

Utilization of computerized probe-microphone real-ear measurements in hearing aid selection, fitting, and management has added a magnitude of science to the evaluation of personal amplification previously not available. During the decade of the 1980s we saw the introduction of this important technology advance to a desktop clinical instrument that could easily be included in the typical clinical hearing aid evaluation protocol. For the first time, dispensers of hearing aids had clinical equipment and procedures that permitted precise measurement of amplification characteristics of the hearing aid from within the patient's ear canal. Early advocates of computerized probe-microphone real-ear measurements recognized the magnitude of the contribution of this new technique as a means of turning the "art" of hearing aid fitting into an improved "scientific" approach.

The explosive growth of utilization of computerized probe-microphone real-ear measurements by audiologists speaks well for the value of the technique. On the other hand, this explosive growth has created confusion in sorting out terminology, definitions, and procedures. Clinicians and students, in order to gain information, have had to search numerous journals (including international publications) to keep up with the rapid development of probe-microphone research and clinical applications. While only three manufacturers' systems were available in 1986, we can now choose from nearly twenty different commercial probe-microphone systems. With each system comes a slightly different approach to measurements.

Thus, the need for a text devoted to probe-microphone real-ear measurements in hearing aid fitting is clear. Moreover, a text that combines the large body of research with state-of-the-art procedures would be a valuable asset

in the field of audiology. As clinicians, we use probe-microphone measures on a daily basis in our clinical practices, and we believe that a text which also provides practical guidelines will be useful to other clinicians.

The purpose of *Probe-Microphone Measurements: Hearing Aid Selection and Assessment* is to provide a comprehensive review of the utilization of probe-microphone measurements that will be readable and understood by the wide variety of hearing specialists concerned with hearing aids for persons who are hearing impaired. This text will be useful in academic training programs to increase the knowledge of graduate students as they study and learn the complexities of hearing aid selection and evaluation.

The information contained in this text covers a variety of technical topics. You will find general introductory information, historical development, definitions and terminology, as well as specific discussion of such problem topics as pediatric applications and information regarding custom in-the-ear or in-the-canal hearing instruments. We have also included technical areas such as prescriptive approaches to hearing aid fitting, correction factors and transfer functions, as well as how to use probe-microphone systems to measure maximum output and assess telecoil and assistive listening devices. Since this text is aimed at clinicians, ample information is provided on basic measurements, sample test protocols and procedures, and descriptions of current instrument systems.

This text has been under development for nearly two years, but every effort has been made to ensure that the information is current and represents state-of-the-art clinical practice. Although our primary purpose has been to detail the applications of computerized probe-microphone measurements, it is also our hope that this text will stimulate new thoughts and improved practices in the fascinating area of personal amplification for the person who is hearing impaired.

Gus Mueller
Fort Collins, Colorado

David Hawkins
Columbia, South Carolina

Jerry Northern
Denver, Colorado

CHAPTER 1

Introduction to Computerized Probe-Microphone Real-Ear Measurements in Hearing Aid Evaluation Procedures

JERRY L. NORTHERN, PH.D.

The challenge of developing scientifically based methods of selecting, evaluating, and fitting hearing aids moved a giant step forward with the advent of computerized probe-microphone real-ear technology. Although measuring the amplified output of a hearing aid in the patient's ear canal had been attempted since the early 1970s, successful clinical applications were dependent on the culmination of a number of technological innovations achieved dur-

ing the 1980s. These developments included the microprocessor-based desktop computer, the miniaturization of an appropriate microphone, and the utilization of a special, flexible, silicon tubing that could be inserted under the earmold or the in-the-ear (ITE) hearing aid and into the ear canal without interfering with sound transmission (Figure 1–1).

J. Donald Harris (1971) concluded that the purpose of clinical hearing aid work is to "pre-

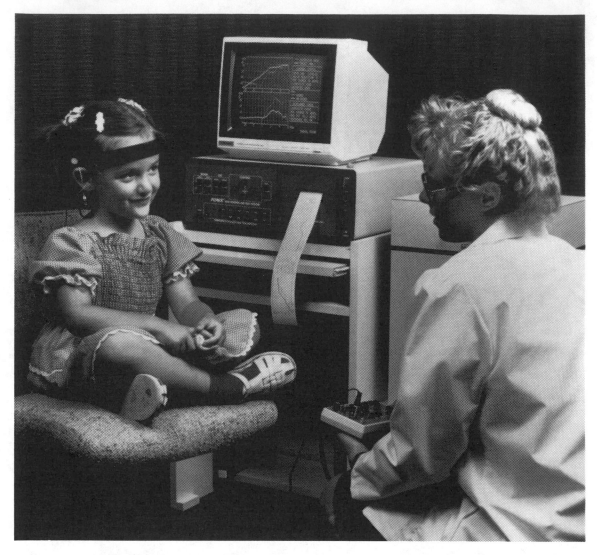

Figure 1–1. Clinical probe-microphone real-ear hearing aid system. Note video monitor, computer, and printout of measurements from the probe-microphone apparatus in child's right ear. Velcro headband holds microphone assembly in place. (Photograph courtesy of Frye Electronics, Tiregard, OR.)

sent to the ear as faithful a representation of the acoustic world as if the aid were in fact not present." Historically, the road to successful hearing aid fitting has been rough, with numerous divergent and digressive trends. It is difficult even to describe the development of a routine clinical hearing aid evaluation procedure due to our lack of standardized terminology and procedures. In fact, the only agreed-on concept in fitting personal amplifi-

cation devices is our understanding that it is difficult to validate the benefits of one fitting procedure over another, so that no one evaluation method seems to be consistently superior to any other evaluation method. The search for a universally acceptable approach to hearing aid selection continues to this day, and the solution, to a certain extent, continues to be elusive (Libby, 1985). We find ourselves with a myriad of fitting methods that have been utilized with varying degrees of commitment. Hearing instrument evaluation procedure ranges from formal mathematically based techniques to nonstandardized, informal methods based on the intuition of the audiologist or the subjective impression of the patient.

The literature abounds with research on the various techniques of hearing aid selection. The many variables that must be considered to produce successful hearing aid fittings include the motivation and personality of the patient. Since these variables must also have some relationship to the characteristics of the hearing loss, it is impossible to predict accurately amplification success with any degree of certainty. Curran (1988) described the hearing aid evaluation as a three step process: (a) a careful patient hearing history is obtained and a detailed hearing evaluation is completed; (b) some procedure is used to select, to recommend or provide, and then to fit the most appropriate hearing instrument(s) with minimal difficulty and time and effort; and (c) a unique interaction takes place among the patient, the hearing instrument(s), and the audiologist. This process may include adjustments and/or modifications to the amplification system to satisfy the person with impaired hearing. **It is this interactive process of adapting the hearing instrument(s) to a particular individual that challenges the expertise of every audiologist**.

The actual choice of procedure for selecting and fitting the hearing aid is the domain of the audiologist and varies considerably among professionals as a function of education, clinical circumstance, patient requirements, setting, philosophy, skill, and motivation. In this chapter, commonly utilized methods of hearing aid evaluation procedures are described and compared to the central theme of this book: real-ear computerized probe-microphone measurements in hearing aid fitting. According to Libby (1985) ear canal measurements performed with a computerized probe microphone assembly have introduced a new dimension of auditory research and should lead to improvement in the quality of hearing aid fittings. Before discussing the various hearing aid fitting procedures, it is relevant to review briefly the different electroacoustic measurements used with hearing aids.

ELECTROACOUSTIC MEASUREMENTS

The one aspect of the hearing aid selection procedure that leads to absolute measurement is the electroacoustic performance of the amplification system itself. Knowledge of the electroacoustic performance of the hearing aid system is essential to the understanding of each specific hearing aid's capabilities. Standard test procedures have been developed and used for the measurement of each electroacoustic parameter of the hearing aid to permit comparison among similar hearing aid models and instruments produced by different manufacturers. A hearing aid may appear acceptable under one method of electroacoustic measurement but unacceptable when another procedure is employed, conditions of measurement change, or variables are not well-controlled. Although a standardized measurement procedure has existed since 1960, it was the revised set of standards put into federal regulation by the Food and Drug Administration in 1977 (American National Standards Institute [ANSI], 1977) that required the hearing aid industry to measure and express hearing aid performance results according to a standardized set of rules and tolerances. The current version of the federal standard is ANSI S3.22, 1987.

The specification data provided by the manufacturers of hearing aids are, in fact, averaged performance measurements taken from many samples of the same hearing aid model. Thus, these data do not specifically describe the performance of the hearing aid under evaluation unless the aid is an ITE or in-the-canal (ITC) instrument that is furnished with its own performance curves. Furthermore, the response-curve tolerances permitted by ANSI S3.22 are fairly wide, permitting two models of the same hearing aid to be as much as ± 6 dB different at the same point on the specification sheet graph and still be within acceptable tolerance (Curran, 1988). That is, **two models of behind-the-ear (BTE) hearing aids can be different by as much as 12 dB and still "meet specs."**

Finally, it is now well-recognized that the electroacoustic characteristics of the hearing aid instrument are modified considerably by the "plumbing" of the system, which includes the earhook and tubing of BTE instruments, as well as all the earmold variables created by the fit, or "seal," in the external ear canal and concha, the length of the earmold canal, the diameter of the canal bore, the presence or absence of vents, and their specific physical diameter in the earmold. When the actual hearing instrument is coupled to the patient's ear, whether it is a BTE model or an ITE or ITC aid, the electroacoustic characteristics noted in the patient's ear canal are the result of the contributions of all these factors *plus* the physical features of the pinna, concha, external ear canal, and middle ear. Until the advent of the computerized probe-microphone real-ear measurement systems, **this acoustic result was impossible to predict with accuracy.**

Beck (1991) has pointed out that there has been a consistent evolution of measurement procedures progressing from the 2-cm^3 coupler to the Zwislocki coupler to the Knowles Electronics Manikin for Acoustic Research (KEMAR) to the hearing aid user directly, resulting in a level of realism that cannot be duplicated by any laboratory coupler measure. She stated that the dilemma that exists between using **in situ measures (that is, measurements taken with the hearing aid on the ear or in the ear canal)** and 2-cm^3 coupler data is analogous to speaking in two different languages. While correction factors can be applied to resolve differences between the two procedures, this mathematical solution is only an approximation of real-ear human performance.

THE 2-CM^3 CAVITY

The ANSI S3.22 standard requires electroacoustic hearing aid measurements to be made in a hard-walled 2-cm^3 coupler (Figure 1–2). The output of the hearing aid is delivered

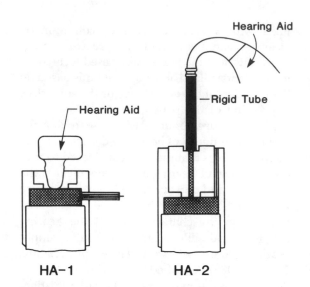

HA-1   HA-2

Figure 1–2. Standard 2-cm^3 couplers for electroacoustic measurement of hearing aid output. The HA-1 coupler, shown on the left, is used with ITE hearing aids and other hearing aids attached to an earmold. The HA-2 coupler, shown on the right, is used with standard tubing attached to a BTE hearing aid.

through a standard connector to the specific dimensions of the 2-cm^3 cavity while a condenser microphone measures the sound pressure level within the hard-walled cavity. The signal from within the cavity is amplified and recorded on a graphic or digital readout system. Results can be plotted across the frequency spectrum or at any specific frequency as a function of signal input level. The 2-cm^3 cavity technique was proposed by Romanow (1942) as a convenient coupler for hearing aids to readily produce standardized electroacoustic measurements. Thus, **this cavity was really never intended to simulate the adult ear canal, but was designed for use for quality-control purposes by hearing aid manufacturers** (Nielsen & Rasmussen, 1984). Romanow suggested, however, that correction factors could be applied to the measurements obtained in the 2-cm^3 cavity to simulate results in the human ear canal. It is ironic that this **2-cm^3, originally designed as a temporary solution, is still in use nearly 50 years later!**

The 2-cm^3 cavity obviously differs from the real human ear in terms of impedance and volume — particularly the amount of air space between the tip of the earmold and the eardrum, which varies considerably from person to person. It is well-recognized that the 2-cm^3 cavity lacks human realism. Pinna, head, and body baffle effects, plus the natural resonant properties of the ear canal, are absent from measurements made in the coupler. Therefore, curves obtained from a 2-cm^3 cavity are not accurate representations of a hearing aid placed in a human ear canal. This particular fact continues to be a source of real difficulty for clinicians when selecting personal amplification devices based only on manufacturer's specifications as measured in an acoustic coupler. In actual use, a hearing aid's performance will vary as a function of the size, shape, and impedance of the ear canal and middle ear, the manner in which it is coupled to the cavity, the setting of the volume control, the level of the input signal, and the position of the microphone. Electroacoustic measurements performed in accordance with ANSI S3.22 are best viewed as a method for ensuring baseline performance and product uniformity and not necessarily for purposes of selecting and fitting a hearing aid.

Preves (1984) suggested a technique to obtain a more realistic level of hearing aid performance assessment with the 2-cm^3 cavity by using the client's actual earmold with the HA-1 coupler. Although the precise effects of earmold characteristics cannot be accurately assessed with this technique, variations in the electroacoustic response with various earmold styles were shown by Northern and Hattler (1970). The problem with attempting to evaluate earmold venting effect in the 2-cm^3 coupler is that the hard-walled coupler has no resistive component, causing vent resonances (increases in sound pressure level [SPL] in the low frequencies due to the vent itself resonating) to be far larger when measured in the coupler than in the real ear. A number of studies (Cox, 1979; Preves, 1977; Studebaker, Cox, & Wark, 1978; Studebaker & Zachman, 1970) have shown that measurement of venting effects in a 2-cm^3 coupler will not be representative of what occurs in the real ear.

Madsen (1987) concluded that, from a clinical point of view, real-ear gain measurement is more desirable than coupler gain measurement. Real-ear gain describes the change in hearing conditions for the patient while wearing the hearing aid. Madsen also summarized the main reasons for differences that are found between real-ear and coupler gain as follows:

1. In clinical use, the hearing aid is mounted on the head or the body of a patient, which changes the gain and response characteristics of the hearing aid, due to diffraction effects;
2. The actual dimensions of the sound channel in the earmold may differ from the dimensions of the channel in the earmold simulator of the 2-cm^3 coupler;
3. During clinical use, the earmold will not always be a tight fit in the ear canal, thereby creating "slit-leak" of acoustic energy and creating change in the amplified low-frequency response;
4. The acoustic impedance of the volume between the earmold eardrum, combined with the impedance of the middle ear, will not be equivalent to the impedance of a simple, hard-walled cavity; and
5. The insertion of an earmold into the ear canal changes the resonance pattern of the ear canal.

THE ZWISLOCKI EAR-SIMULATOR

Other attempts to develop standard physical cavities that more closely resemble the human ear have been made. The Zwislocki ear-simulator (1970, 1971) represents more faithfully the mean impedance across the frequency range of various middle ears than do the 2-cm^3 couplers. However, this method still does not include consideration of the deviation of individual ear canals and diffraction effects caused by the body and head in hearing aid measurements.

KEMAR

The next major technical development was an effort to produce a realistic manikin to represent adult anthropomorphic values (Burkhard & Sachs, 1975). **KEMAR (an acronym for Knowles Electronics Manikin for Acoustic Research)** incorporates the Zwislocki occluded ear-simulator in the manikin's ear canal, to allow in situ hearing aid performance measurements that more closely approximate hearing aid performance during real life. The limitation to this physical representation of the human ear, however, is that the anthropomorphic values were taken from median adult human measurements, over the frequency range of 100–10,000 Hz; therefore KEMAR does not provide specific ear data for any particular individual. However, the use of KEMAR in engineering laboratories has contributed substantially to the understanding and objectifying of hearing aid performance in light of the effects of the torso, head, pinna, ear canal, microphone position, and acoustic coupling characteristics.

CORRECTION FACTORS

Since electroacoustic techniques for measuring hearing aid performance result in values that are substantially different from those obtained in human real-ear measurements, procedures for applying correction factors to data from 2-cm³ couplers, ear-simulators, or ear-simulators with KEMAR were developed. These correction factors enable researchers to make measurements on one type of electroacoustic system and predict results for any of the other systems. The problem with correction factors, however, is that the formulae are derived from average data and thus cannot represent absolute real-life situations.

Killion and Monser (1980) introduced the concept of **CORFIG (an acronym for Coupler Response for Flat Insertion Gain)**, which is a set of correction factors to predict insertion gain from coupler performance. The CORFIG correction factors are derived from a combina-

tion of (a) the unaided SPL produced at the eardrum, (b) the SPL produced at the in situ hearing aid microphone inlet, and (c) the difference between hearing aid output in the real ear and the 2-cm³ coupler. Thus, the CORFIG response is basically the correction that is subtracted from a coupler curve to predict insertion gain of a hearing aid, or the correction that is added to the insertion gain measurement to obtain the coupler response. The **insertion gain of the the hearing aid is simply defined as the difference in SPL produced by the hearing aid at a point in the ear canal and the SPL at the same point in the ear canal without the hearing aid**.

The 1970s brought development and utilization of physical substitute methods based on mathematical constructs, which were attempts to produce hearing aid measurements that would represent real-life situations. Although the limitations of these techniques were readily recognized, their purpose was, in part, to provide standardized procedures by which to evaluate hearing aid performance. Important advances in knowledge were made with these techniques, but the search continued into the 1980s to find a means by which real-ear measurements could be obtained while hearing aids were being worn. Figure 1–3 shows a comparison of full-on gain response curves obtained with the various electroacoustic measurement techniques as reported by Hawkins and Schum (1984). (For a more detailed description of correction and conversion factors from couplers to real ears, see Chapter 12.)

HEARING AID EVALUATION AND FITTING METHODS

Probably no single topic relative to hearing aids has been discussed as often, or written about more, than hearing aid evaluation procedures. Hearing aid evaluation implies the use of some clinical procedure for selecting the best instrument for each patient from among the many choices available to each hearing aid dispenser. Although each dispen-

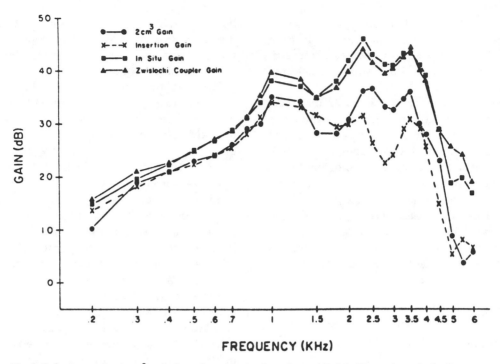

Figure 1–3. Curves for 2-cm³ gain, insertion gain, in situ gain, and Zwislocki coupler gain for the same BTE hearing aid. Curves were obtained in an anechoic chamber with the signal source at 0 degrees azimuth. (Reprinted from Hawkins, D., & Schum, D. 1984. Relationships between various measures of hearing aid gain. *Journal of Speech and Hearing Disorders, 49*, 109, with permission.)

ser has developed his or her own specific selection procedure(s), some general principles and procedural categories exist that permit descriptions of various approaches. The categories that divide the various hearing aid evaluation procedures are rather artificial, and most clinical procedures actually combine parts of more than one evaluation protocol. Some hearing aid selection procedures are related to the type of patient, that is, child or adult, verbal or nonverbal, and so on, or the type of hearing aid being fitted, that is, postauricular or in-the-ear. That hearing aid evaluation is still such a controversial subject after more than 50 years of exploring various techniques reflects the complexities of hearing aid selection and evaluation.

Curran (1988) wrote that no single hearing aid evaluation procedure can withstand close scrutiny because limitations to each method can be identified. Some methods require too

much time to complete while other methods depend on skillful subjective responses. Often the final decisions regarding hearing aid selection are a direct function of the dispenser's insight and experience. Many clinicians depend on some type of speech-based measurement to determine differences between hearing aids, although speech discrimination testing is well-noted to be generally unreliable; that is, speech discrimination test-retest reliability is too large to differentiate among hearing aids, since the test-retest variability of the speech discrimination test exceeds inter-hearing aid differences. A number of hearing evaluation problems must be dealt with in each selection procedure: (a) the measurement should permit rapid re-evaluation each time the hearing aid is adjusted electroacoustically; (b) the measurement should be sensitive enough to note small changes in hearing aid characteristics created when acoustic modifications are made in acoustic coupling system; (c) high objectivity and good reliability of measurements are desirable in the hearing aid evaluation procedure; and (d) some estimate of the validity of the hearing aid selected would be valuable.

Davies and Mueller (1987) wrote that most audiologists employ hearing aid evaluation protocols that can be described as a either *comparative* speech-based approaches or theoretical *prescriptive* fitting techniques, or perhaps a combination of the two. To be sure, other techniques such as *mirror-fitting, subjective preference,* and use of a *master hearing aid* are often incorporated into the evaluation, but the major component of the selection procedure can usually be described as either comparative or prescriptive.

THE COMPARATIVE HEARING AID EVALUATION

The essence of the comparative hearing aid selection technique is to evaluate a number of hearing aids on the patient with hearing impairment, conduct some type of formal or informal speech-based measurement with each hearing aid, and then pick the best performing hearing aid for fitting. This technique is a direct descendant of a well-known procedure described by Raymond Carhart following World War II in 1946. During Carhart's day, the challenge for clinicians was to identify the best brand of hearing aid to fit on soldiers with service-connected hearing loss. An important aspect of this procedure was that it is not necessary to know the absolute real-ear gain or the frequency response of each hearing aid utilized in the procedure, since this information was not readily available in a standard format at that time. The Carhart comparative procedure goal was to select the best hearing aid based on the percentage of correctly identified monosyllabic words. As part of a 12-step fitting procedure conducted over a 6-week period, comparison of speech recognition scores with different brands of hearing aids was made at equivalent sensation levels. The

hearing aid that produced the highest speech-discrimination score was selected and fit, even though the scores may have differed by only a few percentage points.

Jerger (1987) has pointed out that we now know monosyllabic word scores will not rank-order different hearing aid systems in a sufficiently reliable fashion to demonstrate that one hearing aid is significantly better than another. Mueller and Grimes (1983) showed that the variability of the speech materials used in comparative hearing aid evaluations may actually be greater than the differences among the hearing aids under evaluation. Mueller and Grimes tested a group of listeners with impaired hearing three separate times with the same hearing aid and found mean speech-recognition score differences of 5–7% with equally large standard deviations. They concluded that these findings caution against selecting the "best hearing aid" based on small percentage-correct word score differences.

There has been cyclic interest in the use of speech materials in the hearing aid evaluation procedure during the past four decades. Even as Carhart was describing his recommended formal speech-based comparative evaluation, the so-called Harvard Report strategy was published (Davis et al., 1946); this report proposed that the utilization of hearing aids having either a flat frequency response or a rising 6 dB per octave frequency response was sufficient for *all* persons with impaired hearing requiring amplification. A few years later, Shore, Bilger, and Hirsch (1960) attempted to use speech discrimination scores to identify differences among hearing aids with various acoustic parameters. They found that speech discrimination testing using monosyllabic words, in quiet or background noise, did not reveal differences among the hearing aids and that the lack of reliability of these measures did not justify the investment of the large amount of clinical time required to perform these procedures. These findings were confirmed by Jerger, Malmquist, and Speaks (1966), who concluded that **hearing aid performance measures based on single monosyllabic word lists** are sufficiently contaminated by error that they do not necessarily reflect meaningful differences between various hearing aids.

There are a number of well-recognized limitations to the comparative hearing aid selection procedure. A pure comparative procedure that matches every hearing aid against every other possible hearing aid would extend the time required beyond all reasonable means for any clinical procedure. Therefore, each audiologist selects only a few hearing aids for the listener to compare, thereby limiting the number of comparisons to a few preselected instruments. The speech-based test results can easily be contaminated by the order in which the hearing aids are presented and the lack of practice listening time by the patient with each trial hearing aid. Final measurement results are related to the actual technique utilized in the comparison procedure, and of course, there is no real measurement of reliability and fitting validity. Nonetheless, the comparative hearing aid evaluation procedure was reported to be the most popular method used by audiologists as recently as 1980 (Smaldino & Hoene, 1981).

THE PRESCRIPTIVE HEARING AID EVALUATION

The prescriptive hearing aid evaluation method is based on the assumption that given either a patient's pure-tone auditory thresholds, most-comfortable listening levels, and/or loudness discomfort levels, the appropriate amount of gain for each frequency can be calculated mathematically and optimum aided speech intelligibility can be obtained through a predetermined formula.There are numerous prescriptive formulae available and in use in the United States, as described fully in Chapter 5 of this book. For this discussion, however, it should be pointed out that the prescriptive method of selecting hearing aids has become the preferred method among audiologists for fitting ITE and ITC custom hearing aids; true comparative measurements are not feasible with these aids since only one custommade instrument is ordered for an individual.

To be sure, the prescriptive method of hearing aid evaluation also has its limitations. Most of the formulae are based on auditory threshold measurements, yet listeners with impaired hearing do not use their hearing aids at threshold audibility. Each fitting formula gives a different gain and frequency spectrum prescription so that selection of the proper formula becomes an issue among audiologists. The user is not personally involved in this selection method and therefore does not know what to expect until the hearing aid arrives from the manufacturer. And, once again, there really are no validity data relative to this hearing aid selection procedure.

FUNCTIONAL GAIN AS A HEARING AID EVALUATION PROCEDURE

Preves (1984) commented that the highest level of "realism" attainable in hearing aid measurement techniques is that of soundfield audiometry for obtaining functional gain — that is, the amount by which the hearing aid improves the patient's hearing threshold levels. This is a real-ear technique of evaluating hearing aid performance based on behavioral measurements. Functional gain measurements are commonly used by most audiologists, in one way or another, during the hearing aid selection if only to demonstrate improved hearing provided by the new hearing instrument compared with unaided performance. It may be questioned whether functional gain evaluation is actually a hearing aid fitting procedure, as some suggest that the procedure is best utilized as a method to verify a prescription fitting within some theoretical framework.

By definition, **functional gain is the difference in listener performance between aided and unaided threshold measures obtained in a soundfield**. On an informal basis, this procedure is often used to show the listening advantages gained while wearing the hearing instrument. The technique is also used in clinical procedures whereby actual soundfield unaided auditory thresholds are established for speech and warble tones (or narrow bands of noise), and compared with the same measurements obtained with a hearing aid turned on and in place. **The relative decibel difference between the two measurements, unaided and aided, is the functional gain.** Functional-gain measurements are generally easy to obtain and are therefore popular techniques to use with young children, elderly clients, and uncooperative patients.

At the same time, however, because this technique is used in the soundfield, a constant concern for accurate calibration without standing waves must be given consideration. Should the patient move even slightly between the aided and unaided condition measurements, the results of the hearing aid evaluation may be altered. Functional gain measurements usually differ from 2-cm^3 coupler data because of the influence of the ear canal resonance, the body and head baffle influence, and the normal variations expected from behavioral threshold measurements. Hawkins, Montgomery, Prosek, and Walden (1987) showed that a >15 dB difference between two sets of aided soundfield thresholds is necessary for the measurements to be statistically different, which suggests a major limitation in terms of test-retest variability in the same subject. Humes and Kirn (1990) studied the test-retest reliability of unaided and aided soundfield thresholds and the functional gain values derived from these measurements by testing 24 adults with sloping sensorineural hearing loss. They found that test-retest standard deviations were significantly larger for the derived functional gain values than for the unaided thresholds but only slightly (and nonsignificantly) larger than for the aided thresholds. When these functional gain data were compared with insertion gain results obtained with probe-microphone results, **the conclusion was reached that functional gain is the less reliable of these two methods of real-ear gain measurement.**

The functional-gain hearing aid evaluation has certain limitations. Since the technique is based on behavioral measurements, all the well-known factors leading to variability noted in behavioral auditory tests will influence functional gain test results as well. As functional gain testing is conducted in the soundfield, considerable attention must be given to careful calibration of the test stimuli and masking of the nontest ear to eliminate contamination of results when attempting to evaluate hearing aid performance. Since functional gain measurements are often made with acoustic signals at octave intervals, only the general characteristics of the frequency response will be noted, while interoctave spikes and valleys in the frequency response will be overlooked. Small changes in the electroacoustic output of the hearing instrument or acoustic modifications created by manipulation of the acoustic coupling system may create alterations in the frequency response and gain characteristics of the hearing aid that will not be noted with functional gain measurement.

HISTORY OF REAL-EAR PROBE-MICROPHONE MEASUREMENTS

It has always been clear that the optimal measurement of hearing aid performance should somehow be taken near the tympanic membrane while the amplification system is being worn and used by a human subject. Unoccluded probe-microphone measurements along the external ear canal were reported as early as 1946 by Weiner and Ross. A number of subsequent studies were reported by many authors using various fixed probe-microphone measurement techniques and equipment systems to evaluate earmold acoustics and hearing aid amplification. The Europeans produced many of the early studies including work reported by Ewertsen, Ipsen, and Nielsen (1956), Dalsgaard and Dyrlund-Jensen (1976), Johansen (1975), and Ringdahl and Leijon (1984). In North America, research efforts with probe-microphone measurements and hearing aids were published by McDonald and Studebaker (1970), Studebaker and Zachman (1970), Schwartz (1982), Preves (1982), and McCandless (1982).

In the United States, the development of the clinical application of real-ear probe-microphone measurements in the late 1970s must be credited to the efforts of Earl Harford, then an audiology professor at Northwestern University, and David Preves, who worked at that time as an acoustic/electronic engineer at Starkey Laboratories. During a 1979 conference, Harford (1981) first presented his results in measuring in situ hearing aid performance in clinical patients. Harford credited Preves with the development of an impedance-matching network that interfaced a new miniature microphone with acoustic laboratory equipment. This new equipment array permitted sound pressure measurements to be conducted within a patient's external auditory canal while a hearing aid and earmold were in place and operating (Figure 1–4).

Probe-microphone measurements of hearing aid amplification had been available since the classic work of Weiner and Ross (1946) some 30 years earlier. However, in the early years, the available equipment limited application of the technique to only laboratory envi-

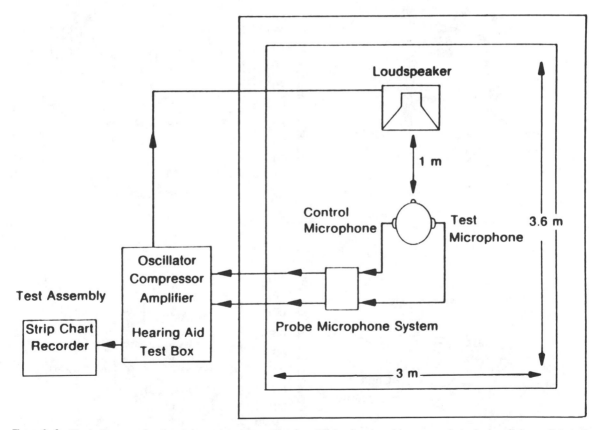

Figure 1–4. Block diagram of early equipment and apparatus for verifying hearing aid response in typical audiology clinic test suite. A miniature microphone is placed in each ear canal approximately 12 mm. The regulator microphone located in the non-test ear leads to a test box containing a compressor, amplifier, and oscillator which drives a loudspeaker. The test microphone leads to a strip chart recorder that prints out the SPL of the pure tone signal that reaches the test ear canal. (Reprinted from Harford, E. 1981. A new clinical technique for verification of hearing aid response. *Archives of Otolaryngology, 107,* 462, with permission.)

ronments. The early in situ hearing aid measurements were made by inserting a small hollow metal tube through the earmold into the external ear canal, which led to an external microphone located outside the canal — a situation Harford described as "cumbersome instrumentation and not very applicable to a clinical situation" (1981, p. 121).

The Harford-Preves technique utilized an exceedingly small (4 × 5 × 2 mm) Knowles electret microphone with a wide, flat frequency response. This microphone was so small that it could actually be placed within an adult's ear canal while a hearing aid was being worn. A sweep frequency oscillator and am-

plifier was placed in an acoustically treated sound chamber, and a compressor circuit was utilized to maintain a constant preselected sound-pressure level at the location of the miniaturized test microphone. This system was designed to record the sound-pressure level of a sweep-frequency test signal, amplified through a hearing aid, from within a subject's external ear canal (Figure 1–5).

The initial clinical protocol with this equipment utilized relative measurements and compared aided with unaided data. The measurements were obtained from a similar miniature microphone placed in the opposite (unaided, nontest) ear canal. The technique required the

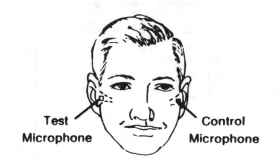

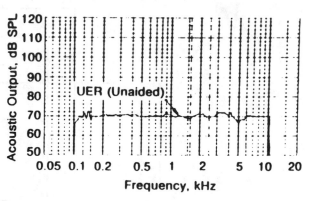

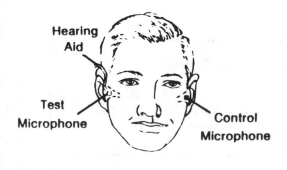

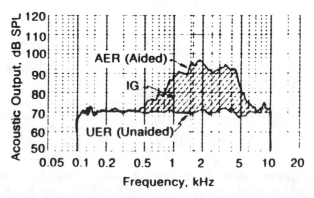

Figure 1–5. Schematic diagram of insertion gain measurement showing miniature microphones in ear canals and unaided equalization references (top) and aided equalizations response (bottom). The difference between the two measures is the hearing aid gain. (Reprinted from Harford, E. 1981. A new clinical technique for verification of hearing aid response. *Archives of Otolaryngology, 107,* 463, with permission.)

establishment of an unaided baseline known as the *unaided equalization reference.* Then a hearing aid was placed on the test ear and turned on, with the miniature test microphone in the ear canal, and a second recording was obtained known as the *aided frequency response.* **The difference between the two recordings was called the hearing aid insertion gain, a term originated by Ayers in a 1953 publication.** This actual hearing aid evaluation procedure was described by Romanow as early as 1942.

The frequency response and linearity of this early testing system had been previously established by Preves at the ·Starkey Laboratories (Harford, 1981). Preves showed on KEMAR that there was no significant difference in the recorded ear canal amplified signal with or without the miniature microphone in place. Harford's early clinical experience with this procedure proved that this real-ear probe-microphone system could be used effectively to quantify objectively the effect of earmold acoustics and the performance of the then relatively new, custom-made, ITE hearing aids. In personal correspondence during 1990, Harford admitted that his initial manuscript describing this equipment and clinical procedure was originally rejected by the *Journal of the Acoustical Society of America* as being "too superficial, trivial and unscientific."

Harford and his colleagues continued to develop and describe the clinical application of this real-ear in situ measurement technique (Harford, 1980a, 1980b, 1984; Harford, Leijon, Liden, Ringdahl, & Dahlberg, 1983; Leijon, Harford, Liden, et al., 1983; Wetzell & Harford, 1983). Dalsgaard and Dyrlund-Jensen (1976) compared real-ear probe-microphone measurements in unoccluded and occluded ear canal conditions with the earmold and hearing aid in place. Their results demonstrated that the 2-cm³ coupler response of a BTE hearing aid and earmold overestimates gain between 2000 and 4000 Hz by 12–18 dB, while in the low-frequency range the 2-cm³ coupler response *underestimates* the real-ear gain by 5–7 dB as shown in Figure 1–6.

These publications clearly established the value of in situ real-ear verification of the ear canal amplification measurements obtained in routine clinical settings. Although it was often noted that the procedures and instrumentation warranted additional refinement, clinicians and researchers used these valuable new data regarding the aided frequency response and insertion gain characteristics to reevaluate previous concepts of hearing aid design, selection, and fitting. The real-ear probe-microphone measurements were easy and quick to establish, objective, noninvasive, relatively inexpensive, and required only passive cooperation from patients. Harford (1980a) concluded, in what can now be regarded as considerable understatement, that

In our judgement, the utilization of these tiny precision microphones has the potential for improving the current state of the art of selecting and monitoring wearable amplification for the hearing-impaired. (p. 337)

CONTEMPORARY REAL-EAR PROBE-MICROPHONE SYSTEMS

Ear canal measurements performed with probe-tube microphone instrumentation introduced a new dimension to the knowledge, quality, and expertise of hearing aid fittings. Acoustic measurements performed in the ear canal, with and without the earmold and hearing aid in place, provide valuable information regarding the total combination of influences on the amplification device, including the impedance characteristics of the ear anatomy itself, as well as the acoustic plumbing (the tubing and earmold attached to the hearing aid) and the natural resonance of the individual's ear canal (Libby & Westermann, 1988). Sound-pressure measurements are taken with, and without, the fitted hearing aid in place, and insertion gain is determined as the difference in decibels between the two response curves (Figure 1–7). This technique is a considerable advance over previous efforts to make real-ear

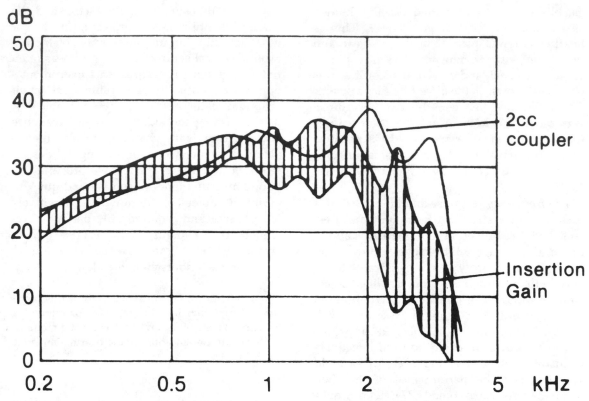

Figure 1-6. Comparison of typical test results in insertion gain measures with 2-cm³ coupler and probe-microphone measurements from a BTE hearing aid. It may be seen that the 2-cm³ coupler overestimates aided high-frequency response and underestimates low-frequency gain when compared to probe-microphone real-ear measurement.

microphone measurements, requiring only modest cooperation from the patient and minimum of testing time, with good data reliability provided appropriate care is taken in obtaining the measures. Hawkins (1987) noted that **the use of these real-ear probe-microphone measurements alone does not result in a better hearing aid fitting.** The critical feature of this method is that the professional have a goal to achieve with the hearing aid fitting; then real-ear probe-microphone measurements can be used to validate and verify the specific advantage provided by the amplification system under evaluation.

The routine clinical application of real-ear probe-microphone systems showed promise following the development of an equipment system that used an external microphone con-

nected to a soft silicone tube inserted into the ear canal through the vent of the earmold, thereby eliminating the need for a miniature microphone in the ear canal. Along with the new silicone tubing, which could be inserted into the ear canal under the earmold or custom ITE hearing aid for noninvasive measurements, was the application of desktop microprocessor technology. The first commercially available probe-microphone real-ear hearing aid measuring system was developed by Steen B. Rasmussen (the Rastronics CCI-10) in Denmark during 1983 and described the following year in the American literature (Rasmussen, 1984). Three additional manufacturers developed similar instrumentation by 1985, and three more new instruments were introduced in 1986 (Mahon, 1986).

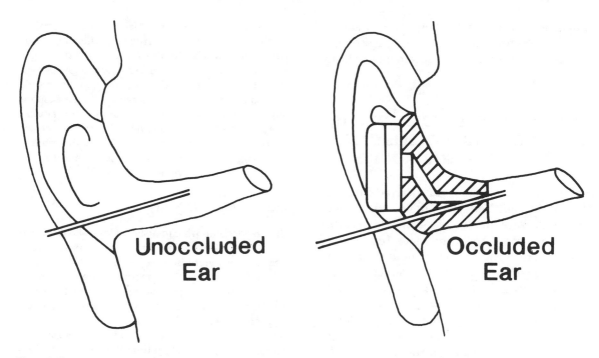

Figure 1–7. In real-ear probe-microphone measurements, the natural resonance of the ear canal is determined with the canal open (unoccluded), and then measurements of amplification from the hearing aid can be measured with the ear canal occluded. (Adapted from Dalsgaard, S., & Dyrlund-Jensen, O. 1976. Measurements of the insertion gain of hearing aids. *Journal of Audiologic Technique, 15,* 170.)

Essentially, each real-ear system consists of a signal generator and soundfield speaker, probe-tube and reference microphone, a computerized microprocessing unit, a video terminal, and/or hard-copy printout of frequency response curves (Chapter 2). The instruments vary in the type of input/output signals available, placement of the reference and probe microphone assemblies, memory, analysis, readout, and graphic display capabilities. The specialized equipment is available in a wide variety of models and prices ranging from packages that can be added to existing personal computers in the $2,000 level to sophisticated freestanding comprehensive systems that also serve as full office business systems with prices ranging beyond $12,500. Current systems continually undergo software improvements, which can be added to existing hardware components for easier menu-driven operation, improved color video graphics, portabil-

ity, mouse hand controls, and improved storage capabilities and hard-copy printing systems (see Chapter 2 for more information on computerized probe-microphone instrumentation).

According to a 1986 survey reported in the *Hearing Journal,* there were some 300–350 real-ear probe-microphone systems in use in the United States (Mahon, 1986); the Europeans had embraced this new technology more quickly than clinicians in North America. Over the next 3 years, however, the use of real-ear probe-microphone measurements in the United States grew to include some 36% of the entire dispenser population (Gallagher, 1989). The heaviest users in the 1989 report were dispensing audiologists who worked in settings other than private practice (49.5%) and private-practice dispensing audiologists (40.8%); only 14% of hearing instrument specialists responding to the survey used real-ear probe-microphone systems. The latest American Speech-

Language-Hearing Association (ASHA) survey in 1991 reported that 45% of audiologists utilize probe-microphone measurements in hearing aid selection.

RECOMMENDED COMPONENTS OF A HEARING AID SELECTION PROCEDURE FOR ADULTS

An important document was derived from the 1990 Vanderbilt/Veterans Administration Second Conference on Amplification held in Nashville, Tennessee. The conference brought together a large group of clinicians and scientists to discuss current considerations regarding all aspects of hearing aid technology and applications. Following the conference, a small group of selected committee members met to develop a consensus statement on hearing aid selection procedures for adults. For the first time, all the various aspects that comprise the hearing aid selection and fitting procedure were put into a format and published for all to read and consider. This document brings to the forefront a number of issues that previously had only been dealt with on a superficial level. The consensus statement is sufficiently important that it is presented here.

AMPLIFICATION FOR THE HEARING IMPAIRED:

Recommended Components of a Hearing Aid Selection Procedure for Adults 1990 Consensus Statement

Introduction

Significant changes have occurred in hearing aid circuitry, the measurement of hearing aid performance and hearing aid selection procedures in the ten years since the first *Vanderbilt/VA Hearing Aid Report*. Although much of this new technology has been integrated into the clinical setting, there still is no universally accepted protocol for selecting an appropriate hearing aid for a given individual. Certain aspects of the selection procedure, however, can be agreed upon by most individuals familiar

with both the research literature and the constraints of clinical practice. The purpose of this consensus statement is to outline the recommended components of a hearing aid selection procedure which meets the following five criteria: (1) it is defensible based on current research literature; (2) the responsibility for decision-making rests with the audiologist; (3) the goals for hearing aid performance are clearly stated; (4) these amplification goals are measured and verified; and (5) counseling and follow-up procedures are viewed as essential.

Hearing Aid Candidacy

The first decision which must be addressed is whether a person is a candidate for hearing aids. It is inappropriate to determine aid candidacy by referring only to hearing sensitivity as represented by thresholds for pure-tone signals or scores on word recognition tests. Anyone who describes hearing difficulties in communicative situations should be considered a potential candidate for hearing aids or other assistive devices. Unless clear contraindications exist, binaural hearing aids should be considered the preferred fitting for the prospective hearing aid user.

Determination of Initial Electroacoustic Characteristics

Selection of SSPL90

Some accepted type of suprathreshold judgement (e.g., loudness discomfort levels, uncomfortable loudness levels, or highest comfortable levels) should be used to determine an appropriate maximum output of the hearing aid. If the person is unable to perform such judgments, a data-based prediction method should be used to determine the SSPL90 setting. For instance, Cox (1979) has suggested that SSPL90 could be determined by the equation 100 + 1/4 HL. Other recommendations for selecting SSPL90 based upon pure-tone thresholds can be found in Cox (1988), Seewald and Ross (1988) and Skinner (1988).

Selection of Gain/Frequency Response

The 2-cm^3 coupler gain should be determined which will yield desired real ear performance as specified by a published gain/frequency response selection procedure (e.g., Berger, Hagberg, & Rane, 1988; Byrne & Dillon, 1986; Cox, 1988; Libby, 1986; McCandless & Lyregaard, 1983; Schwartz, Lyregaard, & Lundh, 1988; Seewald, Ross, & Stelmachowicz, 1987; Skinner, 1988). Many procedures provide corrections from desired real-ear gain to 2-cm^3 coupler gain for the average person. The best approach would be to obtain corrections on an individual basis rather than relying upon average values incorporated into the prescription procedure. An example of such a correction procedure can be found in Punch, Chi, and Patterson (1990). The particular corrections will depend upon the style of hearing aid used. (Use of certain programmable or newer hearing aid circuitry may obviate the need for some 2-cm^3 coupler real-ear conversions.)

Selection of Special Circuit Options

Decisions concerning limitation options, special circuitry needs, etc. should be made at this point.

Determination of Important Hearing Aid Features

Considerations of a variety of important hearing aid features must be incorporated into the decision making process. A needs assessment should be determined for a number of options or features, such as style of hearing aid, telecoil, direct audio input, raised volume control wheels and directional microphone.

Selection of Hearing Aids(s) Which Meet Desired Electroacoustic Characteristics

For behind-the-ear (BTE) hearing aids, the audiologist must select a hearing aid with the appropriate electroacoustic characteristics and options from available specification sheets. For in-the-ear (ITE) hearing aids, the audiologist should order the instrument by either (a) specifying the desired SSPL90 and full-on 2-cm^3 coupler gain (assuming a reserve gain of 10–15 dB); or (b) selecting an appropriate specific circuit designation described by the manufacturer.

Verification of Selected or Ordered Electroacoustic Characteristics

Upon receipt of the hearing aid and prior to delivery to the hearing aid user, electroacoustic measurements performed according to ANSI standards (S3.22 1987) should be completed to verify that the hearing aid functions according to the manufacturer's specifications. Additionally, in the case of an ITE hearing aid, the 2-cm^3 coupler gain and SSPL90 should be examined to determine if an appropriate circuit was delivered from the manufacturer.

Performance Assessment of Hearing Aid Characteristics on the User

Setting and Verification of SSPL90

The SSPL90 should be set to an appropriate level based upon earlier measurements. Verification of the chosen SSPL90 setting for prevention of loudness discomfort and over amplification should be performed for each ear. This determination can be accomplished through a variety of methods, such as Real-Ear Saturation Response (RESR), or presentation of controlled signals or intense environmental sounds to saturate the hearing aid.

Verification of Desired Real-Ear Gain/Frequency Response

The hearing aid should be adjusted to approximate as closely as possible the previously determined target values for each ear. Verification methods may include functional gain, aided sound-field thresholds, Real Ear Aided Response (REAR) or Real Ear Insertion Response (REIR). A determination that adequate reserve gain is available at the chosen use volume control position should be made as well.

Other Assessments

Some type of assessment, formal or informal, should be made of special features of the hearing aid, such as determination of whether adequate telecoil strength is available for the use of the telephone. The person's subjective reactions to amplified sound should be included in the evaluation. An assessment of the person's ability to understand amplified speech should be made. A number of different approaches, such as speech recognition scores, speech intelligibility ratings, or informal subjective responses, can be used for this purpose.

Counseling and Follow-up Procedures

Regardless of the selection strategy employed, proper counseling during the fitting and orientation and careful follow-up procedures are necessary if hearing aids are to be used successfully. During the initial stages of adjustment to amplification, electroacoustic characteristics may need to be altered based upon reactions and experiences of the hearing aid user. In addition, questions may arise which were not considered at earlier sessions and misunderstandings about information provided earlier and expectations may need to be clarified. Finally, other concerns about communicative strategies, remaining difficulties, and use of other devices may need to be explored. Without adequate counseling and follow-up, a well-selected hearing aid can be used improperly, inadequately, or not at all. (p. 321–323)

FUTURE DIRECTIONS

Audiology is a technology-driven field; that is, engineers often design and develop new circuits, new equipment, and new instruments and introduce them into the commercial marketplace before we have developed clinical applications. History is replete with examples, including acoustic immittance meters, evoked-response signal averagers, noise-canceling circuits, and the various types of compression circuitry found in today's hearing aids. Usually the introduction of this new technology is followed by a period of time during which clinicians and researchers use trial-and-error methods to ascertain the usefulness of the new equipment or circuit design. Sometimes the trial-and-error period produces substantive evidence for the incorporation of the new technology into everyday clinical practice; at other times, the evaluation of the new technology does not live up to the engineer's promises, and the scheme is abandoned. Nonetheless, seldom do audiologists set out to develop new technology to improve previous operations — rather we tend to be reactive in attempting to find ways to apply new technical systems.

Probe-microphone real-ear measurement equipment systems were readily available before we had developed clinical protocols, and standardized terminology or conducted the appropriate research studies to know exactly what information we wanted in terms of hearing aid fitting and evaluations. The past 5 years have seen an explosion in our literature with articles dealing with various hearing aid applications of real-ear probe-microphone measurements. Many audiologists comment that the world of hearing aid dispensing has suddenly become more scientific with the use of probe-microphone measurements and that we can now more fully appreciate the intricacies of fitting hearing aids.

Some clinicians believe that we have just begun to scratch the surface in terms of potential future applications of this specialized instrumentation. Klar and Trede (1986) suggested an innovative potential application of this instrumentation in terms of "real-ear audiometry." Their concept was that clinical audiometry (i.e., pure-tone air-conduction testing) could be done with a transducer with the probe tube at the tympanic membrane used to record behavioral auditory threshold in decibels SPL. Stuart, Durieux-Smith, and Stenstrom (1991) described a procedure to determine loudness discomfort levels in children using insert earphone receivers and probe-microphone monitoring of real-ear sound pressure as a means to compare real-ear audiometric measures and hearing aid performance. In fact, according to Beck (1991) of the U.S. Veterans Administration, the future is bright and we are on the threshold of significant changes in technology and the service delivery of hearing aids.

New directions for probe-microphone applications include the use of new and different stimuli as input signals for hearing aid performance measurement; auditory directionality and localization research; the utilization of extended-frequency amplification; in situ measurement of compression and noise reduction circuitry; evaluation of hearing protection devices, assistive listening devices, and telecoil circuitry; calibration of earphones; and a means to investigate new amplification-coupling systems. Other possible uses might include objective analysis of in situ transient-distortion applications, including the use of the real-ear probe-microphone systems for establishing in situ hearing threshold measurements to produce sound pressure level audiograms that will have immediate transference to hearing aid fittings.

CONCLUSION

Without doubt, computerized real-ear probe-microphone applications are among the most important advances in the history of hearing aid technology. Every aspect of the hearing aid evaluation procedure from instrument selection, fitting, electroacoustic adjustments, and acoustic modification can involve computerized real-ear probe-microphone measurements. Consideration of these digital measurements can provide information for audiologists to diagnose hearing aid problems and permit objective evidence for in-office modifications, setting trimmer adjustments, and providing immediate repairs, resulting in better service. Understanding real-ear probe-microphone measurements will provide information previously unavailable to the audiologist, and enable us to control better the amplified hearing aid gain and output and frequency response shape, smoothness, and bandwidth and to evaluate the effect of compression circuits. This specialized instrumentation may also be used in a wide number of audiologic procedures yet to be developed.

CHAPTER 2

Probe-Microphone Instrumentation

JERRY L. NORTHERN, Ph.D.

Although probe-microphone measurements at the tympanic membrane have been done since the mid-1940s, it has only been within recent years that clinically acceptable instrumentation has been commercially available. In 1983, a highly sophisticated, Apple computer-based probe-microphone system, which featured a self-calibrating microphone and soft silicone tube that could be placed under the earmold of the hearing aid into the patient's ear canal was introduced in Europe by Steen B. Rasmussen and H. Birk Nielsen. This instrument was designed to be clinically easy to use and did not require a typical sound-treated booth to reduce environmental noise. The instrument was programmed to perform many of the necessary measurements with minimal manipulation by the audiologist (Rasmussen, 1984).

This new instrument utilized techniques that were safe and comfortable for the patient, and offered a reliable, simple, and objective measurement of hearing aid performance from within the ear canal. Such measurement verified the performance characteristics of the hearing aid and also the interaction of amplification and impedance of the auricle, ear canal, and tympanic membrane. For the first time, audiologists **could easily measure the natural resonance of the unoccluded ear canal, which could then be included into the fitting rationale used to select an appropriate hearing aid** (Figure 2–1).

Klar and Trede (1986) commented that the "development of a practical real-ear (probe-microphone) hearing aid analyzer may be the most important step forward in the hearing health care industry since the advent of the semiconductor in 1953" (p. 15). They justified their statement with the prediction that the routine use of real-ear probe-microphone measurement procedures would lead to increased market penetration because of improved new user satisfaction through better fit and adjusted hearing aids.

The new instrumentation was rather slowly accepted by clinicians in the United States.

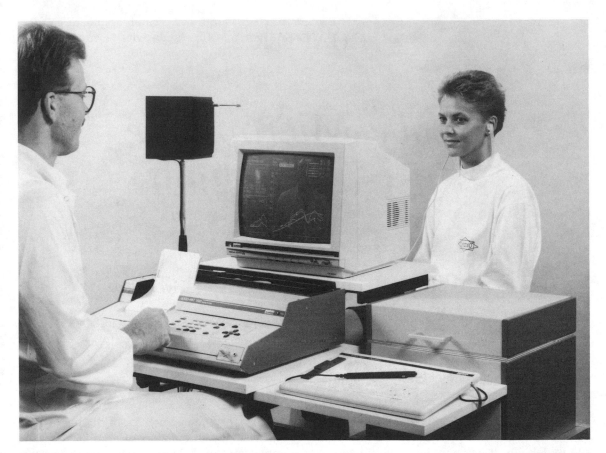

Figure 2-1. Example of a dedicated computerized probe-microphone real-ear hearing aid measurement system (Madsen IGO System). (Photo courtesy of Madsen Electronics, Mississauga, Ontario, Canada.)

However, there were intermittent delivery problems from Denmark, leaving numerous early orders for the equipment largely unfilled. This delay in delivery over the next few years provided an opportunity for other manufacturers to develop their own probe-microphone systems that were immediately available to eager purchasers. By 1987, four manufacturers had practical and reasonably priced real-ear probe-microphone systems, and three other manufacturers had announced their intention to have such systems available within the immediate future (Skadegard, 1987).

The acceptance of probe-microphone instrumentation in Australia and Europe was ahead of that in the United States. Skadegard (1987) reported that some 60% of Australian

hearing aid fittings were made with real-ear probe-microphone measurements. He added that in France, Denmark, Sweden, and Germany real-ear probe-microphone hearing aid fittings were the standard rather than the exception and that overseas the question was no longer "Should I consider real-ear probe-microphone techniques?" but "Which brand, which operations, and how much?" Skadegard concluded that in 1987, hearing aid dispensers in the United States trailed far behind the other industrialized nations with only 8% utilizing probe-microphone instrumentation.

Simon and Harlow (1987) believed that the hesitancy about using probe-microphone equipment in the United States revealed a lack of understanding about the benefits of such measurements. They suggested that many dispensers were confident about the success of their hearing aid fittings and saw no immediate need for incorporating this advanced (and expensive) new technology into their practice. Simon and Harlow added that real-ear probe-microphone equipment actually offered dispensers three major benefits: (a) increased marketing value, (b) improved hearing aid fittings, and (c) cost-effective benefits.

In terms of marketing and sales, Simon and Harlow (1987) suggested that probe-microphone technology offers hearing aid dispensers a new slant for advertising, which might include descriptions such as "computerized fittings" and "individualized" or "personalized" fittings with the latest technology. Probe-microphone systems provide immediate visual and acoustic verification of the hearing aid fitting to the patient and family members who might be present. Certainly, **the use of the video display and direct listening (monitoring) capabilities of the equipment provide an extremely interesting educational experience for all those present at the hearing aid fitting.**

Probe-microphone systems provide an efficient and objective means of verifying hearing aid fittings before the wearer leaves the office. Sullivan (1987) pointed out that the probe-microphone system permits virtually any hearing aid test procedure that can be performed in a 2-cm^3 coupler (ANSI S3.22 1976) or manikin with ear-simulator (ANSI S3.35 1985) to also be performed in the wearer's ear. The instrumentation can be used to verify that the hearing aid meets the audiologist requested characteristics (especially with ITE and ITC models) supplied by the hearing aid manufacturer. Hard copy of the hearing aid real-ear electroacoustics can be made to serve as a baseline in the event of later complaints about performance of the amplification instrument(s). Real-ear probe-microphone measurements can be used to verify acoustic and electroacoustic modifications as well as evaluate the need for repairs. Heide (1991) pointed out that real-ear probe-microphone mea-

surements more accurately estimate gain requirements for clients with normal or near-normal hearing sensitivity. Finally, this new technology offers the dispenser a more effective means to achieve success with difficult-to-fit persons with impaired hearing.

Another advantage is that real-ear probe-microphone measurements are faster than traditional repeated functional gain threshold measures (Heide, 1991). The real-ear probe-microphone measurement procedures (as described in Chapter 3) require a relatively short period of time, thereby leaving more time for patient counseling about the use and care of the hearing aid. The visual display of the amplification characteristics of the hearing aid often proves very useful in the counseling session to demonstrate the capabilities and performance of the selected aid. In addition, careful use of the probe-microphone system allows more accurate hearing aid fittings, with fewer returns, more satisfied clients, and, possibly, generates an increase in future customer referral and return patterns. According to Heide (1991) the use of real-ear probe-microphone measurements provides an increased degree of confidence in fitting adjustments as well as in the accuracy, validity, and reliability of amplification measurements (Figure 2–2).

Of course, in recent years, the variety of real-ear probe-microphone systems available includes products from nearly every major manufacturer of audiometric equipment. **As of 1991, we have nearly 20 different computerized probe-microphone systems from which to choose.** This wide range of equipment includes less expensive units and fully loaded, top-of-the-line systems, so the new consumer has a difficult task deciding which system to buy. A collection of commonly asked questions about real-ear measurement equipment was written by Mauldin and Trede (1991); and, of course, each system has its own pros and cons. Although differences among the various instrument systems are to be expected, each includes some basic and generic parts, which are described in the following text.

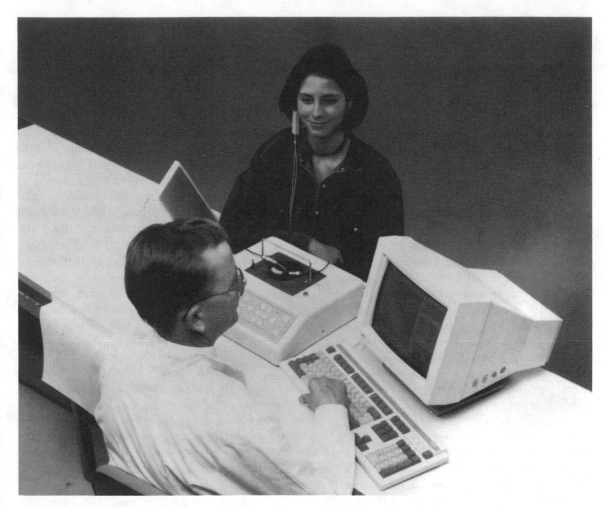

Figure 2–2. General computer-based probe-microphone real-ear hearing aid measurement system (Madsen CAS). (Photo courtesy of Madsen Electronics, Mississauga, Ontario, Canada.)

COMPUTERIZED PROBE-MICROPHONE INSTRUMENTATION

GENERAL COMPUTER-BASED SYSTEMS

General computer-based real-ear probe-microphone equipment may be used for other applications such as word processing, office management, patient data storage and retrieval, and even more technical procedures such as pure-tone and/or speech audiometry. Consid-eration should be given to the availability of useful software, desktop space requirements, ease of use and clinical efficiency, training provided by the computer manufacturer or sales office, and service and technical support access. File storage systems may be available for complete hearing aid office operations including mail merge programs; personalized form letters; inventory of hearing instruments by make, model, and serial number; sales and pricing information; accounts receivable and invoice capability; employee payroll; hearing aid repair records; and battery sales and battery club information.

DEDICATED-COMPUTER SYSTEMS

Dedicated computer probe-microphone systems are designed specifically for real-ear hearing aid measurements only. Often the keyboard or input device is specific to the needs of the hearing aid analysis. Some dedicated real-ear probe-microphone systems are compatible with general computers such as IBM-based systems, which can then be used to generate the other applications described above.

PROBE-TUBE MICROPHONE

Most contemporary real-ear systems utilize a miniaturized, self-calibrating microphone with a very soft silicone probe-tube extension for making measurements near the tympanic membrane. Some means of marking the silicone probe-tube microphone extension should be available (such as a sliding sleeve around the tube or other holding device) to permit reliable replacement of the tube if necessary.

REFERENCE MICROPHONE

The electret reference microphone, used in the comparison method of signal calibration (see Chapter 4), maintains the stimulus level near the patient's ear at a constant sound pressure level (SPL) during the test signal presentation. The main purpose of the reference microphone is to act as a standard against which the probe signal is compared. The reference microphone eliminates most of the influence created by patient movement and poor environmental acoustic conditions; it also eliminates the need for testing to be conducted in a sound-treated test booth or room. Most real-ear measurement systems locate the reference microphone somewhere near the test ear pinna, although if the reference microphone is located too near the microphone of the hearing aid under evaluation, feedback conditions may exist when sufficient hearing aid gain is determined.

COMPRESSOR MICROPHONE

Some manufacturers use a high-performance compressor microphone system rather than a reference microphone. The compressor microphone controls the intensity of the stimulus coming from the soundfield speaker, keeping the stimulus at a constant intensity level regardless of the distance of the speaker from the patient.

STIMULUS SIGNALS

A variety of stimulus signals are available on most real-ear probe-microphone systems. The effects on measurement of real-ear amplification in probe-microphone systems have been considered by several researchers including Hawkins and Mueller (1986), Hawkins (1987), and Mueller and Sweetow (1987). A thorough discussion of stimulus signals may be found in Chapter 4. Brief descriptions of various stimuli that may be found in probe-microphone instrumentation follow.

Clicks

A click is a broad frequency spectrum transient of short duration characterized by an instantaneous onset. The actual acoustic spectrum, however, is heavily influenced by the transducer capabilities. Clicks are difficult to calibrate precisely because of the inability to define, or limit, the frequency spectrum. In addition, the rapid onset of the click stimulus may activate the automatic gain suppression circuit of the hearing aid, thereby giving erroneous performance results of the amplification system under evaluation.

Composite Noise

Composite noise is composed of a large number of individual sinusoidal signals summed for simultaneous presentation. The result is a "noise-like" stimulus with controlled spectral characteristics. Composite noise stimuli are commonly used in probe-microphone measurements because they can be generated to mimic the spectrum of spoken speech, which is the signal of most interest to hearing aid wearers. Some system manufacturers provide a predefined composite signal, whereas other systems permit the user to synthesize varying signal spectra for custom applications (Frye, 1986).

Narrow-band Noise

Narrow-band noise stimuli are generally produced by one-third-octave band filtering of broad-band white noise. The narrow-band noise stimuli may automatically track the sweep frequency of the measurement or may be individually selected for specific frequency analysis of the hearing aid.

Pure Tone

A pure tone is a continuous sinusoid of a single frequency typically available at any specific point within the test frequency range. Because of the well-known standing wave problems caused by reflective surfaces, continuous pure tone stimuli are not recommended for real-ear probe-microphone measurements.

Warble Tone

Warble tones are created by a frequency modulation of a single frequency continuous sinusoid stimulus. Warble tones are typically not easily influenced by standing waves from reflective surfaces, and therefore they are commonly used in real-ear measurements.

ANALYSIS OF MEASUREMENTS

Probe-microphone systems generally use one of three forms of signal analysis: swept filter analysis, Fast Fourier Transform, and real-time measurement.

Swept-Filter Analysis

In this analysis system, used in most probe-microphone systems, a one-third-octave nar-

row-band filter tracks the sweep-frequency test signals. Background noise will contaminate the probe-microphone measurements, so the effect of the narrow-band filter on the measurement is to eliminate, as much as possible, influences from the unwanted sounds of the environment. The probe-microphone measures the output of the narrow-band filter and monitors the SPL of the stimulus signal. This analysis technique enables the probe-microphone systems to be used outside of traditional sound-treated booths.

Fast Fourier Transform

Schwietzer (1986) described the application of Fast Fourier Transform (FFT) computations to hearing aid analysis in probe-microphone instrumentation. This mathematical principle is used to separate a complex wave into its constituent frequency and intensity components. In addition, the technique also permits analysis of the time dimension of the complex sound wave. Schwietzer compared the FFT analysis of a complex waveform into its various frequency components to the manner in which a prism separates light into its various spectral colors. Instruments that use real-time analysis techniques can show all three dimensions of acoustics (frequency, amplitude, and time) on one video or graphic display.

Real-Time Measurement

Frye (1986) commented that we normally listen to a mixture of sounds mixed with noise, and therefore it is unrealistic to use pure tones to evaluate hearing aids. He pointed out that a hearing aid might have a different saturation response for pure tones than for noise and that it is difficult to test the gain and frequency response of automatic gain control (AGC) hearing aids with pure tones. Frye described a technique designed with time domain signal processing that can produce frequency response tests of a hearing aid at the rate of about two per second, thereby permitting nearly immediate measurement of the changes in response to adjustments.

VIDEO DISPLAY

A wide variety of video display equipment is available with real-ear probe-microphone systems, both in color and monochrome formats. With the monochrome displays, multiple frequency-response curves are presented with different line patterns (solid line, broken line, dots, dashes, and so on), or different densities are used for each result to allow for differentiation of several curves when presented on the screen at the same time. With color video display, each frequency response curve is likely to be presented in its own color. The use of a color video monitor has great appeal to patients and may make explaining results easier.

Although most probe-microphone systems use a cathode-ray tube (CRT) video display, some manufacturers use a liquid crystal display screen. The major problem with the liquid crystal display screen is that reading the screen may be somewhat difficult under certain conditions, such as when the screen reflects light.

A valuable feature is a movable cursor, or arrow of some sort, to measure specific points along the frequency response curves or determine the exact difference in decibels between two curves at a certain frequency.

PRINTER

The routine use of a printer to produce hard copy records of real-ear probe-microphone measurements is extremely valuable. The real-ear measurement graphs become an important part of every client's file. The printer may also be used to record the 2-cm^3 results of electroacoustic hearing aid analysis. Usually, the format of the printed record mirrors the video graphic display. In general terms, printers provide three print formats for hearing aid graphs: (a) thermally treated paper printout in strip format; (b) dot matrix printer output on computer paper; or (c) color print on specially prepared and treated paper.

Many printers are computer driven from video screen menus, which may permit rotating the printout 90° or printing the video graph information in numerical format.

Hard copy of the hearing aid's initial fitting performance will serve as a permanent record against which to compare later amplification performance — especially when the client returns with complaints about the hearing aid. Hard copy data also permit comparison of pre- and post-repair alterations in the performance of the hearing aid. Printout paper should provide space for the date, hearing instrument model, model number, patient's name, and special comments to be written in by hand or automatically inserted by the computer.

TEST CHAMBER

Many probe-microphone systems include a sound treated contained test chamber that permits 2-cm^3 coupler measurements in accordance with the ANSI standards. Some manufacturers sell the acoustic treated sound chamber as an optional external accessory to the system. Many systems will manually, or automatically, perform the complete test battery, or specific segments of the test battery, as described by ANSI S3.22 1987. Some probe-microphone systems provide a "free-field" 2 cm^3 coupler test rather than a test chamber per se; other systems provide for both test arrangements.

PORTABLE SYSTEMS

Numerous real-ear probe-microphone hearing aid analysis systems are now available in units that are compact and easily transportable. These systems may be moved among offices or used at the bedside of an institutionalized client. These systems often include an attractive, relatively lightweight, self-contained carrying case. If you intend to use the probe-microphone system in more than one location, a portable unit may fit your needs.

PROBE-MICROPHONE INSTRUMENTS

ACOUSTIMED HA-2000II

The Acoustimed HA-2000II is an IBM computer-based real-ear and 2-cm³ coupler system. Speech shaped complex, pure tone, and sweep-tone test signals are synthesized in the computer and presented through the speaker for testing in the patient's ear and in the 2-cm³ couplers provided with the system.

The use of the computer with hard drive storage allows the saving of test results for comparison with follow-up tests. The software provided with the HA-2000II includes a comprehensive database for client, hearing aid, and audiometric record-keeping. The full-sized color monitor provides assistance in counseling patients regarding their hearing loss and the results of the real-ear measurements.

Additional test capabilities with the HA-2000II include the measurement of Real Ear Aided Responses (REARs) with the speech shaped complex signal, the sweep tone, and real voice or telephone signals. Transient responses and phase shift of hearing aids may be measured. Soundfield thresholds may be tested with the *Acoustometry* programs, using the probe-microphone to measure the levels at which the patient responds. Speech may be digitized and played back for testing and for simulation of hearing loss.

The software may be upgraded as the technology changes to ensure that the system will not become obsolete (Figure 2–3).[1]

AUDIOSCAN RM500

The Audioscan RM500 Real-Ear System is the smallest and lightest of the portable systems. While it performs all the essential functions of

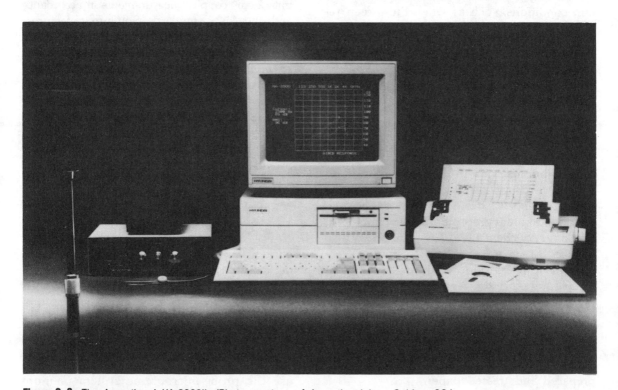

Figure 2–3. The Acoustimed HA-2000II. (Photo courtesy of Acoustimed Inc., Golden, CO.)

[1]For more information, contact Acoustimed, Inc., 2801 Youngfield, Suite 178, Golden, CO 80401.

the larger, more-expensive units, it has been developed with special attention to ease of use and elimination of sources of error. All functions are accessed directly from a keyboard by means of clearly labeled single-function keys, with on-screen instructions providing appropriate guidance. A true two-channel system (with a warbled stimulus and optimized tracking filters) and extensive self-test diagnostics ensures hardware accuracy while expert software checks for blocked probe tubes, speaker overdrive, and hearing aid nonlinearity.

The RM500 is unique in its ability to display real-ear data either as SPL insertion gain or aided thresholds on an audiogram. All thresholds are accompanied by an articulation index calculation. These tools not only provide a new level of assistance in fitting optimization, but also are valuable counseling aids.

In addition to its real-ear measurement capabilities, the RM5000 also contains a test chamber, couplers, and software for single-button hearing aid tests in accordance with ANSI S3.22 1987 (Figure 2–4).[2]

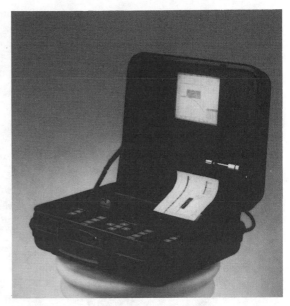

Figure 2–4. The Audioscan RM500 Real Ear system. (Photo courtesy of Audioscan, Dorchester, Ontario, Canada.)

BIO-LOGIC SYSTEMS

Bio-logic's Real-Ear Probe is an add-on package to their evoked potential instruments, the Navigator and Traveler Express. This probe package is also available as a kit to convert an IBM-compatible computer to a real-ear measurement system. Full keyboard, color monitor, menu-driven software, and floppy disk storage make this system user friendly. Since this system is IBM-compatible, many other software packages can be utilized with it by hearing aid dispensing facilities.

The FFT algorithm produces data points in the frequency responses every 125 Hz. There is a "zoom" feature that expands desired sections of the curves. Two microphones are used in the pressure mode normally, but the reference microphone may be turned off to permit the substitution method of equalization. The reference microphone also may be placed directly over the hearing aid microphone inlet for a true pressure soundfield equalization via Velcro or a headband strap.

Either a pseudorandom noise or a click is used for input stimuli, with external inputs being accepted as well. Hard copy is available with a standard built-in color ink-jet printer.

Threshold values may be entered and stored for each patient's audiogram for use with several stored hearing aid prescription methods. Up to 10 curves may be displayed simultaneously on the CRT.

An automatic mode permits real-ear and unaided measurements with a minimum of operator interaction. Several target formulae are available, including POGO, Libby, and NAL. There is also a manual mode that allows you to create your own target curve (Figure 2–5).[3]

---

[2]For more information, contact Audioscan, 41 Byron Avenue, Dorchester, Ontario, Canada N0L 1G0.

[3]For more information, contact Bio-Logic Systems Corp., One Bio-logic Plaza, Mundelein, IL 60060.

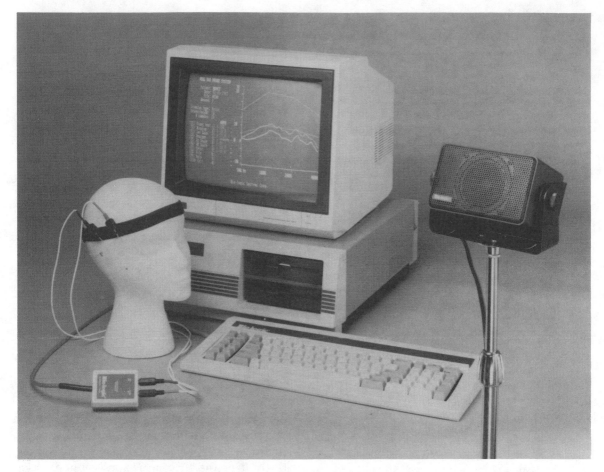

Figure 2–5. The Bio-Logic Real Ear Probe System. (Photo courtesy of Bio-Logic Systems Corporation, Mundelein, IL.)

ENSONIQ

The ENSONIQ Sound Selector Fitting System combines ear-calibrated audiometry with real-ear measurement by the substitution method using an electronically simulated diffuse field.

Ear-calibrated audiometry provides a common point of reference for measuring thresholds and real-ear gain. It eliminates the SPL variances caused by differences between a calibration cavity and the individual ear. Additionally, it minimizes the effects of headphone placement, interaural crossover, and collapsed canals.

A diffuse field represents the "real world" environment. The substitution method includes diffraction effects of the head, torso, and instrument; coupling acoustics; and angle of incidence. The conditions needed to produce a diffuse field and use the substitution method are impractical at most sites. ENSONIQ controls these conditions by electronic simulation, making them repeatable from office to office.

Probe microphones (accurate within tenths of a decibel) measure the SPL generated in the ear canals by calibration signals. The signals represent a diffuse field and are delivered electronically through the instruments. The measured SPL is the REAR. The real ear insertion response (REIR) is computed by subtracting the real ear unaided response (REUR) of the average unoccluded ear in a diffuse field from the measured REAR of the patient. As

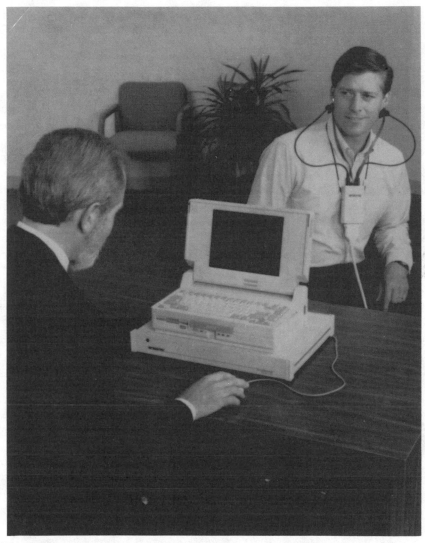

Figure 2–6. The Ensoniq Sound Selector Fitting System. (Photo courtesy of Ensoniq Corporation, Malvern, PA.)

the instrument matches an insertion gain target, it "corrects" the external ear effects to the average REUR (Figure 2–6).[4]

FRYE ELECTRONICS

The FONIX 6500 with Quik-Probe II uses a multifrequency, speech shaped, composite sig-

nal that displays a complete real-ear curve in less than 0.5 sec, with continuous updates several times. This method is called *real-time analysis*. The composite signal is designed as a voice-like signal, but pure tone tests with smoothing (similar to warbling) are selectable. With the signal turned off, the spectrum of any external signal, live or recorded, is measured. This permits real-time analysis of a person's

[4]For more information, contact Ensoniq Corporation, 155 Great Valley Parkway, Malvern, PA 19355.

own voice in the ear canal or of the real-ear response under environmental conditions.

Target insertion gain is calculated from a choice of six fitting formulas. A 2-cm^3 full-on gain (FOG) prescription is calculated from any of the forumulas — not just NAL. An SSPL90 prescription is calculated from dB HL loudness values. The FOG prescription can be compensated not only for the subject's unaided ear but also for the effects of ear impedance.

The FONIX 6400 is a real ear only version of the complete Fonix 6500 Hearing Aid Test System. The FP40 makes available in a portable unit many of the features of the 6500, including the speech shaped composite signal. The FP30, also a portable, performs real-ear

and coupler measurements and printouts, but has no video monitor (Figure 2-7).[5]

MADSEN ELECTRONICS

The Madsen IGO-HAT series was introduced in 1985 as a complete system to offer either real-ear measurements, hearing instrument analysis, or both, in a single integrated system. Its outstanding features are speed, accuracy, and repeatability. These are achieved by random access memory (RAM) for all control functions (with virtually instantaneous color screen updates) by using a two-channel approach (for realistic stimuli and tracking filter),

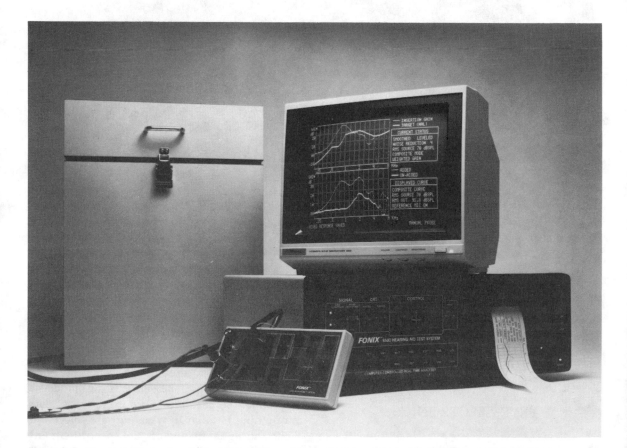

Figure 2–7. The Frye Electronics Fonix 6500 System. (Photo courtesy of Frye Electronics Inc., Tigard, OR.)

[5]For further information, contact Frye Electronics, Inc., 9826 SW Tigard Street, P.O. Box 23391, Tigard, OR 97223.

making real-time display possible with minimal effects from ambient noise, and by making far-field working possible to minimize head and shoulder diffractions and movement effects.

These instruments provide a wide variety of test parameters, with easy user programmability for three commonly used tests. The test box is large enough to test auditory trainers as well as the largest body aids, and it has telecoil and auditory stimuli (Figure 2-8).

The Computer Analysis System (CAS) was introduced by Madsen Electronics in 1990. This personal computer-based menu-driven system will perform all the routine real-ear and measuring instrument tests. Test sequences are user selectable and will run automatically.

The software included may be mouse driven if desired and will support EGA or VGA color video graphics.

The probe system is the modified pressure type, with on-line equalization. Gain rules can be programmed as can all test sequences and coupler to real-ear conversion calculations. Real-time analysis is possible through repeating warbled pure tone sweeps. The CAS can be portable when used with a laptop or notebook PC.

The outstanding feature of this system is that the software has been structured so that the operating PC can be used to store and retrieve not only CAS results, but also audiometric data from a Madsen 602 or 622

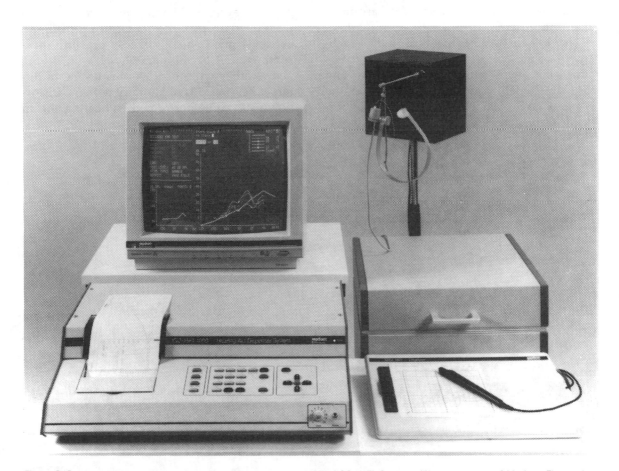

Figure 2–8. The Madsen Insertion Gain Optimizer-Hearing Aid Test (IGO-HAT) System. (Photo courtesy of Madsen Electronics, Mississauga, Ontario, Canada.)

Audiometer, as well as impedance test results from Madsen's Zodiac 901 Middle-Ear Analyzer. Further, all data can be merged with *HearWare* — a software package developed by Software and Systems. *HearWare* is an office-management, report-writing, marketing, and financial package for dispensers of hearing instruments (Figure 2–9).[6]

MAICO SYSTEM 2400 MODULAR AUDIOMETRIC SYSTEM

The Maico System 2400 is an IBM computer-based instrument consisting of a clinical two-channel audiometer and a real-ear hearing aid analyzer, available separately or together. The system also includes a patient database management system.

The system utilizes user friendly touch-screen technology; that is, menus on the screen allow the operator to perform programs and tests by merely touching selections on the screen. The System 2400 responds immediately by displaying the chosen selection.

Features of the system include (a) a patient database which makes it possible to store and display all patient file information in the System 2400 (patient data or tests can be viewed any time); (b) sweep, real-time, and calibration modes; (c) extensive ability to compare curves; (d) complete audiogram retrieval from the patient database; and (e) stimulus types including narrow-band noise, pure tone, warble tone, pink noise, and composite tone.

The System 2400 Real-Ear Insertion Gain module does standard tests, insertion gain and in situ gain, with comparison to NAL, Berger, Most Comfortable Level (MCL), POGO, and Lybarger, 1/3, 1/2, and 2/3 gain prescription techniques.

Three microphones are standard on the real-ear system. The probe microphone is positioned on an earhook that also contains an ear level microphone for easy pressure measurements. A barrel microphone, with Velcro, allows other types of tests plus testing of different hearing aids or auditory trainers. Distortion tests can be performed on hearing aids in the ear (Figure 2–10).[7]

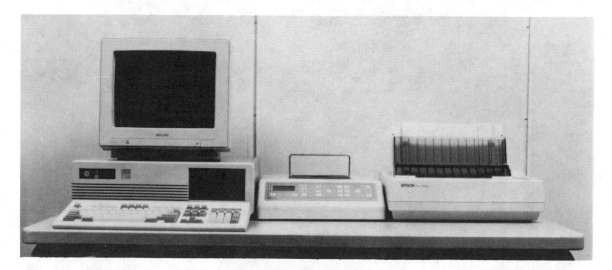

Figure 2–9. The Madsen Computer Analysis System (CAS). (Photo courtesy of Madsen Electronics, Mississauga, Ontario, Canada.)

---

[6]For more information, contact Madsen Electronics, Inc., 5090 Orbitor Drive, Unit 8, Mississauga, Ontario, Canada L4W 5B5.
[7]For more information, contact Maico Hearing Instruments, Inc., 7375 Bush Lake Road, Minneapolis, MN 55439-2029.

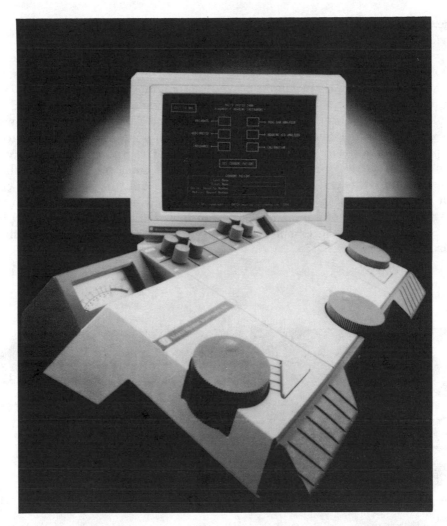

Figure 2-10. The Maico System 2400 Audiometer and Real-Ear Hearing Aid Analyzer. (Photo courtesy of Maico Hearing Instruments, Inc., Minneapolis, MN.)

RASTRONICS porta-REM 2000 DIGITAL REAL-EAR SYSTEM

The Rastronics porta-REM 2000 Digital Real-Ear System from Starkey Labs is a compact, portable real-ear measurement system that offers a user friendly comprehensive approach to hearing aid fitting utilizing the most advanced digital technology available. The system is designed to operate on menu driven and procedure-oriented software programs that guide the user through each step in the fitting process. The user identification (ID) function permits up to 10 different operator-designed setups allowing operators to make their own fitting protocols. Pull down windows permit the operator to simultaneously display a variety of measurement curves, program steps, articulation index calculations, and on-line system prompts to quickly assess the test parameters. The port-REM 2000 Digital offers a true complex-noise source along with a two-channel real-time FFT digital processing analyzer to accurately measure hearing aid performance. Digital signal-processing techniques provide updated measurements up to five times per second, with a resolution of 2048 data points on the screen. The 2000 is a stand-alone system that includes a built-in 5-in. monitor, hearing aid test chamber, auto-programmable battery simulator, seven-color plotter for hard copies of test measurements, RS-232 computer interface, and external outputs for speaker and VGA color monitor. Optional features include wireless remote control; built-in audiometer; *Trilogy* hearing aid programming module; and software releases for IEC, ANSI, and other measurement standards (Figure 2–11).[8]

SIEMENS RT450

The Siemens RT450 is designed for comprehensive hearing aid analysis and probe-microphone measurement in a compact, transportable unit. A large, backlit, black-on-white liquid crystal display allows complete tabular and graphic information to be viewed at once. The system is menu driven for ease of use. A quiet, fast, high-resolution thermal printer is built in, so that hard copy of test results can be easily made. Also included is an interface and software to display graphic test results in VGA graphics via IBM-compatible computers.

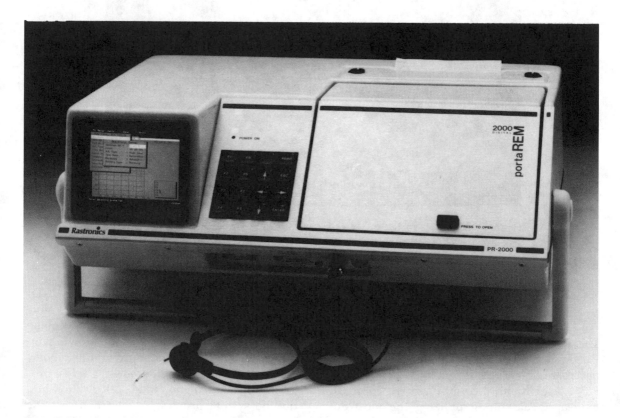

Figure 2–11. The Rastronics Porta-REM 2000 Digital Real-Ear Measurement System. (Photo courtesy of Starkey Labs, Inc., Minneapolis, MN.)

[8] For more information, contact Starkey Laboratories, 6700 Washington Avenue South, Eden Prairie, MN 55344.

The RT450 features an automatic hearing aid analysis mode in which a full range of tests in accordance with ANSI standards can be run in approximately one minute. An open test chamber with sweeping filters is included, making the adjustment of the volume control for reference test adjustments easier; an optional external test chamber is available for use in noisier surroundings. The RT450 also includes battery "pills," providing for measurement of battery drain in hearing instruments. A manual hearing aid analysis mode allows in-depth testing of specific parameters of hearing aid performance.

The probe-microphone section of the RT450 has a variety of competitive features. Calibration of the system is done by means of a menu selection, and a quick calibration check feature is provided. Audiometric data can be input and the target insertion response can be generated using 1/3 Gain, 1/2 Gain, POGO, NAL, Berger, or IDM formulas which are built in; alternately, the clinician's own target curve can be inserted. The type and level of test signal can be selected by the user. The system provides for REUR, REAR, REOR, and REIR tests, a hearing aid fitting mode, and real-ear harmonic distortion and input/output test protocols. An "analyze" function is available, allowing determination of the exact test value at any point along the frequency-response curve. Up to three REUR curves can be displayed, and the KEMAR curve can also be displayed during testing. In REIR and hearing aid fitting modes, the target insertion gain curve and fitting rule are displayed. The hearing aid fitting mode provides a continuous signal so that the effects of modifications can be monitored (Figure 2–12).[9]

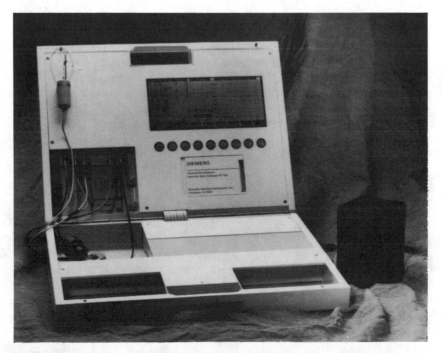

Figure 2–12. The Siemens RT 450 Hearing Aid and Insertion Gain Analyzer. (Photo courtesy of Siemens Hearing Instruments, Inc., Piscataway, NJ.)

---

[9] For more information, contact Siemens Hearing Instruments, Inc., 10 Constitution Ave., P.O. Box 1397, Piscataway, NJ 08855-1397.

VIRTUAL MODEL 340 PROBE-MICROPHONE SYSTEM

The model 340 Probe-Microphone System is a computer controlled hearing aid fitting workstation. It integrates all functions needed to characterize and fit hearing aids, print test results, and store test data for future use. The 340 computer screen displays a complete and immediate picture of all the information necessary for hearing aid adjustment within the patient's ear. It provides immediate, real-time waveform updates based on FFT calculations of complex waveform stimuli.

Measurements are easily captured and stored on the computer hard disk for later retrieval and analysis. Waveforms may be displayed in SPL or gain; waveform cursors read precise values from the plot; and waveforms may even be computed and displayed. To make testing even simpler, the 340 software directly reads audiograms saved from Virtual's Model 320 Clinical Audiometer, eliminating the need to re-enter audiogram information.

The probe-microphone test utilizes a reference microphone to ensure an accurate presentation in SPL of the pure-tone or composite signal. Eight waveforms may be saved and displayed in this test. Two waveforms may be subtracted to display an insertion gain waveform. Seven different prediction algorithms may be called on for calculating the estimated target insertion gain. The patient's audiogram can also be displayed next to the measured frequency response. Digital listings, as well as the waveform output, may be reported.

The full battery of ANSI tests can be done in the optional sound chamber. These tests include linear and AGC aids (with and without EIN). Telecoil evaluation is a standard feature. Tests similar to those done in the probe-microphone test may be performed on a hearing aid

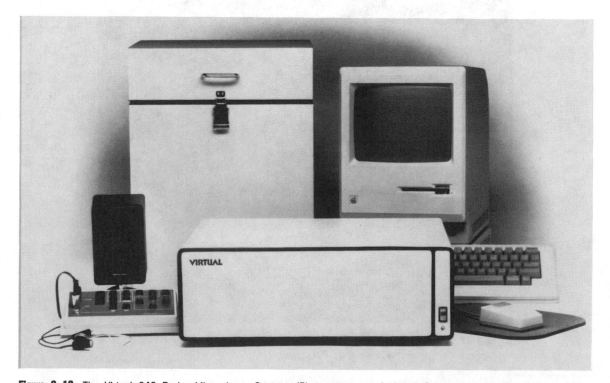

Figure 2–13. The Virtual 340 Probe Microphone System. (Photo courtesy of Virtual Corporation, Portland, OR.)

in the sound chamber. This feature is very useful for evaluating the hearing aid with other than simple ANSI tests. Full reference signal level versatility and waveform manipulation provide a quick way to characterize a hearing aid.

The 340 prints hard copy of the test results on a dot matrix or laser printer attached to the computer, with the option of saving the test results to a report form. When all the testing is done, the report form is printed on a convenient, standard size page. Operator comments can easily be added using the built-in word processor (Figure 2–13).[10]

---

[10]For more information, contact Virtual Corporation, 521 S.W. 11th Street, #400, Portland, OR 97205.

CHAPTER 3

Terminology and Procedures

■ H. GUSTAV MUELLER, Ph.D. ■

The development, introduction, and clinical acceptance of probe-microphone measurements for selecting and fitting hearing aids has led to much new terminology and many new procedures. The terminology has evolved over the years, as manufacturers, researchers, clinicians, and dispensers have struggled to decide what terms from the past should be retained, and what new terminology is needed to compliment this rapid technology advancement. Specific procedures also have been established, although refinement, modification, and further development continues. As illustrated in the next few pages, however, the new terminology and procedures follow a logical transition, can be learned easily, and do not present a major hurdle to the routine clinical use of probe-microphone measurements.

For the past few years, the American National Standards Institute (ANSI) Working Committee S3.80 has been developing procedural and terminology standards, and some preliminary reports of their work have been published (Mueller, 1990; Schwietzer, Sullivan,

Beck, & Cole, 1990). Many of the terms recommended by this group have gained popular use among researchers, clinicians, and dispensers, and these terms frequently appear in current publications related to probe-microphone measurements. At this writing, however, no ANSI standard on this topic has been published, or even formalized. In the absence of a standard, therefore, this chapter offers guidelines based on current theory, clinical practice, and common usage, with portions adapted from the preliminary work of the ANSI S3.80 Committee.

PREMEASUREMENT PROCEDURES

Prior to using probe-microphone equipment for assessing the performance of hearing aids, it is first necessary to conduct a series of premeasurement procedures to prepare both the equipment and the patient. These preliminary procedures are critical in assuring that all subsequent measurements are valid and reliable.

EQUALIZATION

The first procedure performed when conducting probe-microphone measures with most types of equipment is the soundfield equalization. This is the process of controlling the acoustic signal at a specific point in space so that the amplitude remains at the desired level across frequencies. There have been two commonly used methods of soundfield equalization, the *substitution method* and the *pressure method*. At one time it was suggested that the pressure method is more appropriately referred to as the modified comparison method (Preves, 1987; Preves & Sullivan, 1987). In the most recent version of the proposed ANSI standard, however, the term *modified pressure* is recommended, and this term will be used throughout this text.

The differences between the substitution and modified-pressure equalization methods are illustrated in Figures 3–1 and 3–2, taken from Madsen (1986). These figures illustrate the use of each method for measuring the gain of a hearing aid.

Figure 3–1 illustrates the **substitution method.** Observe that in the top panel, the **soundfield equalization occurs without the patient in the room** (or at least near the measurement location in the soundfield). The middle panel shows the unoccluded ear testing conducted with the patient present. Note that the center of the patient's head is now placed in the precise location previously occupied by the microphone in the top panel (referred to as the *subject reference point*). The microphone (probe tube) is located in the ear canal. The bottom panel shows the aided measure, conducted in a similar manner to the unaided testing.

Figure 3–2 illustrates the same hearing aid measurement procedure utilizing the modified-pressure method. **Two major differences** are apparent. First, there is **no equalization conducted with the patient absent,** and second, there is a **second regulating microphone present** for all measurements. For the modified pressure method, the regulating microphone is used to control the signal delivered from the speaker and to maintain this signal at

a constant level (as determined by the audiologist). This approach differs significantly from the substitution method, where the level is determined for the equalized empty field, and no monitoring is conducted during the evaluation of the patient. As stated in the ANSI S3.80 draft standard, the **field reference point** (controlling or reference microphone) must be:

■ Near the surface of the head.
■ Close to the hearing aid.
■ Not positioned within the acoustic influence of the test ear or the hearing aid.

The exact location of the controlling or reference microphone does influence the results of the probe-microphone measurement, and we will discuss this in detail in Chapter 4.

There are distinct advantages and disadvantages of each of the two equalization procedures. The primary limitation of the substitution method is that the patient's head must be fixed in the exact position where soundfield calibration was conducted. For most clinical testing, therefore, where patient movement and slight head turns are common, **the advantages of the modified-pressure procedure outweigh those of the substitution method.** An inexperienced or careless clinician is more apt to make serious errors using the substitution method, and for this reason, several probe-microphone systems default to the modified-pressure method, and some manufacturers do not even offer the substitution method as an option.

Not all probe-microphone equipment conducts equalization in the same manner. To help categorize these differences, equalization procedures can be referred to as either *on-line* (real time) or *off-line* (stored).

■ On-line: Equalization based on simultaneous monitoring at the time of the measurement.
■ Off-line: Equalization based on data obtained from a prior measurement of the soundfield (illustrated in Figure 3–1).

When using the substitution method, only off-line equalization is used. **Either on-line or off-line** equalization, however, **could be used**

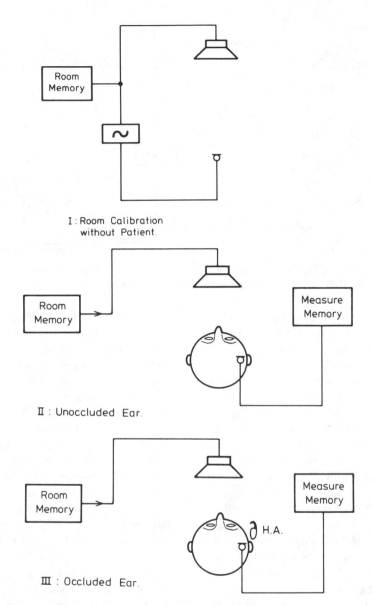

I : Room Calibration
without Patient.

II : Unoccluded Ear.

III : Occluded Ear.

Figure 3-1. Illustration of the substitution method of soundfield equalization for probe-microphone measurements. (Reprinted from Madsen, P. 1986. Insertion gain optimization. *Hearing Instruments, 37*(1). 28–32, with permission.)

for the modified-pressure method (see Chapter 4 for further description).

PROBE CALIBRATION

When using some types of probe-microphone equipment, a second procedure that is necessary prior to probe-microphone testing is the calibration of the probe tube itself. The sili-

cone extension tube is considered part of the microphone; hence, the acoustical effects of passing sound through this tube must be taken into account. The **purpose of this calibration is to make the probe tube acoustically invisible,** so that the measurement will be recorded as if the microphone itself were located in the ear canal near the tympanic membrane (A notable exception to this calibration procedure is the

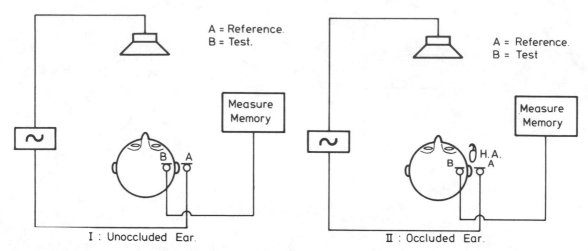

Figure 3–2. Illustration of the modified-pressure method of soundfield equalization for probe-microphone measurements. (Reprinted from Madsen, P. 1986. Insertion gain optimization. *Hearing Instruments, 37* (1), 28–32, with permission.)

Fonix 6500 — this system is designed so that the probe tube, used in conjunction with the probe microphone, has a flat frequency response; therefore, corrections are not needed).

Figure 3–2 showed that the modified-pressure method employs two microphones. To account for the acoustical effects of the probe tube, therefore, one only has to compare the signal recorded from the reference microphone to the simultaneously recorded response of the signal traveling through the probe tube attached to the test microphone. The difference between these two responses reflects the effects of the probe tube. With some equipment, the uncorrected response is displayed on the monitor.

With the above description in mind, it then becomes obvious that the tip of the probe must be placed near the reference microphone for this calibration procedure. Some manufacturers offer a bracket on the probe assembly to hold the probe tube in the appropriate position. Simply holding the tube in place by hand works equally well, assuming one is careful not to obstruct the sound that is entering either the probe tube or the reference microphone. An example is shown in Figure 3–3.

Calibration of the probe tube is critical to the accuracy of all real-ear measures, as the equipment will automatically make a mathematical correction to all subsequent measurements. Whenever a response is questioned, a quick check of probe calibration is advised. The most common subtle problem is cerumen, moisture, or debris in the probe tube that has not completely plugged the tube but has altered the acoustic transmission effects. To quickly check the calibration of the system, simply conduct a repeat measure holding the opening of the tube near the reference microphone as shown in Figure 3–3. Because the acoustical transmission effects of the probe tube already are stored in equipment memory, the measured response should be equal to the response of the reference microphone; that is, there should be a flat response across frequencies at the input level chosen for the calibration check.

Figure 3–4 illustrates the procedure described above. The left panel displays the typical response that is obtained for the probe-tube-reference microphone comparison. Notice that some of the resonant characteristics of the tube are reflected in the response. Following this calibration procedure, a second curve can be generated to assure that the equipment has indeed accounted for the acoustic characteristics of the probe tube. This response is shown in the right panel, and as expected, a flat response is obtained at the level of the input signal, 70 dB. Once the probe tube has been calibrated, it is not necessary to re-calibrate before each measurement. Periodic checks, however, are recommended.

The effects of careless probe calibration are shown in Figure 3–5. In this example, the probe tip was held an inch away rather than adjacent to the reference microphone during the calibration process. Observe that the calibration curve displayed in the left panel differs somewhat from that of Figure 3–4, especially for the frequencies above 2000 Hz. The right panel of Figure 3–5 shows the results of the calibration check. While the measured response is consistent with the input level of 70 dB through 2000 Hz, deviations as large as 5 dB are present in the 2500–4000 Hz region. This decibel error, if undetected at the time of calibration, will be present in all subsequent hearing aid measures.

As mentioned, the primary culprit of altered probe-tube calibration (after the initial calibration) is cerumen lodged in the probe tip. Many manufacturers suggest that a new probe tube be used for each ear, and if the examiner adheres to this advice, clogged probe tubes will be less of a problem. **Probe-tube calibration, however, should be repeated every time a tube is changed.** While the tubes might all look alike, acoustic transmission differences sometimes exist.

For examiners who are not compelled to change probe tubes for every ear, and who experience an occasional plugged tube, it is tempting to simply snip off the plugged end of the tube. While this practice saves time, there is an accuracy penalty if recalibration is not conducted: shortening of 10 to 15 mm will cause 3–5 dB errors. Given the simplicity of replacing and recalibrating a probe tube, there is little reason not to follow this procedure

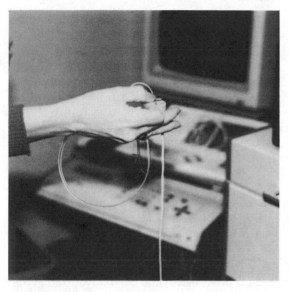

Figure 3–3. Positioning of the probe-tube tip near the reference microphone for conducting soundfield calibration.

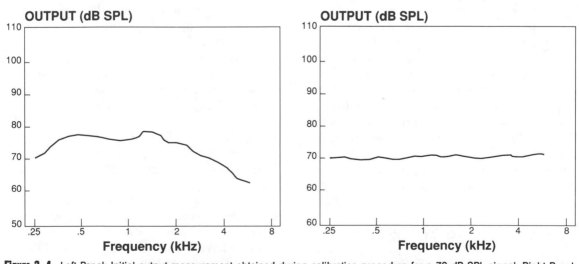

Figure 3–4. Left Panel: Initial output measurement obtained during calibration procedure for a 70 dB SPL signal. Right Panel: Results of repeat measurement after the acoustic effects of the probe tube have been stored in equipment memory.

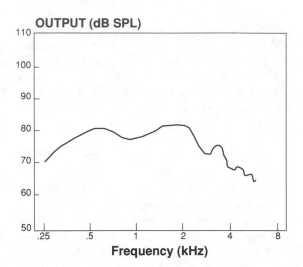

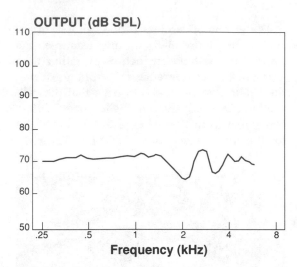

Figure 3–5. Left Panel: Initial output measurement obtained during calibration procedure for a 70 dB SPL signal — tip of probe tube was held one inch away rather than adjacent to the reference microphone. Right Panel: Results of repeat measurement after the acoustic effects of the probe tube have been stored in equipment memory — the deviation from 70 dB SPL in the higher frequencies reflects the error caused by the careless calibration procedure.

(further discussion of plugged probe tubes is contained in Chapter 4).

A final probe-calibration issue concerns the location of the probe assembly during the calibration process. We suggest that the probe calibration be conducted the same distance and azimuth from the loudspeaker as will be used when patient testing is conducted. For example, if hearing aid evaluations will be conducted with the patient seated 0.5 m from the speaker at a 0° azimuth, then the probe calibration should be conducted at this location.

It is important to again emphasize that, for some probe-microphone equipment, portions of the above discussion are not relevant, as the probe tube is part of the overall microphone response, and specific probe-tube calibration is not necessary. With these units, such as the Fonix 6500, it is important to **use the probe tube recommended by the manufacturer.** Also, one must be careful not to cut or stretch the probe tube. Doing so will result in erroneous measurements.

POSITIONING THE PATIENT

Following the field equalization and/or the probe calibration, the equipment is ready for patient evaluation. When seating the patient, both distance from and azimuth to the loudspeaker must be considered. The distance issue is the least controversial of the two decisions. Distances beyond 1 m begin to increase measurement error, and little advantage is obtained by placing the patient closer than 0.5 m. Hence, most manufacturers **recommend a distance of 0.5–1 m** (one manufacturer recommends 12 in.). The positioning of the patient is particularly critical when the substitution method is used, as deviations from the point of calibration will cause significant errors in the probe measurement. When using the modified-pressure method, minor deviations in patient positioning are allowable, as the reference microphone will adjust the input signal accordingly.

Since it usually is desirable to use a relatively low input signal (e.g., 60 dB) when testing a hearing aid, the 0.5 meter distance allows the system to operate more efficiently, as the closer distance reduces the undesirable effects of ambient noise measured by the reference microphone. Many patients find it bothersome to have a loudspeaker positioned 0.5 m from their face, and they usually try to slide their chair back a few inches when the audiologist is not looking. It may be necessary, therefore, to **check the distance periodically during the hearing aid evaluation procedure.**

The azimuth of the loudspeaker relative to the patient is a second issue to be considered. Two choices that are acceptable and used commonly are 0° and 45°. As discussed in Chapter 4, however, somewhat different results will be obtained for probe measurements depending on the azimuth selected. One example is the real ear unaided response (REUR), which can vary by several decibels (above 2000 Hz) as a function of azimuth.

Figure 3–6 illustrates the positioning of the patient using a 0° azimuth. This location has a distinct practical advantage, as the loudspeaker can remain in a single out-of-the-way position for all testing. The audiologist can work behind the patient, going from ear to ear when fitting and adjusting the hearing aids. The patient can see the monitor using their peripheral vision.

If a 45° azimuth is used, the loudspeaker must be moved from side to side as one con-

ducts testing on the right and left ears. Moving the patient around in a swivel chair is a poor second choice, as the patient inevitably will end up with the back of his or her head facing the monitor as you are trying to point out the incredible response that just has been displayed. If the 45° azimuth is used, it is helpful to mount the loudspeaker on a wall boom, as moving a speaker stand back and forth for each patient is tiresome, and encourages mishaps.

Either the 0° or 45° azimuth will result in reasonably accurate probe-microphone measures. Unacceptable errors are obtained at 90° and this azimuth should be avoided. Most manufacturers recommend a specific azimuth and distance for their equipment. Additional issues to consider when selecting the loudspeaker azimuth are reviewed in Chapter 4.

OTOSCOPIC EXAMINATION

As with other audiologic and hearing aid procedures, a careful otoscopic examination is necessary before beginning testing. In addi-

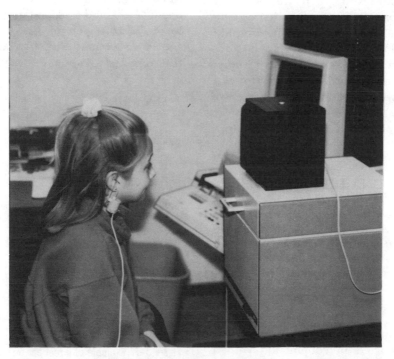

Figure 3–6. Example of a patient positioned at 0° azimuth, 0.5 meter from the loudspeaker for probe-microphone measurements.

tion to assuring that no medical pathology is present, this is also important to assess the amount of debris or cerumen that might be present in the ear canal. If a significant amount of cerumen is present, the audiologist is faced with deciding if this will affect the test outcome, or if testing is even possible. If not restricted by scope of practice or state license, one simple solution is to clean the ear. Presently, most audiologists do not engage in ear cleaning; however, recent articles have urged audiologists to assume a greater role in the management of cerumen (Roeser & Crandell, 1991a, 1991b).

Excessive cerumen, perforations and middle ear pathology do have a significant effect on probe-microphone measurement (see Chapter 4 for specific examples).

REAL-EAR MEASUREMENT PROCEDURES

After the equipment and the patient have been prepared for testing, there are a series of probe-microphone measurements that usually are conducted at the time of the hearing aid fitting. Terminology has been developed to describe these procedures, complete with convenient acronyms all beginning with RE (for real ear). The following section describes the six most commonly used procedures, and some of the clinical applications of each procedure are discussed.

REAL EAR UNAIDED RESPONSE

The real ear unaided response (REUR) is the SPL, as a function of frequency, at a specified point in the unoccluded ear canal for a specified soundfield. This can be expressed either in SPL or a gain in decibels relative to the stimulus level.

Background

The first probe-microphone measurement that usually is conducted in conjunction with a hearing aid fitting is the patient's real ear unaided response (REUR). This unaided re-

sponse has been referred to by several other terms, each of which have enjoyed some degree of popularity:

■ Free field-to-eardrum transfer function
■ Wearer frequency response (WFR)
■ External ear effects (EEE)

As described by Mueller (1990), these three terms all suggest a specific measurement procedure (e.g., either substitution or modified-pressure), which somewhat causes the terms to be user and equipment specific. The term **REUR, however, is not specific to a given manufacturer's equipment or a particular measurement procedure**, and therefore communication among researchers, clinicians, manufacturers, and dispensers is facilitated.

The REUR primarily is a measure of the resonance characteristics of the ear canal and the concha. Other parts of the external ear and the patient's head and body also can influence the REUR measure, and these factors are discussed later in this section. The average adult REUR has a primary peak around 2700 Hz of about 17 dB, and a secondary peak in the 4000 to 5000 Hz region of 12–14 dB. Figure 3–7 shows an average REUR, which is similar to the unaided response obtained from the

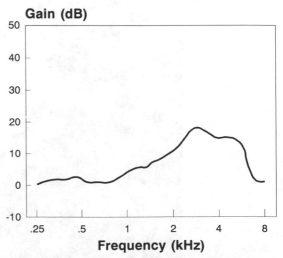

Figure 3-7. Example of a real ear unaided response (REUR) that approximates average values. This response is similar to the manikin unaided measure obtained from the KEMAR.

KEMAR (Knowles Electronics Manikin for Acoustic Research).

Much of the basic research concerning the acoustic characteristics of the external ear was first provided by Shaw (1974) who detailed the physiologic and anatomic correlates to the response now known as the REUR. For example, Figure 3–8, from Shaw (1974) shows the contributions made by five different factors that enter into the final REUR. Observe that the overall response primarily can be attributed to the acoustic properties of the ear canal and the concha.

In the clinic setting, the individual rather than the average REUR is of primary interest, and seldom does the individual REUR equal the average at all frequencies of interest. For example, Figure 3–9 depicts the REUR for the right ear of eight audiologists. Observe that the peak of the response varies from below 2000 to over 4000 Hz, and the maximum intensity varies from 12 to 25 dB. Only the REUR shown in panel 3–9E bears a close re-

semblance to the average unaided response. Notice that the REUR of one audiologist (James W. Hall III, Figure 3–9H) has two prominent peaks while the REUR of another audiologist (Brad A. Stach, Figure 3–9B) has no prominent peaks. Importantly, if these **eight ears were all fitted with the same hearing aid**, the resulting **insertion gain** from that instrument would **vary to the same degree as the REURs** shown in Figure 3–9. This issue is discussed more thoroughly later and also in Chapter 9.

Measurement Procedures

In addition to the premeasurement issues already discussed (e.g., location of the loudspeaker) there are two primary procedural considerations when conducting the REUR:

■ Probe-tube placement
■ Selection of input intensity

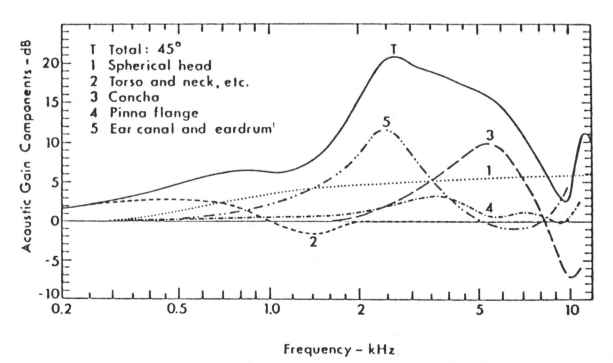

Figure 3–8. Acoustic factors of the external ear which contribute to the real ear unaided response. (Reprinted from Shaw, E. 1974. Transformation of sound pressure from the free field to the eardrum in the horizontal plane. *Journal of the Acoustic Society of America, 56,* 1848–1861, with permission.)

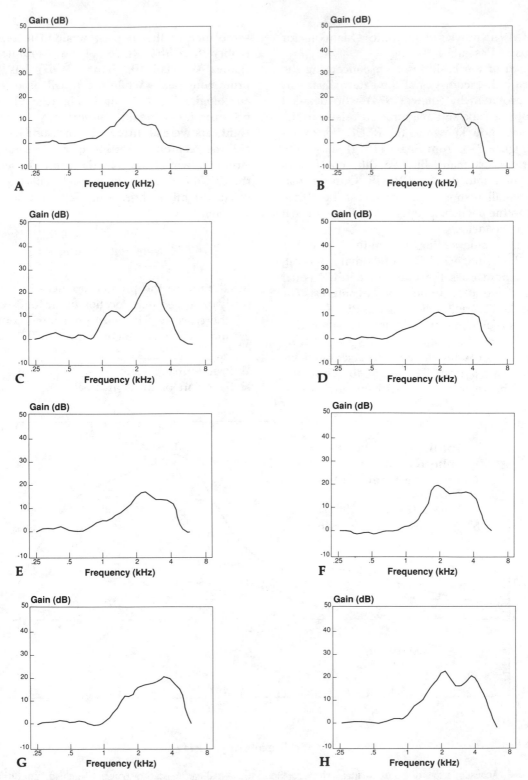

Figure 3–9. The real ear unaided response (REUR) for the right ear of eight different audiologists.

Probe-tube placement is very important, and poor placement for the REUR can have a significant effect on all other measures conducted during the hearing aid fitting. It is important to place the **tip of the tube reasonably close to the tympanic membrane to assure that the high-frequency components of the response are accurately measured**. While several methods are available, the easiest method simply is to set the **ring marker** of the probe tube at **30 mm from the tip**, and then slide the tube down the ear canal until the ring **marker is located at the tragal notch**; a black marking pencil can be used on probe tubes that do not have a ring marker. On occasion, the 30 mm distance will result in the tip of the tube striking the tympanic membrane (not terribly painful, but might cause a reflexive jerk and some eye watering), so a **more conservative approach would be to use a distance of 25–28 mm from the tragal notch** (different rules apply for children; see Chapter 8). The logic of this approach is explained in Chapter 4, where alternative methods of selecting the appropriate placement also are offered.

A **second important consideration** is the selection of the **intensity of the input signal**. If the REUR is conducted separate from the evaluation of a hearing aid, the input level is not very critical; it just must be above the ambient noise floor of the test environment. In most cases, however, the REUR is used as a reference value for the aided response. In such cases, it is best to use an input level that would also be suitable for the subsequent hearing aid assessment. Usually an input **level of 60 dB is appropriate**.

Clinical Applications

The **most common clinical use** of the REUR is to serve as a **reference value for calculation of insertion gain**. Since most prescriptive methods are validated by using the real-ear measure of insertion gain, and a component of insertion gain calculation is the REUR, the REUR is a critical measure for almost all probe-microphone hearing aid assessments. Because there is a straightforward relationship between insertion gain and the patient's REUR, experienced dispensers usually can predict whether the hearing aid's insertion response will meet prescriptive target gain simply by viewing the REUR.

A somewhat **different clinical application** of the REUR is to use these values to assist in **formulating the best 2–cm³ coupler response** for a patient at the time that a custom in-the-ear (ITE) hearing aid is ordered. Based on the patient's REUR, mathematical alterations are made to the prescriptive coupler gain (see Chapter 9). It has been reported that this approach will assist in obtaining the appropriate prescriptive insertion gain when the hearing aid is fitted (Bratt & Sammeth, 1991; Mueller, 1989; Valente, Valente, & Vass, 1991).

Another, less formal, use of the REUR, which reportedly has surfaced as a hearing aid fitting procedure, is to use this curve as a reference and then select a hearing aid real-ear frequency response that follows the same pattern. This fitting strategy is based on the belief that hearing aid-processed speech will sound more natural to the patient if the amplified frequency response closely mimics the configuration of the patient's REUR. This fitting procedure, therefore, assumes that the configuration of the desired gain of the hearing aid is unrelated to the patient's hearing loss — a selection philosophy that is in opposition to the underlying theory of most formalized prescriptive approaches. **Little documentation is available showing that an REUR-shaped hearing aid fitting actually results in better speech quality or intelligibility for the user**.

An indirect clinical application of the REUR is that this measure often reflects abnormalities of the ear canal or the middle ear. It is possible that a **tympanic membrane perforation** that was **missed by otoscopic examination** could **cause an unusual REUR**, which would prompt a closer visual re-examination of the ear.

REAL EAR OCCLUDED RESPONSE

The real ear occluded response (REOR) is the SPL, as a function of frequency, at a specified point in the ear canal for a specified soundfield, with the

hearing aid in place and turned off. This can be expressed either in SPL or as gain in decibels relative to the stimulus level.

Background

The REUR is an individual's natural amplification which the patient has had all of his or her life. One of the first things, however, that audiologists do for (or to) the patient at the time of the hearing aid fitting is to place an earmold or hearing aid in the ear and thereby alter this natural amplification. The effect of the placement of the hearing aid or the earmold in the ear easily can be measured, and it is known as the *real ear occluded response, or REOR.* While the REOR may be very similar to the REUR at some frequency regions for open-ear fittings, for **most hearing aid or earmold styles, the REOR will fall substantially below the REUR.** For earmold or hearing aid styles that **fit tight enough to cause attenuation, the REOR also will reflect this aspect**, along with the alteration of the REUR. Rarely will the REOR be greater than the REUR, except in cases where the vent of the hearing aid causes a resonance effect for a frequency region where the REUR values were small (e.g., 1500 Hz or below).

The difference between the REUR and the REOR provides an *estimate of insertion loss,* which is the difference between the real ear aided response and real ear insertion gain. With a relatively tight-fitting hearing aid, the **REOR usually falls at or below the input signal.** This happens **despite the size of the patient's REUR.** This means that patients with 30-dB peaks in their REURs have the potential to experience 20 dB more of insertion loss than patients with 10-dB peaks in their REURs. This factor interacts significantly with the real ear insertion response (REIR), and will be discussed again later.

For the most part, the REUR–REOR difference is a factor of how the placement of the hearing aid or earmold alters the external ear's resonance and collection properties. Not surprisingly, therefore, **REORs usually become smaller as the size of the earmold or hearing aid placed in the ear becomes larger.** Sullivan (1985) wrote a three-part article in which he uses REOR measures to categorize hearing aid fittings into four different types based on the acoustic coupling. Figure 3–10, taken from Sullivan (1991) shows the relation of the REOR to the REUR (and the real ear aided response, or REAR) for the four different acoustic coupling classifications.

Mueller (1990) conducted REOR measures on 40 ears fitted with three different styles of ITE hearing aids. The mean REOR results, and the mean REUR, are shown in Figure 3–11. Notice that for the IROS-type ITE fitting some external ear resonance effects remained for most frequencies when the hearing aid was placed in the ear; also note that the mean REOR actually was greater than the mean REUR at 1500 Hz — perhaps due to the vent resonance effect discussed previously. In contrast to the IROS-ITE, when a full-concha ITE or an in-the-canal (ITC) hearing aid was placed in the ear, mean REOR values became substantially smaller. The ITE hearing aids used in this study fitted relatively loosely; even more depressed REOR values would occur for tight-fitting instruments (see the Class IV fitting of Sullivan shown in Figure 3–10).

Measurement Procedures

The purpose of the REOR measure is to determine the effect that the placement of the hearing aid or earmold in the ear has on the input to the ear and how such placement alters the patient's REUR. General test procedures, therefore, are similar to those in the REUR measurement protocol:

■ While it is not necessary to conduct an REUR first, it does make interpretation of the REOR more meaningful, and therefore we recommend an initial REUR measurement.
■ After the REUR is completed, the hearing aid is placed in the ear. Remember that the hearing aid remains *turned off.*
■ The same probe-tube depth as used for the REUR is appropriate (25–30 mm from the tragal notch).

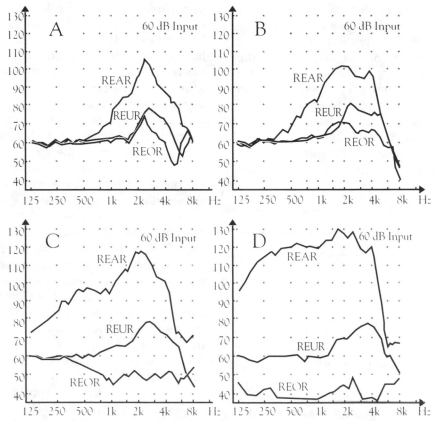

Figure 3–10. Illustration of the relationship between the real ear occluded response (REOR) and the real ear unaided response (REUR) for four different types of acoustic coupling systems. (Reprinted from Sullivan, R. 1990. Acoustic coupling classification system and hearing aids. *Reports on Hearing Instrumentation and Technology, 2,* 15–22, with permission.)

■ The input level is not critical, although typically it is convenient to use the same input as routinely used for the REUR measure (e.g., 60 dB).

The method used to display the REOR on the equipment monitor varies among probe-microphone instruments. Some units will allow you to equalize for the patient's REUR, which becomes the zero reference line. Using this method, the REOR per se would not be displayed, but rather, the resulting curve would represent the differences between the REUR and the REOR. For most fittings, the difference curve falls substantially below the reference line, and the negative effects of placing a hearing aid in the ear are easily observed visually

(see Sweetow, 1991, for an example of this type of display of the REOR).

On other probe-microphone equipment, it is necessary to conduct the REOR measures in the absolute rather than relative scale, so that enough display area is available on the monitor below the input level to show the REOR. Sometimes, raising the input level will help. On some equipment, however, REORs that dip more than 20 dB below the input level cannot be measured accurately.

Clinical Applications

The REOR is directly related to both the real ear aided response and the insertion gain of a hearing aid. In effect, however, this influence is observable in these other measures, and for this reason, most audiologists do not directly measure the REOR at the time of the hearing aid fittings. This is not to suggest that the REOR measure is not useful for modifying a fitting, trouble-shooting a user complaint, or in assisting in the explanation of unexpected insertion gain results.

One example of how the REOR can be used at the time of the hearing aid fitting is shown in Figure 3–12. First, consider the insertion

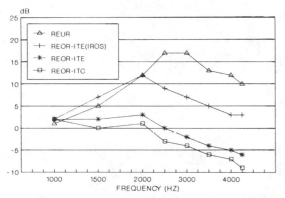

Figure 3–11. Real ear occluded response (REOR) results for three different styles of in-the-ear (ITE) hearing aids. (Reprinted from Mueller, H. 1990. Probe tube microphone measures: Some opinions on the terminology and procedures. *Hearing Journal, 42* (1), 1–5, with permission.)

gain curve shown in the left panel; this was obtained using a custom ITE-IROS. This patient had normal hearing through 1000 Hz; therefore, little or no gain in the low frequencies was desired. Initially, based on the large peak of gain in the 750 Hz region, this response was deemed inappropriate for this patient. An examination of the 2-cm³ coupler results for this instrument, however, made it difficult to believe that this low frequency gain was a function of the hearing aid circuitry. For this reason, an REOR measure was conducted. As shown in the left panel, observe that in the 750 Hz region, an REOR peak of 10 dB was present. Recall that the hearing aid is *turned off* for the REOR measure. We concluded, therefore, that the **unacceptable insertion gain probably was a result of the resonance of the IROS vent** (which was plugged for the 2-cm³ measures) and not due to inappropriate circuitry. Sending the hearing aid back to the manufacturer for circuitry change was not the solution.

While traditionally, we normally would make vents larger to reduce low frequencies, in this case we made the IROS vent smaller, to reduce the resonance effect. The right panel of Figure 3–12 shows the second REOR measurement, which is the result of filling in a portion of the IROS vent. Notice that a large portion of

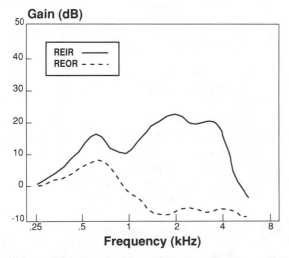

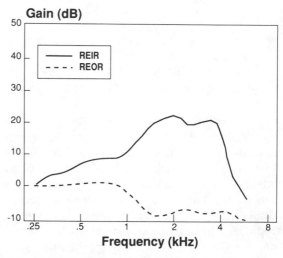

Figure 3–12. Left Panel: The real ear occluded response (REOR) and the real ear insertion response (REIR) obtained from an in-the-ear (ITE) hearing aid with a large vent. Right Panel: The REOR and REIR obtained from the same hearing aid after the vent had been made smaller.

the low-frequency peak is gone. Also notice that the REOR remains essentially the same for the higher frequencies, which suggests that we did not make the vent too small. As expected, this change in the REOR was reflected in the second REIR measure, also shown in the right panel of Figure 3–12. The fitting was now considered acceptable.

This example not only points out the clinical utility of the REOR, but clearly illustrates the value of probe-microphone measures in general — imagine doing the same type of trouble-shooting using functional gain or speech audiometry.

There are some particular clinical applications of the REOR when fitting individuals with upward sloping hearing losses. On occasion, individuals with this hearing loss configuration have excellent hearing thresholds in the higher frequencies, such as 0–10 dB in the 3000–4000 Hz range. One approach of fitting this individual is to place a vent in the hearing aid that is large enough to avoid attenuation at these higher frequencies, yet not so large that low-frequency gain is substantially reduced. **The REOR measure** (combined with insertion gain findings) is helpful in **determining the appropriate vent size** to accomplish this often difficult task.

The REOR also can be used as an indirect measure of the occlusion effect (the direct

measure of the occlusion effect is discussed in Chapter 10). In general, the more the REOR falls below the patient's REUR, the greater the occlusion effect. If someone with normal hearing thresholds through 2000 Hz is being fitted with an ITE-IROS hearing aid, and the REOR falls at or below the input reference, it is probable that this patient will have complaints associated with the occlusion effect. Bryant, Mueller, and Northern (1991) reported on different probe-microphone measurements for a group of individuals fitted with minimal-contact long canal ITE hearing aids, which were specifically designed to reduce occlusion. These authors reported that there was a measurable change in the occlusion effect for these subjects when these special hearing aids were compared with ITE hearing aids with a standard canal length. Significant differences in the REORs also were observed between the two different canal styles. Figure 3–13 shows the right and left ears for one of the subjects from this study. Observe that in both cases, the REOR for standard canal length falls substantially below that of the minimal-contact long canal hearing aid.

Kopun, Stelmachowicz, Carney, and Schulte (1992) used the REOR to examine the attenuation characteristics of different FM system sound delivery options. Figure 3–14 illustrates the attenuation effects for four different options,

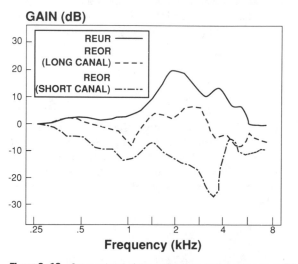
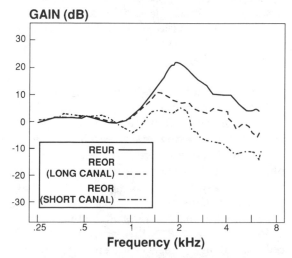

Figure 3–13. Comparison of the real ear occluded responses (REORs) for the right and left ears of a patient fitted with an in-the-ear (ITE) hearing aid with a standard canal and an ITE hearing aid with minimal-contact long canal.

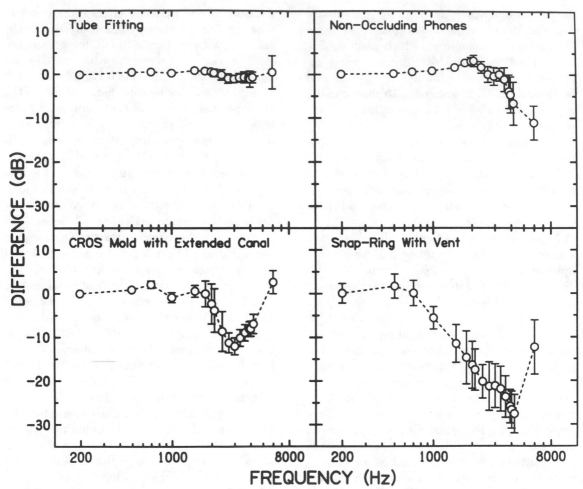

Figure 3–14. Illustration of the difference values between the real ear unaided responses (REURs) and the real ear occluded responses (REORs) for subjects fitted with four different sound delivery options used with an FM system. The degree that the values fall below the zero reference line reflects the attenuation caused by that particular sound delivery option. (Reprinted from Kopun, J. G., Stelmachowics, P. G., Carney, E., & Schulte, L. 1992. Coupling of FM systems to individuals with unilateral hearing loss. *Journal of Speech and Hearing Research, 35,* 201–207, with permission.)

measured on ten adults. The plottings represent the mean differences between the REUR and the REOR. Used in this manner, the **REOR is helpful in selecting an acoustically appropriate sound delivery system.** Notice that the data of Kopun et al. (1992) show that only the tube fitting is truly non-occluding across all measurement frequencies.

Perhaps the most understated clinical application of the REOR is that often, when done unintentionally, it serves as an excellent reminder that we have forgotten to put in a battery or turn the hearing aid on!

REAL EAR AIDED RESPONSE

The real ear aided response (REAR) is the SPL, as a function of frequency, at a specified measurement point in the ear canal for a specified soundfield with the hearing aid in place and turned on. This can be expressed either in SPL or as gain in decibels relative to the stimulus level.

Background

The third new term of the probe-microphone measurement family is the *real ear aided re-*

sponse, or the REAR. REAR can be used either to express the decibels SPL, or the decibels SPL relative to the input, of the output of a hearing aid measured in the ear canal. In the past, the REAR often was referred to as the *in situ response,* or *in situ gain.* The REAR typically is displayed in decibels SPL — unlike the REUR which normally is displayed as a relative value. Examples of REARs are shown in Figure 3–15. The left panel shows the REARs of a hearing aid tested with inputs of 60, 70, and 80 dB. The right panel shows the REARs of the same hearing aid, at the same input and volume control wheel setting, tested in *three different ears.* The significance of the differences among the three curves is discussed later.

The REAR is one of the most straightforward of the real-ear measures, as the test procedures are similar to those employed when 2-cm³ measures are conducted. The difference, of course, is that the ear now serves as the coupler. As mentioned previously, the 2-cm³ coupler is not an accurate predictor of how a hearing aid will perform in a real ear. Average correction factors can be used (see Chapter 12), but they do not account for the specific variances of a given individual. The **REAR allows the audiologist to use the patient's own ear as a coupler**, and make fitting decisions

accordingly. The differences among the REARs obtained with the same hearing aid shown in the right panel of Figure 3–15 clearly illustrate the potential value of this procedure.

Measurement Procedures

If the REAR is conducted immediately after the REUR, which often is the case, the probe tube is already in the ear. If not, the probe tube should be placed according to the recommendations given in the preceding section. With the hearing aid in place, the probe tube should lie under the instrument in the area of the tragal notch. This will allow for continuous monitoring of the ring marker on the probe tube to assure that a consistent and appropriate depth is maintained. While it **sometimes is tempting to place the probe tube through a conveniently sized vent, this is not a suitable alternative**, since this approach may alter one of the very things that you wish to measure: the acoustical effects of venting.

When sliding the hearing aid or earmold into the ear, it is best to hold onto the probe tube with one hand, while pushing in the hearing aid with the other. This will help keep the probe tube in place, as it will want to slide along with the hearing aid (the patient will

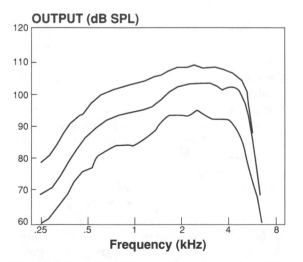

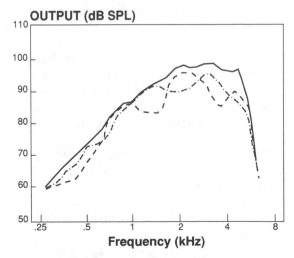

Figure 3–15. Left Panel: The real ear aided responses (REARs) of an in-the-ear (ITE) hearing aid for inputs of 60, 70, and 80 dB SPL. Right Panel: The REARs for the same ITE hearing aid for a single input measured in three different ears.

eagerly inform you if the tip moves down the canal too far!). **This approach will also help assure that you do not lose sight of the ring marker, which easily can be hidden by the hearing aid.** Once the hearing aid has been placed in the ear, two important decisions must be made:

■ The intensity level of the input to the hearing aid.
■ The hearing aid volume control wheel (VCW) setting.

The levels that are selected for each of these two variables are highly dependent on the aspect of the hearing aid fitting that is under consideration. If the REAR measurement is being conducted for the **purpose of calculating insertion gain**, then the **input level should not place the hearing aid in saturation.** Also, unless one is purposely trying to measure the effects of compression, the input should be **below the activation level for an input-compression instrument** (more on this in Chapter 4). With these factors in mind, an input of 70 dB speech-weighted noise or 60 dB swept warble tone usually is satisfactory. If testing is conducted in a typical office, and some background noise is present, it may be difficult to conduct testing using a 60 dB input. It might be necessary to use a slightly higher input to overcome the noise — this varies among probe-microphone units.

As shown earlier in Figure 3–15 (left panel), it is often useful to conduct REARs at different inputs and display the curves together. This will help identify whether the hearing aid has been placed into saturation or if an input-controlled compression instrument is functioning in a linear manner.

There are **no specific rules for setting the hearing aid's volume control wheel (VCW) for REAR measures**, and again, it depends on what feature of hearing aid performance is being measured. Most audiologists use one of four methods:

■ Arbitrarily set the VCW to 1/2 to 2/3 rotation.

■ Set the VCW so that the output equals the prescriptive gain target at a specific frequency.
■ Set the VCW to what the patient says is a comfortable listening level.
■ For experienced users, set the VCW at normal use gain (which should be similar to their most comfortable listening level).

In some instances it is helpful to conduct REARs at different VCW settings. By systematically changing the VCW to specific rotation points, the linearity or taper of the VCW can be assessed by examining the series of REARs. This approach can be useful in responding to user complaints regarding hearing aid gain adjustment problems.

For individuals with severe-to-profound hearing impairments, use gain might be at or near a full VCW rotation. In some cases, the probe tube will cause a slight slit leak, and the resulting **acoustic feedback prevents the measurement of the REAR at this use gain level.** When this happens, it is best to **use a combined real-ear and 2-cm³ coupler approach.** This will provide a reasonable prediction of what the REAR would have been if testing was possible at that VCW setting. This procedure is further detailed later and in Chapter 4.

Clinical Applications

It is possible that the greatest clinical applications of the REAR have yet to be realized. As discussed in Chapter 6, insertion gain, rather than the REAR, is the most popular method of verifying hearing aid performance today. There is a **gradual shift, however, toward greater use of the aided response in the fitting process.** As described in Chapter 8, the application of the REAR seems to have particular appeal for pediatric hearing aid selection. As prescriptive methods, probe-microphone equipment, and hearing aid selection procedures evolve in the next few years, it is **probable that the REAR will surface as the method of choice** for determination of the quality of the hearing aid fitting.

Because of the present popularity of the insertion gain approach, however, **the most** common use of the REAR is to serve as a reference for the insertion gain calculation (the REUR is subtracted from the REAR to obtain the insertion gain value). Since this calculation is conducted automatically by the probe-microphone equipment, the actual REAR assumes a rather passive role and may not even be displayed with some equipment.

There are several clinical applications of the REAR, even for audiologists who rely solely on insertion gain measures for validation of their prescriptive fit. As shown earlier in Figure 3–15, it is sometimes useful to display a family of curves, obtained at different input levels. This is especially useful if intermodulation distortion is suspected. Illustrated in Figure 3–16, are REARs conducted at inputs of 60, 70, and 80 dB. Observe that for the 80 dB input (top REAR), there is a substantial alteration in the response when compared with the other two output curves, suggesting that intermodulation distortion is present in this instrument. Such distortion will occur most prominently in peak-clipping hearing aids when the input plus the gain are saturating the instrument. Because the hearing aid user's own voice often is at or near 80 dB at the hearing aid microphone, the presence of intermodulation distortion for this input level will often prompt the user to lower the VCW setting — a strategy that potentially will reduce the benefit obtained from the hearing aid.

The REAR usually is preferred over insertion gain when measuring certain special hearing aid features, such as directional microphones, compression, or signal-processing circuitry (see Chapter 10 for illustrative cases). On occasion, the **REAR is useful in trouble-shooting user complaints about hearing aid performance.** Sharp peaks in the frequency response, which might cause incipient feedback or unpleasant sound quality, are identified more readily in the REAR than in the insertion gain measures (i.e., if the feedback peak is located at or near the REUR peak, its magnitude would be significantly decreased in the insertion gain response).

A final important use of the REAR is to measure the maximum output in the real ear

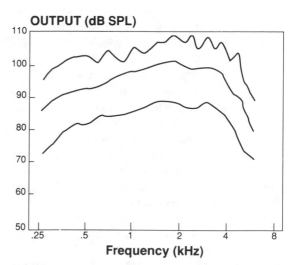

Figure 3–16. Intermodulation distortion was present in this hearing aid for an 80 dB SPL signal, as shown in the top real ear aided response (REAR).

of the hearing aid when it is in saturation. When the REAR is used in this manner, a new term is applied, the *real ear saturation response,* which is discussed next.

REAL EAR SATURATION RESPONSE

The real ear saturation response (RESR) is the SPL, as a function of frequency, at a specified measurement point in the ear canal with the hearing aid in place and turned on. The measurement is obtained with the stimulus level sufficiently intense as to operate the hearing aid at its maximum output level.

Background

As already mentioned, REAR measurements can be conducted at a variety of inputs, and with the hearing aid VCW set at different levels. There are times, however, when it is important to specify that the hearing aid was in saturation at the time of the REAR measure. The REAR then becomes the *real ear saturation response,* or the RESR. This measurement is the **real-ear counterpart to the 2-cm³ measure of SSPL90.**

As the use of probe-microphone measurements developed, it was quickly realized that the actual measurement of saturation sound pressure level in the ear canal was one of the most prominent benefits of this instrumentation. Unlike insertion gain, which has a behavioral analog in functional gain, there is no behavioral equivalent for the RESR. The RESR is especially critical for **children and nonresponsive patients**, when the **maximum output of the hearing aid** must not only **be comfortable, but also safe**. While acoustic trauma or noise-induced hearing loss from hearing aids occurs rarely in children (or at least is documented rarely), all audiologists would agree that one case is too many.

Measurement Procedures

The **measurement procedures** for the RESR are **essentially the same as for the REAR**, except that it is critical to **ensure that the hearing aid is in saturation**. This can be accomplished by:

■ Using a 90 dB SPL input signal.
■ Adjusting the hearing aid's VCW to a point just below feedback.

These procedures will ensure that the RESR measurement represents the highest output that will be delivered to the ear from the instrument under evaluation.

Earlier we discussed that there are several different input signals that can be used when conducting probe-microphone measurements. Most commonly, the choice is between speech-spectrum shaped noise or warble tones. **RESR values can vary significantly as a function of the input stimulus;** lower levels are obtained for noise than for warble tones (Revit, 1991a; Stelmachowicz, 1991). This factor must be considered when RESR measures are conducted, and clinical guidance is offered in Chapter 7.

There is some concern that dangerously high levels can be produced in the ear canal during the RESR measurement. The chances of excessive output in an adult would not seem to be too likely; presumably, the hearing aid will be adjusted prior to the RESR measurement to a reasonable output based on careful unaided audiometric measures, such as

loudness discomfort levels. With children, where responses to unaided measures might be less available or reliable, the potential of producing excessively loud signals in the ear canal becomes more of a concern. Luckily, there is a relatively simple and safe method to obtain a predicted RESR:

■ Conduct an REAR using a 60 dB input with the VCW set at a 50% rotation. Record the REAR values for key frequencies and peaks — print out if possible.
■ Remove the hearing aid from the ear — be sure that the VCW is not moved (tape in place if necessary).
■ Conduct 2-cm^3 coupler measures for the hearing aid using a 60 dB input (record values).
■ Adjust the VCW to a full-on position and conduct 2-cm^3 measurements for a 90 dB input (record values).
■ Subtract the 60 dB input 2-cm^3 values from the 90 dB input 2-cm^3 values.
■ Add the 2-cm^3 difference values to the REAR values obtained at a 60 dB input with a 50% VCW setting.

This procedure will result in a predicted RESR that will be very similar to the actual RESR values obtained in the ear canal (see Chapter 7 for further discussion).

Clinical Applications

The clinical applications of the RESR are directly related to the measurement of the patient's loudness discomfort levels (LDLs). One of the primary goals of the hearing aid fitting procedure is to assure that maximum output of the hearing aid is both comfortable and safe. While this can be accomplished with some degree of accuracy with adult patients without using probe-microphone measurements, by combining the RESR with aided LDLs, a more precise fitting of the hearing aid's output can be obtained. With young children and nonresponsive patients, the RESR can be extremely valuable in choosing an appropriate setting for the hearing aid's output.

As discussed more thoroughly in Chapter 7, the probe-microphone system can be used to measure real-ear SPLs which correspond to the patient's LDLs for specific frequencies. These values then become the target for the RESR fitting and adjustment. An example is shown in Figure 3–17 from Stelmachowicz (1991). Notice in this case the output of the hearing aid was adjusted so that the RESR did not exceed the real-ear LDL (dB SPL) values. In this example, the LDLs and RESR follow a similar pattern, which simplifies the output adjustment process. In some instances, a peak in the RESR will dictate that the overall output is lowered across frequencies, which can result in the RESR falling substantially below the LDLs for some frequency regions. As **multichannel programmable hearing aids** become more widely used, however, it will become easier for the audiologist to **shape the configuration of the RESR to match the real-ear LDL function**.

REAL EAR INSERTION RESPONSE

The real ear insertion response (REIR) is the difference, in decibels as a function of frequency, between the REUR and the REAR measurements taken at the same measurement point in the same soundfield.

The real ear insertion gain (REIG) is the value, in decibels, of the REIR at a specific frequency.

Background

The probe-microphone measurement that normally receives the most attention during the hearing aid fitting is the *real ear insertion response, or REIR*. If gain at only a single frequency is being described, rather than an entire response curve, then the preferred term is the *real ear insertion gain, or REIG*. As the name implies, the REIR refers to the amount of gain that is obtained from the hearing aid when it is inserted in the ear. Unlike the REAR, however, the REIR only refers to the gain that falls above (or below) the patient's REUR. Hence the simple formula: *REAR − REUR = REIR*. Practically speaking, the **REIR is the amount**

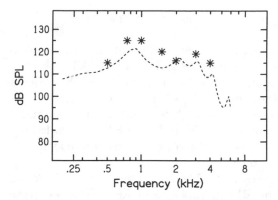

Figure 3–17. Example of the comparison between the real ear saturation response (RESR) and the real ear SPL loudness discomfort levels for a specific hearing aid fitting. (Reprinted from Stelmachowicz, P. 1991. Clinical issues related to hearing aid maximum output. In G. Studebaker, F. Bess, & L. Beck [Eds.], *The Vanderbilt hearing aid report II* [pp. 141–148]. Parkton, MD: York Press, with permission.)

of gain delivered to a patient wearing a hearing aid that he or she did not have before the hearing aid fitting (remember that the REUR was previously present).

The concept of REIR calculation is not unlike the behavioral measurement of functional gain, and real-ear terminology can be substituted accordingly: the patient is first tested unaided (REUR), then aided (REAR) and the difference between the two measures is called *functional gain* (REIR). Intuitively then, the **REIR would be the electroacoustic equivalent (or close equivalent) of functional gain**. Research comparing these two measures has found this to be true (see Chapter 4 for details).

Because the REIR is a relative measure, it is not necessarily a positive value, and unfortunately there are many individuals using hearing aids that result in negative REIG values. Recall from our earlier discussion of the REOR, that when an earmold or hearing aid is placed in the ear, insertion loss occurs. If the gain as measured in the REAR does not adequately compensate for the lost REUR, it is possible that the REUR will exceed the REAR at some frequencies, which then results in a negative REIR. This usually occurs at the 3000 Hz frequency range and is an undesirable outcome, suggesting that an alteration in the fitting is necessary.

Measurement Procedures

The REIR is the mathematical difference between the REUR and the REAR. All probe-tube equipment automatically makes this calculation and displays the REIR on the screen. On some equipment, it is possible to continue to view the REUR and the REAR, which is helpful when attempting to explain unusual peaks or troughs in the REIR.

Figure 3–18 illustrates the relationship among the REUR, REAR, and REIR. The left panel shows the patient's REOR, REUR, and above that the REAR, all shown in decibels SPL. In the right panel, the difference value, the REIR, is displayed. Observe that for this patient, who had an unusually high peak in the REUR, the REAR roughly followed the pattern of the REUR. This explains the relatively flat REIR above 1000 Hz shown in the right panel.

As will be discussed shortly, **the primary purpose of conducting REIR measures is to compare these findings to the desired target gain** that has been derived from some prescriptive fitting procedure. Almost all probe-microphone systems can calculate prescriptive target insertion gain, if a pure-tone audiogram is entered, and then display this curve on the monitor screen. Many audiologists use this feature, as it provides a graphic display of the task at hand. The target REIR curve also can be used for patient counseling, as it provides a visually meaningful display of the goals of the procedure. It is important to keep in mind, however, that rarely is target gain achieved at all frequencies; therefore, the target REIR on the screen also might vividly illustrate the inadequacies of the fit to you and your patient. For the knowledgeable patient, this has the potential to cast some doubt on the quality of the fit (or the fitter); for this reason, some audiologists prefer to compare the REIR to prescriptive target gain in a less obvious manner.

Because the REIR is a relative measure, probe-tube depth is not as critical as when absolute measurements are made. What is important, however, is that **the probe tube is placed at the same depth for both the REUR and REAR measure**. If the 25–30-mm-from-the-tragal-notch method described earlier is used, then REIR measures should be valid, as the following objectives will be met:

■ Probe placement is at a constant location.
■ Probe tip extends beyond the hearing aid/earmold by 4–6 mm.

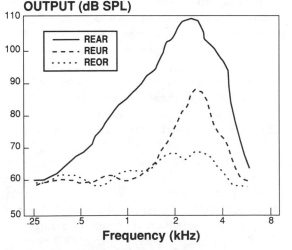
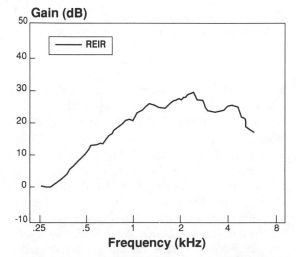

Figure 3–18. Left Panel: Illustration of the real ear occluded response (REOR), the real ear unaided response (REUR) and the real ear aided response (REAR) for a patient fitted with a vented in-the-ear (ITE) hearing aid. Right Panel: The resulting real ear insertion response (REIR) for the measurements shown in the left panel.

■ Probe tip is within 10 mm of the tympanic membrane.

If, for some reason, however, it is not possible to obtain a deep placement, a shallow placement for both the REUR and REAR will still provide reasonably accurate results, as described by Hawkins and Mueller (1986) and illustrated in Figure 3–19. The zero reference point refers to the insertion gain obtained when both REUR and REAR measures were conducted with a deep placement (which we will consider the clinical gold standard). Observe that when either the REUR or the REAR measures were individually conducted with the probe at a shallow position, significant errors occur in the higher frequencies. When *both* measures were conducted with the probe at the shallow position, however, REIR values were very similar to those obtained when a deep placement was used.

Beginning students of probe-microphone measurements sometimes fail to recognize the **direct and important relationship that the REUR measurement will have on the REIR result**. Before a hearing aid is rejected because of an unacceptable REIR, it might be wise to go back and review (or repeat) the REUR, to assure that this measure is valid. In some cases, an undesirable REIR can be predicted before the hearing aid is even taken out of the box simply by viewing the REUR. Otherwise stated, dispensers who desire good REIRs in the 2500–4000 Hz region yearn for patients with small REURs. All experienced users of probe-microphone equipment remember the time that they obtained the unbelievably good REIG at 4000 Hz — for a patient whose REUR at 4000 Hz was at or near zero!

The relationship between the REUR and the REIR is graphically displayed in Figure 3–20. Shown in the left panel is the REUR of the right ear of two different people; both have gradually sloping high-frequency hearing loss. Note that the REURs are quite different; patient A's is relatively average, whereas patient B's REUR is abnormally small in the mid-frequencies, with a large peak in the 4000 Hz region (patient B has a very narrow ear canal).

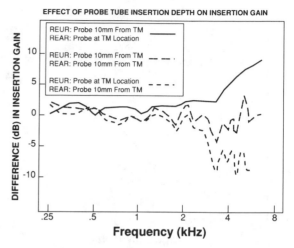

EFFECT OF PROBE TUBE INSERTION DEPTH ON INSERTION GAIN

Figure 3–19. Illustration of the variation in the real ear insertion response (REIR) that will occur when various probe-tube depths are used for the real ear unaided response (REUR) and the real ear aided respone (REAR) measurements. The zero reference represents the REIR obtained when a deep placement was used for both the REUR and the REAR. (Adapted from Hawkins & Mueller, 1986.)

The right panel shows the REIR that was obtained for these two people when they were fitted with the *same in-the-canal hearing aid.* Notice that patient B has an undesirable peak in the REIR in the mid-frequencies and significantly less gain than desired in the high frequencies. The REIR for patient A, on the other hand, is reasonably close to prescriptive target gain across all frequencies of interest. In some dispensing practices, patient A would be fitted with the instrument, and patient B would not, yet in this example, the same hearing aid was used for both individuals.

Some procedural considerations regarding the input stimulus for REIR measurements deserve a brief mention (see also Chapter 4). First, as described in the REAR section, most probe-microphone equipment requires that for accurate REIR calculations, the same input is used for the REUR and REAR measurements. If different input intensity levels are used, it is necessary to include the difference value when REIR calculations are made. Second, it is **best to use a relatively low input**

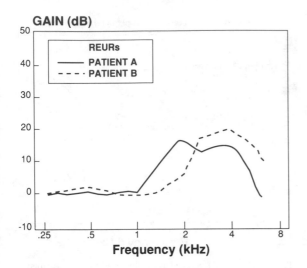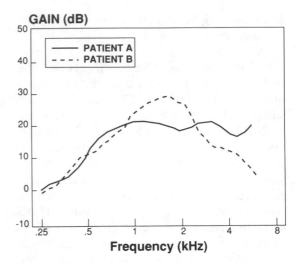

Figure 3–20. Left Panel: The real ear unaided response (REUR) for two different patients. Right Panel: The real ear insertion response (REIR) for the same two patients fitted with the same in-the-canal hearing aid.

(e.g., 60 dB) to assure that the hearing aid is not in saturation when the REAR is obtained (when the hearing aid is in saturation, less gain from the hearing is recorded, while the "gain" of the REUR remains unchanged — resulting in a reduced REIR value). The level of the input also must be considered when testing input-activated compression instruments (see Chapter 4). The **type of stimulus input** (e.g., warble tone, noise, etc.) does **not appear to be a major concern for REIR measures**, as researchers have found relatively equal REIRs when different input signals (from different equipment) have been compared (Humes, Hipskind, & Block, 1988; Mueller & Sweetow, 1987).

Clinical Application

The clinical application of the REIR is to verify that a predetermined prescriptive target insertion gain has been achieved. In fact, **without a theoretical target, REIR measures become rather meaningless**. It could (and has been) argued that the *REAR* should be the real-ear response that is the basis for the pass/fail criterion of the hearing aid fitting. This argument has merit and will surface several times in this text. For the present, however, and probably for the near future, the REIR is the most commonly used real-ear measure among audiologists to assess the acceptability of a hearing aid fitting.

The clinical popularity of the REIR can be traced to the use of functional gain, which was directly tied to the 1980s shift to prescriptive fitting approaches. As recent as 1988, almost all audiologists who used a prescriptive fitting approach were using a threshold/gain-based procedure (Martin & Morris, 1989). These procedures (e.g., POGO, NAL, Berger; see Chapter 5) were all devised and validated using functional gain. As functional gain's real-ear replacement, the REIR quickly was adopted. Today, because most probe-microphone equipment only conducts target gain calculations for threshold-based prescriptive methods, dispensers are encouraged to continue, or in some cases begin, using the REIR fitting strategy. Extensive discussion concerning the use of the REIR as a pass/fail criterion for hearing aid fittings is contained in Chapter 6.

REAL EAR COUPLER DIFFERENCE

The real ear coupler difference (RECD) is the difference, in decibels, as a function of frequency, between the outputs of a hearing aid measured in a real ear versus a 2-cm³ coupler.

Background

While it is tempting to refer to this final term as the real ear coupler *response* or *ratio*, to maintain the consistency of acronyms ending in *R*, the fact is that this measure is neither a single response or a ratio, but a difference; hence the acronym *RECD*. The RECD term was not included in the published article from ANSI S3.80 working group, but has been included in recent draft proposals.

The RECD is a measure that **solves some of our problems of correcting responses from the 2-cm³ coupler to the real ear**. The REAR offers the opportunity to use the ear as a coupler; therefore, direct comparison to 2-cm³ coupler values on an individual basis is possible. Factors that cause the hearing aid to perform differently in the real ear, such as residual ear canal volume, resonance, and middle ear impedance all can be accounted for by establishing an individual correction factor for the ear being fitted (see Chapter 12 for a discussion of these factors and their effect on the magnitude of the RECD).

Measurement Procedures

It is possible to calculate the RECD using either insert earphones or a hearing aid. The procedure using a hearing aid is described here, as this has the widest clinical application:

- The first portion of the RECD procedure is to measure an REAR. It is important that the hearing aid is not in saturation or compression, so a relatively low input should be used (e.g., 60 dB SPL).
- The VCW setting should be at a 1/2 to 2/3 rotation setting. If a low SSPL90 hearing aid is used, it is important that the VCW setting is not set too high, as saturation could occur even for a 60 dB SPL input signal.
- Once the REAR has been obtained, the hearing aid is removed from the ear and a 2-cm³ coupler response is obtained. It is

important to assure that the VCW is not changed, and that the same input is used.
- The 2-cm³ coupler values are then subtracted from the REAR, and the difference is the RECD.

Clinical Applications

The RECD serves as an individual's personal correction factor, and its values can be applied at times when average correction factors ordinarily would be used. The primary example would be in the selection of an appropriate hearing aid based on 2-cm³ information, whether it be a behind-the-ear hearing aid from a specification sheet, or when designing a custom ITE hearing aid order. Logic would suggest that the application of the **RECD, rather than average correction values, would allow a hearing aid to be selected that would more closely approximate the prescriptive target**, be it REIR or REAR. The same RECD values also would apply to the selection of SSPL90. (Further discussion of the RECD is presented later in this text.)

CONCLUSION

By now, the acronyms should start to sound familiar, and gradually they might even be finding their way into your casual clinical conversations. As mentioned in the introducory remarks of this chapter, many of the definitions presented here were taken from working drafts of a proposed standard from the ANSI S3.80 Committee studying probe-microphone measurements of hearing aid performance. While some of this terminology is new, there is considerable similarity with the terminology used in the ANSI S3.35 (1985) standard. Table 3–1, from Hawkins (1991), serves as a good summary of the terminology discussed thus far, as it shows a comparison of the ANSI S3.35 terms from manikin measurements and the consensus terms from the ANSI probe-microphone committee. The far right column includes other terms that

TABLE 3–1. COMPARISON OF THE TERMINOLOGY USED IN THE MEASUREMENT OF HEARING AID PERFORMANCE.

Measurement	ANSI S3.35 (In situ standard)	ANSI S3.80 (Probe-Tube Committee)	Other Terms
SPL near TM unaided	Manikin unoccluded ear gain (1 frequency) Manikin frequency response (curve)	Real ear unaided response (REUR)	FF eardrum TF Wearer unoccluded gain (1 frequency) Wearer frequency response (curve) Ear canal resonance External ear resonance External ear effects Open ear response Unaided response
SPL near TM aided		Real ear aided response (REAR)	In situ output response
Difference (dB) near TM between unaided and aided	Simulated insertion gain (1 frequency) Simulated insertion gain frequency response (curve)	Real ear insertion gain (REIG) (1 frequency) Real ear insertion response (REIR) (curve)	Insertion gain Real ear gain Insertion gain frequency response Real ear response
Maximum output of hearing aid near TM	Simulated in situ SSPL90 frequency response	Real ear saturation response (RESR)	Real ear SSPL90

Source: Reprinted from Hawkins, D. 1991. Acoustic measures of hearing aid performance. In G. Studebaker, F. Bess, & L. Beck (Eds.), *The Vanderbilt hearing-aid report II* [pp. 123–139]. Parkton, MD: York Press, with permission.

are commonly used or have appeared in the literature.

The advancement of new technology is not possible without the concurrent development of appropriate terminology and procedures. This chapter has provided some introductory information which will be expanded on in subsequent chapters. In Chapter 4, we provide more detailed insight and guidance regarding many of the procedural variables surrounding probe-microphone measurements.

Procedural Considerations in Probe-Microphone Measurements

■ DAVID B. HAWKINS, Ph.D. ■

■ H. GUSTAV MUELLER, Ph.D. ■

A major advantage of probe-microphone measurements is that the variability so characteristic and inherent in the behavioral audiometric response is removed. It has been well-documented that substantial variability is present in functional gain (FG) and aided soundfield threshold measurements (see Chapter 1). Hawkins, Montgomery, Prosek, and Walden (1987) found that differences in two sets of aided soundfield thresholds must exceed 15 dB to be considered significant at the .05 level.

Probe-microphone measurements, however, are not without their own distinct sources of variability, and many decisions concerning how probe-microphone measurements will be performed can affect both reliability and validity. In Chapter 3, some of the variables were discussed that can affect probe-microphone measurements. The purpose of this chapter is to describe further some of these procedural considerations and, when appropriate, how they can affect the reliability and validity of probe-microphone measurements.

PROCEDURAL CONSIDERATIONS

ABSOLUTE ACCURACY OF THE MEASUREMENT

Before addressing procedural considerations that affect measurements, it is useful to examine whether a commercial probe-microphone system can accurately measure sound pressure level (SPL) in an ear canal. Two studies (Dirks & Kincaid, 1987; Hawkins & Mueller, 1986) compared probe-microphone measured SPLs to the output SPLs from a Zwislocki ear simulator in a Knowles Electronics Manikin for Acoustic Research (KEMAR). Figure 4–1 from Dirks and Kincaid (1987) shows the real ear unaided response (REUR; Figure 4–1A), real ear aided response (REAR; Figure 4–1B) and real ear insertion response (REIR; Figure 4–1C) measured with the Rastronics system (solid lines) and with the KEMAR (dashed lines). The probe tube was placed 4 mm from the microphone in KEMAR's ear canal, thus representing a location close to the tympanic membrane of a real person. Notice that agreement is good among all three measurements. It may be concluded that when careful procedures are followed, the probe-microphone clin-

ical systems allow the user to make **measurements that agree well with standard manikin values.** Although data of this type have not been published for all manufacturer's probe-microphone units, it is logical to assume that similar accuracy exists, as several studies have found **good agreement among different instruments** (Humes, Hipskind, & Block, 1988; Mueller & Sweetow, 1987).

TEST ENVIRONMENT

One of the first decisions that the audiologist must make is where to conduct probe-micro-

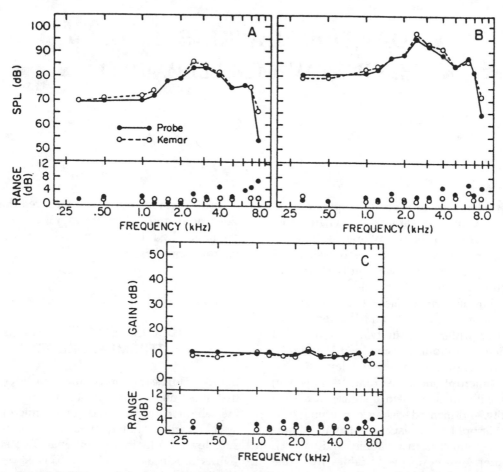

Figure 4–1. REUR (A), REAR (B), and REIG (C) measured with a Zwislocki ear simulator in a KEMAR (open circles) and with a probe tube in the KEMAR's ear canal (solid circles) located 4 mm from the eardrum location. (Adapted from Dirks & Kincaid, 1987.)

phone measurements for clinical hearing aid evaluations. There are two possible choices: inside or outside of a sound-treated room. Given the very short reverberation time, few reflective surfaces, and low noise levels of the sound-treated booth, this location has some clear advantages and is probably ideal. However, space in sound-treated booths is often at a premium, and when the probe-microphone system is located in the sound-treated booth, the probe-microphone equipment itself becomes a reflective surface. Therefore, locating the probe-microphone equipment outside of the sound-treated booth is an attractive alternative. The important issue then becomes whether the probe-microphone measurements can be made outside the sound-treated booth with the same reliability and validity as inside.

Two studies reported comparisons of probe-microphone measurements in a sound-treated booth and in a reverberant room. In one study, Hawkins and Mueller (1986) found large differences between the two environments that were variable with retest. The reverberant room used in that study, however, had many reflective surfaces that were close to the measurement location. In contrast, Tecca (1990) reported close agreement between real ear insertion gain (REIG) measures made in a sound-treated booth and in a reverberant room.

While testing in a sound-treated booth is preferred, **probe-microphone measurements in a reverberant room are acceptable** if the following conditions are met:

■ the loudspeaker is located at an appropriately close distance to the listener,
■ the background noise floor in the room is not excessive given the output levels from the loudspeaker, and
■ no reflective surfaces are near the measurement location.

METHOD OF SOUNDFIELD EQUALIZATION

As discussed in Chapter 3, all probe-microphone systems utilize some method to create a

desired SPL in the soundfield where the probe measurements will be made. Two major instrumentation methods are currently in use, both of which have advantages and disadvantages.

The first procedure for soundfield equalization is the **substitution method**. As shown in Figure 3–1, the exact point in the room where the person will be seated is identified. Without the person present, a microphone is placed at the location the person will occupy for the measurements. A signal is produced by the loudspeaker, measured by the microphone, and deviations from a flat free field are calculated. The person is then placed in the exact location, and the unit delivers a signal that has the desired spectrum in the vacant field.

The advantage of this method is that it incorporates all head and body diffraction effects into the measurement. Although these effects tend to be relatively minor, they will be present in measurements that have used the substitution method of soundfield equalization. The loudspeaker can be placed at any azimuth and the effects of the sound source orientation will be observed accurately. Any measures of actual SPL in the ear canal are accurate because all diffraction and transformations of sound are included in the measurement. Preves and Sullivan (1987) listed three advantages to using the substitution method of equalization: (1) feedback effects can be examined when a nonoccluding earmold or large vent is used, (2) azimuth effects and hearing aid orientation can be evaluated, and (3) the effect of head and body diffraction can be observed. In actual practice, these three points are often not of major clinical importance, as the first rarely occurs, the second is a fact of life and need not be measured routinely, and the third represents fairly minor effects.

The disadvantage of the substitution method is that the **person must be located in the exact reference location** and cannot move in any direction during the measurement. If the person's head moves toward the loudspeaker during the measurement, more SPL will be measured in the ear canal; if the person leans back, less SPL will be present. These effects are shown in Figure 4–2. Notice that move-

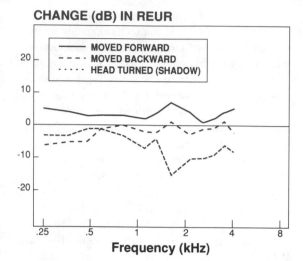

CHANGE (dB) IN REUR

Figure 4–2. The effect of head movement forward, backward, and to the side when the substitution method of soundfield equalization is used.

ment of the head with the substitution effect can alter the hearing aid output by up to 7 dB. Head movements in the horizontal plane affect higher frequencies if the aided ear is turned away from the loudspeaker, resulting in a head shadow. The dotted line in Figure 4–2 shows the effect when the person turns 45° to the side. If the substitution method is selected, a **head restraint should be used.** As this is not practical with children, the substitution method is not recommended with the pediatric population.

The other procedure for soundfield equalization is the **modified-pressure or modified-comparison method** (Preves, 1987; Preves & Sullivan, 1987). In this method, there are two microphones, one that measures SPL in the ear canal and one that is placed at some location on the head and measures and/or regulates the SPL being generated by the loudspeaker. In one approach to this procedure, the external microphone monitors the loudspeaker SPL and keeps it constant at the regulating microphone location during the measurement process. This modification of the loudspeaker output is typically done on line or in real time. The audiologist can verify this loudspeaker adjustment by moving the probe assembly closer and further away from the loudspeaker and listening to the SPL change

as the system achieves equalization. The SPL from the loudspeaker increases as the probe assembly is moved further from the loudspeaker and decreases as the probe is moved closer.

Ideally, the regulating microphone is located next to the hearing aid microphone, thereby maintaining a constant SPL entering the hearing aid. Current commercial units utilizing this method suggest placement of the regulating microphone either over the test ear, on the cheek, or off to the side of the test ear. By keeping a constant SPL at these regulating microphone locations, much of the head and body diffraction effects are subtracted from the measurements. As a result, actual SPL measurements in the ear canal are slightly different from those obtained with the substitution method. Relative measures of gain, such as REIG, will not be affected. With the modified-comparison or -pressure method, it is important that the regulating microphone not be so close to the ear canal that sound leakage (such as through a vent) is processed and the loudspeaker output modified as a result.

A variation of the modified-pressure method utilizes a second microphone, used as a **reference microphone** rather than a regulating microphone. An initial calibration procedure is accomplished (called *leveling*), during which the reference microphone measures the output levels of a broad-band noise and determines the corrections necessary for appropriate loudspeaker output. During the probe measurements, the reference microphone does not modify the loudspeaker output, but simply measures the loudspeaker output and compares it to the probe-microphone measured output; in this way, hearing aid gain is computed. In this system, the effects of head and body movement are measured by the reference microphone and corrected for in the final values.

The major advantage of the modified-pressure or -comparison method is that **minor movements of the head do not affect the measurement.** In most units the regulating microphone is always active (Preves & Sullivan, 1987, call this a real time method) and thus holds the SPL constant regardless of head movement forward, backward, or to the side. As a result, unless the head can be fixed in place, we **recommend the modified-comparison method** of soundfield equalization over the substitution method.

LOUDSPEAKER AZIMUTH

The exact location of the loudspeaker relative to the client is another procedural variable that the audiologist must consider. Most manufacturers recommend either a 0° or 45° azimuth; in addition, we have observed clinicians using a 90° azimuth.

Killion and Revit (1987) investigated a variety of loudspeaker locations to determine the position that produced the best test-retest variability. Figure 4–3 shows the test-retest variability for the four locations that they evaluated. In Figure 4–3, the first number in each notation represents the orientation in the vertical plane, and the second number in the notation represents the horizontal plane. For instance, 90,0 is directly over the subject's head, and 0,45 is in the horizontal plane 45° off to the side. The least variability is noted for the 45,45 position, closely followed by the 0,45 position. If the audiologist is unable to locate the loudspeaker at the 45,45 position, the reliability data from this study suggest the 0,45 loudspeaker location as next best. However, the audiologist must consider two other factors: first, practical considerations may dictate a preference for 0° (as discussed in Chapter 3), and second, a 0° loudspeaker location with the modified-pressure method (probably the most common clinical procedure) will produce values that most closely resemble those obtained with the substitution method (Ickes, Hawkins, & Cooper, 1991).

Whatever loudspeaker azimuth is adopted, the audiologist must be aware that **different SPLs will be measured in the ear canal depending on which location is chosen**. For instance, Figure 4–4 shows portions of the classic data from Shaw (1974), in which the REUR

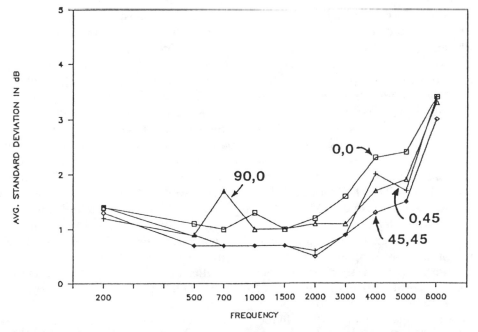

Figure 4–3. Average standard deviations of the test-retest differences for REIG with four loudspeaker locations: 90,0; 0,0; 45,45; and 0,45. (Reprinted from Killion, M. & Revit, L. 1987. Insertion gain repeatability versus loudspeaker location: You want me to put my louspeaker WHERE? *Ear and Hearing, 8* (Suppl. 5), 68S-73S, with permission.)

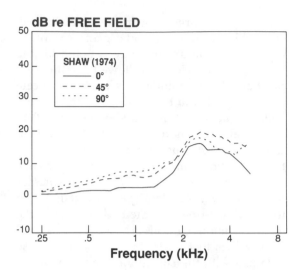

dB re FREE FIELD

Figure 4–4. Field-to-eardrum transfer function from three loudspeaker azimuths: 0°, 45°, and 90°. (Adapted from Shaw, 1974.)

was measured from a variety of loudspeaker azimuths. The 0°, 45°, and 90° REURs were obtained with a substitution method. The effects of head diffraction and head baffle are clearly seen as the signal source moves from 0° to 90°. If the substitution method is used and corrections are made to a prescription formula for deviations from the average REUR, it is important that the average REUR was obtained with the same loudspeaker azimuth.

Given that few audiologists use the substitution method clinically, a more relevant question is whether the REUR, REAR, and REIR will change with different loudspeaker locations when the modified-pressure method of soundfield equalization is utilized. Ickes et al. (1991) measured the REURs, REARs, and REIRs with loudspeaker azimuths of 0°, 45°, and 90° and an over-the-ear reference microphone location. Figure 4–5 shows these results for a behind-the-ear (BTE) hearing aid. It is apparent that differences in all three measurements can occur as loudspeaker azimuth is changed. This is particularly important to consider when attempting to match a target REIR. In the high frequencies, it might be possible to match the target REIR quite well with one loudspeaker azimuth, but not as well with another loudspeaker azimuth.

REGULATING OR REFERENCE MICROPHONE LOCATION

Probe-microphone measurement systems that utilize the modified-pressure method of sound-field equalization have a variety of potential locations for regulating- or reference-microphone placement. The most common locations are over the ear, on the cheek, and at the ear, perpendicular to the plane of the head about 1 inch from the pinna. A recent study by Feigin, Nelson, Barlow, and Stelmachowicz (1990) compared the SPLs at the microphone of a BTE hearing aid when the SPL was regulated by a microphone over the ear and on the cheek. Large differences were found between the resulting inputs to the hearing aid microphone with the regulating microphone in the two locations. For instance, the SPL at the hearing aid microphone was 9.5 dB higher than at the cheek regulating-microphone location in the 1200 to 2000 Hz region. Such large differences were not present with the over-the-ear regulating microphone location. If absolute measures of SPL in the ear canal are being made, **substantial differences can be observed depending on the location of the regulating microphone**.

Ickes et al. (1991) expanded the Feigin et al. (1990) study by examining the effect of three loudspeaker locations (0°, 45°, and 90°) and three reference-microphone locations (over the ear, on the cheek, and at the ear) on the REURs, REARs, and REIRs of both in-the-ear (ITE) and BTE hearing aids. A Frye 6500 probe-microphone system was used with a KEMAR. **All sizeable differences that resulted from reference-microphone location and loudspeaker azimuth were restricted to frequencies above 2000 Hz.** Figure 4–6 shows the REURs for the three microphone locations and three azimuths. Shaw's curves (1974) using the substitution method are shown for comparison. The largest variations are seen at the 90° loudspeaker azimuth and with the at-the-ear microphone location. Figure 4–7 shows the REIRs for the same conditions with an ITE. The differences among the three reference-microphone positions are reduced when the REIR is

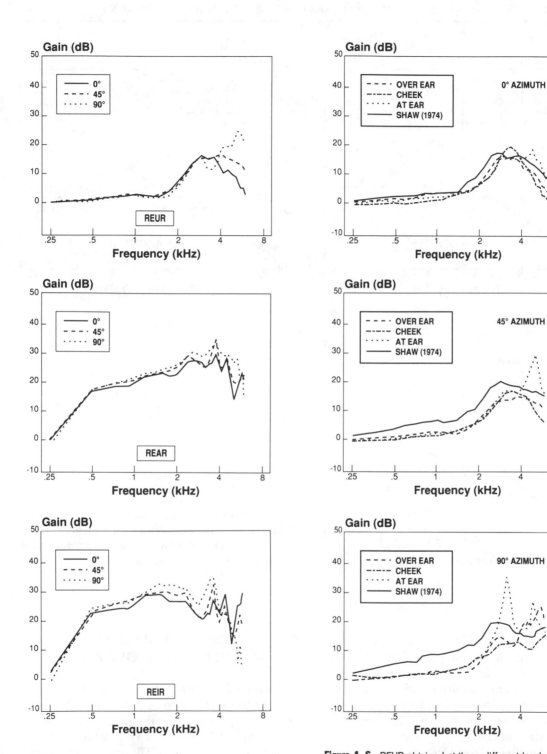

Figure 4–5. REUR, REAR, and REIR obtained on a KEMAR with three loudspeaker azimuths (0°, 45°, and 90°) with an over-the-ear regulating-microphone location and a BTE hearing aid. (Adapted from Ickes et al., 1991.)

Figure 4–6. REUR obtained at three different loudspeaker azimuths (0°, 45°, and 90°) with three different regulating-microphone locations (over the ear, at the cheek, and at the ear). Data from Shaw (1974) using a substitution method are shown for comparison. (Adapted from Ickes et al., 1991.)

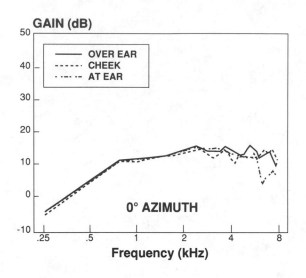

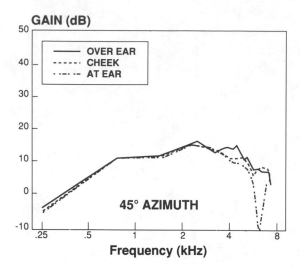

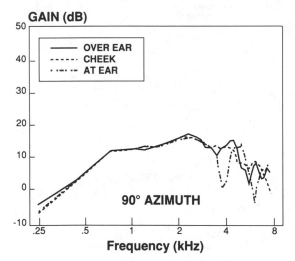

Figure 4–7. REIRs for an in-the-ear hearing aid at three loudspeaker azimuths (0°, 45°, and 90°) and three regulating-microphone locations (over the ear, at the cheek, and at the ear). (Adapted from Ickes et al., 1991.)

measured, since the REIR is a difference curve, and the variations among the different reference-microphone REURs are also present in the REARs. There are significant differences in the REIRs, however, for the 90° azimuth and with the at-the-ear regulating-microphone position.

These data, in combination with those of Killion and Revit (1987) and the practical concerns mentioned earlier, would suggest that a **0° or 45° loudspeaker azimuth with either an over-the-ear or cheek regulating-microphone location is the preferable measurement condition.**

PROBE-TUBE INSERTION DEPTH AND MOVEMENT

Location of the probe tube in the ear canal is one of the most important procedural aspects in making accurate probe-microphone measurements. It is particularly important in the establishment of the REUR and REAR, where measures of absolute SPL in the ear canal are determined.

Figure 4–8 from Dirks and Kincaid (1987) shows the situation that exists in a transmis-

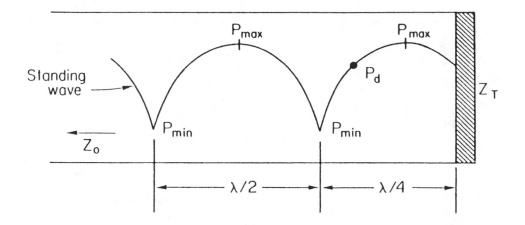

Standing Wave in Lossless Transmission Line

Figure 4–8. Representation of standing wave patterns, where Z_o is the acoustic impedance of the transmission line, Z_t is the termination impedance, P_{max} is the maximum, and P_{min} is the minimum pressure of the standing wave for a sound of wavelength lambda. P_d is the sound pressure developed at distance d from the termination. (Reprinted from Dirks, D., & Kincaid, G. 1987. Basic acoustic considerations of ear canal probe measurements. *Ear and Hearing, 8* [Suppl. 5], 60S–67S, with permission.)

sion line equivalent to the ear canal. Since the termination impedance (Z_t) is not equal to the impedance of the transmission line (Z_o), sound is reflected back from the end (tympanic membrane), causing standing waves, with pressure maxima (P_{max}) and pressure minima (P_{min}). The maxima and minima will be in different places in the ear canal depending on the frequency of the input signal. The first minima occurs for each frequency at a distance equal to one fourth of its wavelength. For example, the wavelength of a 4000 Hz tone is 8.6 cm, and one fourth of 8.6 is 2.1 cm (21 mm). Therefore, if the probe tube is 21 mm from the tympanic membrane, a very low SPL reading at 4000 Hz will be measured due to the probe tube being located at a pressure minima for this frequency. That is, the measured SPL reading will be much lower than that actually occurring at the tympanic membrane.

An example of the error at 3000 Hz as a function of probe-tube location is shown in Figure 4–9 (Dirks & Kincaid, 1987). Plotted on the abscissa is the distance from the tympanic

membrane, while the ordinate shows the difference between the SPL that the probe-microphone measures and the SPL that is actually present at the tympanic membrane. The negative numbers indicate that the probe measurement underestimates the actual SPL at the tympanic membrane. As the probe microphone is located further and further from the tympanic membrane, the error increases until it reaches a maximum error at about 25 mm, close to the one fourth of the wavelength for a 3000 Hz tone. It should be noted that the **impedance of the middle ear has an effect** on the magnitude of the error and the specific location of the minima.

Figure 4–10 from Dirks and Kincaid (1987) shows the errors that will be present for frequencies from 1000 to 8000 Hz as the probe tube is located at varying distances from the tympanic membrane. When the probe tube is located 10 mm from the tympanic membrane, the error is approximately 10 dB at 8000 Hz, 5 dB at 6000 Hz, 3 dB at 4000 Hz, 2 dB at 3000 Hz, 1 dB at 2000 Hz, and less than 1 dB at

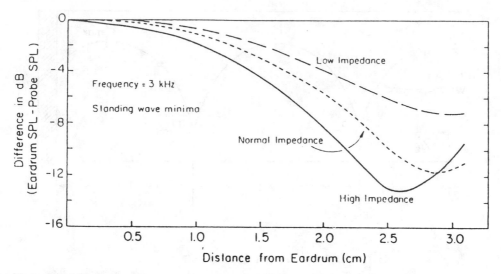

Figure 4–9. Difference between eardrum- and probe-measured SPL at 3000 Hz for average, low-normal, and high-normal impedance transmission lines as a function of distance of the probe from the eardrum. (Reprinted from Dirks, D., & Kincaid, G. 1987. Basic acoustic considerations of ear canal probe measurements. *Ear and Hearing, 8* [Suppl. 5], 60S–67S, with permission.)

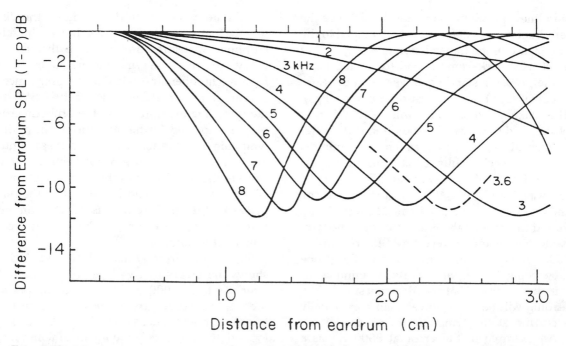

Figure 4–10. Difference between eardrum- and probe-measured SPL at eight frequencies as a function of distance of the probe from the eardrum. (Reprinted from Dirks, D., & Kincaid, G. 1987. Basic acoustic considerations of ear canal probe measurements. *Ear and Hearing, 8* [Suppl. 5], 60S–67S, with permission.)

1000 Hz. When a 5-mm location is achieved, the accuracy of the probe measurements is within 2 dB through 8000 Hz. There is a direct relationship between distance of the probe from the tympanic membrane and the accuracy of the measurement in the high frequencies; **the closer to the tympanic membrane the probe tube is placed, the more accurate will be the high-frequency measurement**.

An example of the importance of this issue of insertion depth in clinical practice is shown in Figure 4–11. Three REAR curves were obtained with the probe tube inserted 2 mm, 6 mm, and 13 mm past the tip of the earmold on a person wearing a BTE hearing aid. Notice that differences in SPL in the ear canal begin to appear above 1500 Hz. The differences between the two extremes, 2 mm and 13 mm, are 5 dB at 3000 Hz and 10 dB in the 4000 to 6000 Hz region. These curves demonstrate the importance of probe-tube placement for accurate measurement in the higher frequencies.

In clinical practice, there are two basic considerations in deciding where to place the probe tube in the ear canal. First, the probe tube should be close enough to the tympanic membrane to achieve the desired accuracy in

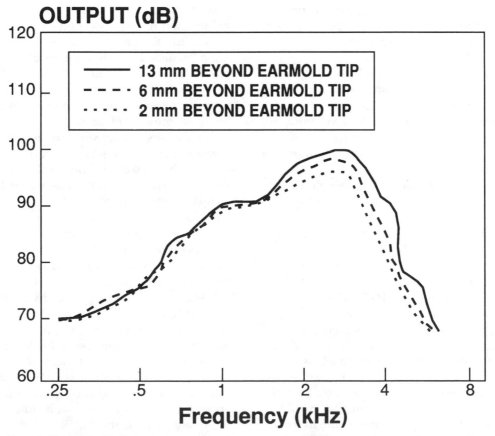

Figure 4–11. REARs obtained with three probe tube insertion depths into the ear canal: 2 mm, 6 mm, and 1 mm past the tip of the earmold.

the high frequencies. A location of **5mm or closer to the tympanic membrane is ideal**, since this location will yield absolute SPL measurements with an accuracy of within 2 dB through 6000 Hz. Second, it is important that the probe tube extend at least 5 mm past the tip of the canal portion of the earmold or ITE hearing aid. Burkhard and Sachs (1977) have shown that inaccuracies can occur in the higher frequencies if the probe tube is too close to the tip of the earmold. Given these considerations, there is a variety of methods for placement of the probe tube at an appropriate insertion depth in the ear canal. One common, but somewhat tedious, method consists of the following steps:

1. before insertion into the ear, place the probe tube next to the earmold or ITE and extend it at least 5 mm past the tip,
2. mark the probe tube with a pen (or place a collar) next to the outer edge of the earmold,
3. place the earmold and probe tube in the ear and determine an anatomical landmark where the mark or collar rests,
4. remove the hearing aid and earmold; replace the probe with the mark or collar at the appropriate location and measure the REUR, and
5. replace the earmold or ITE, being careful to keep the mark in the same location.

A good alternative method is to place the probe at a **constant insertion depth** past the tragus or the intratragal notch. The length of the average adult ear canal is 25 mm (Zemplenyi, Gilman, & Dirks, 1985). The typical distance from the ear canal opening to the tragus or intratragal notch is 10 mm, yielding a total distance from this external location to the tympanic membrane of 35 mm. Hawkins, Alvarez, and Houlihan (1991) have recommended using an insertion depth of **30 mm past the tragus**, resulting in a placement that should be 5 mm from the tympanic membrane in the average adult. A more conservative approach, to avoid ever touching the tympanic membrane, is to place the probe 25–27 mm past the tra-

gus, resulting in a placement 8–10 mm from the tympanic membrane. Such placement will yield absolute SPL measurements with an accuracy within 3 dB through 4000 Hz. This approach is quick, reproducible, and yields reliable results (Hawkins, Alvarez, & Houlihan, 1991). Procedures for probe tube placement in children are discussed in Chapter 8.

A third alternative for placement of the probe tube was suggested by Sullivan (1988). Based on the pressure maxima and minima principles described above and illustrated in Figure 4–8, a 6000-Hz warble tone is introduced and the SPL is monitored as the probe tube is slowly inserted into the ear canal. When the lowest SPL reading is obtained, it is surmised that the distance from the tympanic membrane at that location should be between 13 and 16 mm, based on the calculated pressure minima. The probe is marked at an external location for this insertion depth, 10 mm is added, and the probe is reinserted, thus yielding a predicted insertion depth of 23–26 mm, which should be within 3–6 mm of the tympanic membrane according to Sullivan. This procedure can be cumbersome and is affected by hand movement around the ear.

Finally, several newer probe-microphone measurement systems have incorporated procedures that make estimates of the probe tube distance from the tympanic membrane through acoustic measurements. While the accuracy of such measurements has not been verified, this type of procedure represents an interesting development, as it holds promise for an accurate method of placement and replacement of the probe tube in the ear canal.

If the primary interest is not in the absolute SPL in the ear canal, but instead in measuring the REIG, the exact location of the probe is not as important as the necessity for the probe to stay **exactly** in the same location for both the REUR and REAR measurements. Since the REIR is a difference value (REAR minus REUR), an error in probe placement can be tolerated if it is present in **both** the REUR and REAR measurement. Figure 4–12 from Dirks and Kincaid (1987) demonstrates this point. In Figure 4–12A, the REUR is shown as measured in a KEMAR

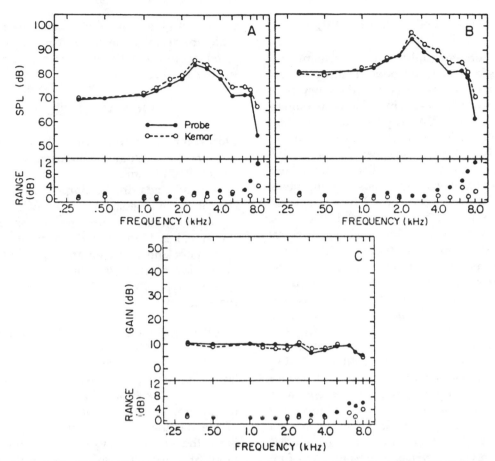

Figure 4-12. REUR (A), REAR (B), and REIG (C) measured with a Zwislocki ear simulator in a KEMAR (open circles) and with a probe tube in the KEMAR's ear canal (solid circles) located 14 mm from the eardrum location. (Reprinted from Dirks, D., & Kincaid, G. 1987. Basic acoustic considerations of ear canal probe measurements. *Ear and Hearing, 8*[Suppl. 5], 60S–67S, with permission.)

and as measured with a probe tube in KEMAR's ear located 14 mm from the tympanic membrane location. At this distance, the probe microphone will measure less SPL than is actually present in the higher frequencies. Notice that the probe-microphone values (solid line) fall below the KEMAR values above 3000 Hz. Figure 4–12B shows the REAR; again, because of the 14-mm location, the probe-microphone measured values are too low. Because REIG is a difference between the REAR and REUR, Figure 4–12C shows no error present in the REIG values. Since the probe tube was in the same location for both the REUR and REAR, the error was the same for both measurements and the REIG values are accurate.

In summary, for accurate SPL measurements in the higher frequencies, it is necessary to locate the probe tube **at least 5 mm past the tip of the earmold or ITE hearing aid and within 5–10 mm of the tympanic membrane**. For REIG measurements, it is necessary that the probe tube stay in the **same location** for both the REUR and REAR. Since many applications of probe-microphone measurements may involve the assessment of both absolute SPLs and REIG, the clinician should try to satisfy both the depth and constant-location criteria. **Our clinical recommendation to satisfy these criteria in adults is to use a constant location, placing the probe tube 25–30 mm past the tragus.**

STIMULUS SIGNAL TYPE

When probe-microphone measurement systems were initially introduced, the only test stimulus signals were sweep-frequency pure tones or warble tones. Since that time, numerous other signals have appeared on various instruments, including clicks, wide-band noise, narrow-band noise, and speech-shaped noise. Many instruments have multiple signal options and the audiologist can choose among them. There is a clear trend toward having speech-shaped noise available on most instruments.

It is not obvious at this point which signal will dominate future instruments or prove to provide more valid measurements. There are, however, **clear advantages to a speech-shaped noise signal** for measuring the REAR and REIR. The noise signal is capable of measuring more accurately the response of hearing aids whose compression circuits are activated over a range of typical inputs (e.g., 40–80 dB SPL) and of hearing aids that automatically reduce the low-frequency gain in the presence of more intense low-frequency input or as a function of input level (e.g., many "noise reduction" and "ASP" circuits). In addition, use of a noise signal can allow a visual representation of intermodulation distortion with higher input levels (see Figure 3–15). Finally, the use of speech-shaped noise allows the audiologist to rapidly adjust the hearing aid until the speech spectrum is amplified to certain target values in the ear canal. However, while the speech-shaped noise does have these advantages, for typical linear hearing aids, the REAR and REIR should be the same regardless of the signal type if the hearing aid is operating within the linear portion of its response.

The Real Ear Saturation Response (RESR) will differ with some probe-microphone units depending on whether a narrow-band signal (such as a pure tone) or broad-band signal is used. The issue of ideal signal types with RESR measurements is discussed in Chapter 7.

In summary, while we believe acceptable and valid clinical REARs and REIRs can be obtained for most hearing aids with either a warble-tone or a broad-band noise signal, the latter will give more realistic results for the wide spectrum of newer and more sophisticated hearing aid circuits that are appearing on the market.

SIGNAL LEVEL

Most commercial probe-microphone units can deliver signals from the loudspeaker over a 50–90 dB SPL range. The signal level that is chosen depends on the purpose of the measurement. For assessment of the REUR, the signal level is relatively unimportant as long as the signal is high enough to be above the noise floor and low enough to prevent loudness discomfort. Signal levels of 60–70 dB SPL are typically sufficient to meet both of these criteria.

Signal Level for REAR and REIR Measurements

In contrast, the choice of signal level can be important for certain REAR and all REIR measurements. One application of the REAR is determination of the maximum saturation output of the hearing aid in the real ear, or RESR. Since the purpose is to determine the maximum SPL that the hearing aid can deliver to the ear, it is important that the hearing aid be saturated during this measurement. In other words, the signal level must be sufficiently high so that, when combined with the gain of the hearing aid, the maximum output is achieved. If the hearing aid volume control wheel (VCW) is rotated to its maximum point before feedback, then an input level of 85–90 dB SPL will typically cause the hearing aid to saturate, and an accurate measure of the RESR can be obtained.

When making REIR measurements, the level should probably approximate a typical input to the hearing aid. With this criterion, a **70 dB SPL speech-weighted noise** (which would have lower level per cycle values across frequency) or a 60 dB SPL swept-warble tone would be most appropriate. Typical input levels such as these should not saturate the hearing aid (i.e., a 60–70 dB SPL input plus the gain should not equal the SSPL90). If saturation does occur, which may be the case when a low SSPL90 is combined with a rather high amount of gain, or when an excessively high input level is used (e.g., 75–80 dB SPL), the gain of the hearing aid will be reduced. An example of how the REIR can be affected by an inappropriately high signal level is shown in Figure 4–13 from Hawkins and Mueller (1986). In this figure, REIRs are shown for a hearing aid with a relatively low SSPL90 when the input is 60 and 80 dB SPL. Notice that the REIG is substantially greater with the 60 dB SPL input. When attempting to match certain target REIG values, the choice of input level is important. The 80 dB SPL input would be too high here and would result in inappropriate findings. This problem of a high SPL input causing reduced and misleading REIG values will typically occur in low SSPL90 hearing aids where more than minimal amounts of gain are being used. This reduction in gain is not an artifact; it is a true representation of the gain present in the hearing aid for that input signal level.

Signal Levels for Special Circuits

The input level issue is also important when assessing hearing aids with compression circuitry. Figure 4–14 from Hawkins and Mueller (1986) shows the REIRs of a hearing aid with an input-compression threshold of 65 dB SPL when the input level is 60 and 80 dB SPL. Notice that the REIG is substantially higher for the 60 dB SPL input as the hearing aid is producing full gain and the automatic gain reduction circuit has not been activated. With the 80 dB SPL input, the compression threshold of 65 dB SPL has been exceeded and gain reduction has occurred, causing the REIG to be substantially reduced. Again, the results with the 80 dB SPL input are accurate, but the REIR obtained with the 60 dB SPL is probably more representative of how the hearing aid will function under typical listening situations.

Other Signal Level Issues

Several remaining issues concerning signal level should be mentioned before leaving this topic. First, when a complex signal is being employed (such as a noise or click) it is important to know the **crest factor** — that is, the number of decibels by which the peak exceeds the root mean square (rms) level of the signal. The crest factor in actual speech is approxi-

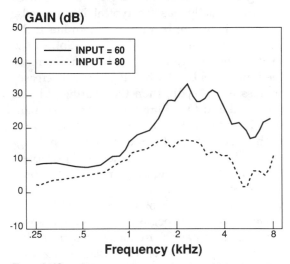

Figure 4–13. REIRs obtained with a hearing aid having a low SSPL90 for an input SPL that did not cause saturation (solid line, 60 dB SPL) and an input SPL that did cause saturation (dotted line, dB SPL). (Adapted from Hawkins & Mueller, 1986.)

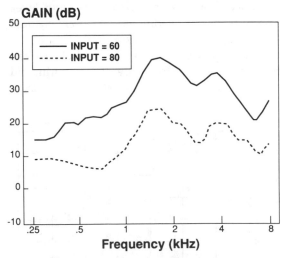

Figure 4–14. REIRs obtained with an input automatic gain control (AGC) (threshold = 65 dB SPL) hearing aid for an input SPL that did not cause the AGC to be activated (solid line, 60 dB SPL) and an input SPL that did cause activation of the AGC (dotted line, 80 dB SPL). (Adapted from Hawkins & Mueller, 1986.)

mately 12 dB, a value that has been designed into some speech-shaped noise signals such as the Frye composite weighted noise. If a higher crest factor is present, as in a click, the peaks of the waveform can cause the hearing aid to saturate at a lower overall signal level (Frye, 1987), giving the impression of less gain than the hearing aid actually has for typical input levels.

There is a simple way to determine if the signal being used is causing saturation of the hearing aid and thus gain reduction. Decrease the input level by 10 dB; if the output decreases by less than 10 dB, then the hearing aid was saturated and functioning in a nonlinear manner. If such is the case, the audiologist may wish to repeat the REIR at a lower input signal level to determine the amount of gain present when the hearing aid is not in saturation.

A second issue concerning signal level involves measurement of REAR and REIR with newer circuits that begin compression at lower levels and/or have a frequency response that varies with input level. For instance, **the gain and frequency response of the K-Amp circuit change with input level**. Figure 4–15 shows the REIRs with the K-Amp for inputs of 40, 60, 70, and 90 dB SPL. Notice that both the amount of insertion gain and the shape of the frequency response change with increases in input level. The REIR of the hearing aid purposely changes as the input level increases. With this newer type of signal processing, the audiologist can best define the performance of the hearing aid by obtaining REIRs at **several input levels**.

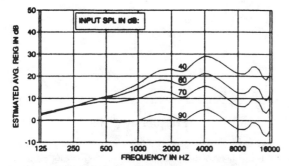

Figure 4–15. REIRs for the K-Amp hearing aid for inputs of 40, 60, 70, and 90 dB SPL. (Adapted from Etyomtic Research K-amp product literature.)

A similar situation is seen with wide-range dynamic-compression hearing aids. This type of circuit has a low compression threshold (e.g., 45 dB SPL), and in some cases an adjustable compression ratio. As a result, the REIG is higher if lower level inputs are used and lower with higher input signals. The amount of gain reduction observed with higher input signals will be related to the compression ratio (i.e., the higher the ratio the more gain reduction and the less REIG will be measured).

To summarize, given that we are trying to assess the REIR available to the user for realistic everyday use, inputs of 60 dB SPL (for warble tones) and 70 dB SPL (speech-shaped noise) are recommended for clinical measurement of REAR and REIR for typical hearing aid circuits. For more sophisticated circuits, several input levels may be necessary.

COMPARISON OF DIFFERENT PROBE UNITS

As discussed in Chapter 2, there are numerous companies manufacturing probe-microphone units, and new instrumentation appears each year. All of the units have not been compared in a single study, and only two studies to date have compared some of the different units. Mueller and Sweetow (1987) compared REIG on 14 ears with the Acoustimed HA 2000, Madsen IGO 1000, and the Rastronics CCI-10/3. Figure 4–16 shows the mean REIRs with the three probe-microphone systems. Although the mean responses are rather close, test-retest variability was different among the units. Mueller and Sweetow concluded that "insertion gain data obtained from one system reasonably can be compared to that obtained on a different system" (p. 57). Humes et al. (1988) compared REIG with the Madsen IGO 1000, Acoustimed HA 2000, and the Frye 6500 on 8 ears. Their mean data are shown in Figure 4–17 and indicate that, for the average ear, **reasonable agreement** is observed among the different systems. As did Mueller and Sweetow (1987), however, Humes et al. (1988) reported differing test-retest reliability with the three units.

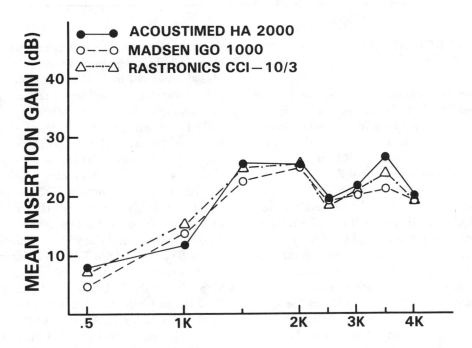

Figure 4–16. Mean REIGs obtained from a group of subjects using the Acoustimed HA-2000, Madsen IGO 1000, and Rastronics CCI-10/3. (From Mueller, H., & Sweetow, R. 1987. A clinical comparison of probe microphone systems. *Hearing Instruments, 38,* 20–21, with permission.)

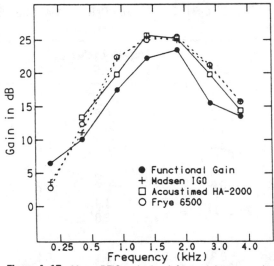

Figure 4–17. Mean REIGs obtained from eight ears using the Madsen IGO 1000, Acoustimed HA-2000, and Frye 6500. Also shown are mean FG values. (From Humes, L., Hipskind, N., & Block, M. 1988. Insertion gain measured with three probe tube systems. *Ear and Hearing, 9,* 108–112, with permission.)

TEST-RETEST RELIABILITY

When consideration is given to all the procedural issues that have been discussed, it is not surprising that considerable variability exists in probe-microphone measurements. In discussing variability, Tecca (1990) stressed that three types of test-retest variability need to be considered in evaluating probe-microphone measurements. The first is **immediate test-retest variability**. In this case, the probe tube is not removed from the ear, calibrations are not repeated, and the system is not turned off. Examples of measurements that would be evaluated in terms of immediate test-retest standards would be repetition of REIRs as the tone control is changed or repeated RESRs as the output control is altered. Although no data are presented, Tecca stated that test-retest differences of greater than 2 dB should be considered significant.

A second type of variability is called **short-term test-retest variability**. In this case, the hearing aid is removed and the probe is reinserted. Several data sets are available that provide information on this type of variability for REIG measurements. Ringdahl and Leijon (1984) reported standard deviations of test-retest differences ranging from 1 dB at 250 Hz to 4.7 dB at 6000 Hz. Revit (1987) calculated similar values from Hawkins (1987a), with results ranging from 1.9 dB at 1000 Hz to 5.9 dB at 6000 Hz. Most recently, Hawkins, Alvarez, and Houlihan (1991) examined short-term test-retest variability for the REUR, REAR, and REIG. The mean test-retest differences, standard deviations, and the 95% confidence intervals (CIs) are shown in Table 4–1. Summarizing these results, it could be concluded that the 95% CIs for the REUR would be ± 2–3 dB at 3000 Hz and below and ± 4–5 dB at 4000 and 5000 Hz. CIs for REAR and REIG would be ± 2–3 dB below 1000 Hz, ± 3 dB in the 1000 to 2000-Hz region, and ± 4–6 dB at 3000 Hz and above.

The third type of variability mentioned by Tecca (1990) was **long-term test-retest variability**. Although no data are available on this type of variability, it is probably slightly larger

TABLE 4–1. MEAN SIGNED TEST-RETEST DIFFERENCES, STANDARD DEVIATIONS (SD), AND 95% CIs (IN dB) FOR THE REUR, REAR, AND REIG

	Frequency (kHz)								
	.25	*.5*	*.75*	*1*	*1.5*	*2*	*3*	*4*	*5*
REUR									
Mean	0.3	0.3	0.4	0.0	−0.2	0.0	0.1	0.4	2.0
SD	0.7	1.3	1.8	1.0	1.1	1.4	1.6	2.7	1.9
95% CI	1.4	2.6	3.6	2.0	2.2	2.8	3.2	5.4	3.8
REAR									
Mean	−1.3	−0.6	−0.6	−0.4	−0.2	−0.2	−0.3	−0.4	−0.2
SD	*	*	*	1.6	1.4	1.7	2.0	2.7	3.0
95% CI	*	*	*	3.2	2.8	3.4	4.0	5.4	6.0
REIG									
Mean	1.4	0.9	−0.9	−0.4	0.1	0.1	−0.3	−0.8	−0.6
SD	*	*	*	1.7	1.5	1.6	2.0	2.2	2.5
95% CI	*	*	*	3.4	3.0	3.2	4.0	4.4	5.0

* Values not reported due to variable leakage around earmold resulting in inflated test-retest variability.

Source: Reprinted from Hawkins, D., Alvarez, E., & Houlihan, J. 1991. Reliability of three types of probe tube microphone measurements. *Hearing Instruments, 42,* 14–16, with permission.

than short-term variability as a result of different calibration values, minor changes in middle-ear pressure, and so on.

There is no doubt that test-retest variability of probe-microphone measurements can be good if care is taken. Probably the major variable affecting the repeatability of these measurements is the exact probe-tube location and the ability to maintain it. The audiologist should pay particular attention to this aspect of the probe-microphone measurement procedure and develop a consistent and reliable method of probe-tube placement.

RELATIONSHIP BETWEEN REIG AND FG

When probe-microphone measurements first became popular, there was some suggestion that REIG might not be the equivalent of FG. The argument was that the REIG measurement took place in the ear canal, whereas the

FG measurement assessed the processed signal through to the central auditory system. Three studies have addressed this issue by comparing REIG and FG on the same sets of subjects. The first study to report such data was by Mason and Popelka (1986). Their data are shown in Figure 4–18. Plotted in this manner, with the ordinate being REIG minus FG, values along the zero line would indicate perfect agreement between the two measurements. Although there were some subjects for whom differences were present, the obvious conclusion from these data is that REIG and FG yield similar values. Results similar to these have been reported by Dillon and Murray (1987) and Humes et al. (1988), and it is possible that the observed differences are a result of variability and not true differences between the measurements themselves.

Although the equivalence of REIR and FG has been established, aided soundfield thresholds should also be obtained for persons with **severe-to-profound hearing loss** in whom thresh-

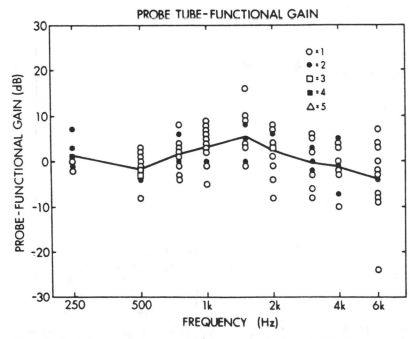

Figure 4–18. Differences between probe-tube measured gain and FG for the same subjects. (Reprinted from Mason, D., & Popelka, G. 1986. Comparison of hearing-aid gain using functional coupler and probe-tube measurements. *Journal of Speech and Hearing Research, 29,* 218–226, with permission.)

olds could possibly be vibrotactile. For instance, Figure 4–19 shows the result from a 4-year-old child presented by Stelmachowicz and Lewis (1988). Unaided responses were obtained only to signals at 250 and 500 Hz and were vibratory. With a high-gain hearing aid, the aided threshold improved by only 10 dB, again suggesting that no hearing was present and that the aided response was also vibrotactile. Probe-microphone measurements showed 50 dB of REIG at 250 Hz and 65 dB at 500 Hz. While this amount of gain was certainly present in the ear canal, for this child the input speech signal was not really being amplified by these amounts. Very different rehabilitative statements would have been made for this child based on the two types of gain measurements. As a result, **aided soundfield thresh-**

olds should also be obtained on persons with potential vibrotactile responses.

SOME FINAL PROCEDURAL ISSUES

Feedback With High-Gain Hearing Aids

A problem that is often encountered with high-gain hearing aids is feedback caused by the slit leak that is produced by the placement of the probe tube between the earmold (or ITE) and the ear canal wall. The feedback can prevent probe-microphone measurements from being obtained at the desired use VCW position. This problem can be approached in three ways. First, if feedback is anticipated as a problem with an ITE, a **vent especially drilled for probe-**

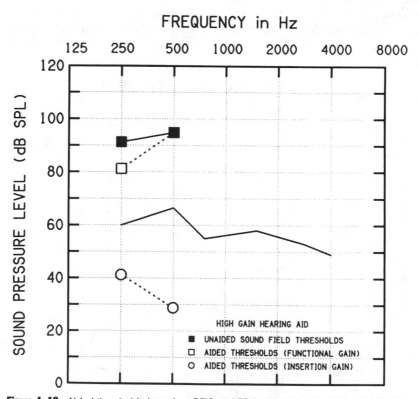

Figure 4–19. Aided thresholds based on REIG and FG for a child with vibrotactile thresholds. See text for further details. (From Stelmachowicz, P., & Lewis, D. 1988. Some theoretical considerations concerning the relation between functional gain and insertion gain. *Journal of Speech and Hearing Research, 31,* 491–496, with permission.)

microphone measurements can be ordered (the vent would be plugged during normal hearing aid use). This probe-tube vent is an option on the order sheet of several custom hearing aid manufacturers. It is important to specify the manufacturer of the probe tube that will be used (or send a tube with the ear impression) as the external diameter of probe tubes varies among manufacturers. The ring marker on the probe tube can be used to help seal the tube in the vent and to ensure that the tip of the tube is extending a predetermined distance beyond the end of the hearing aid or earmold.

A second method to reduce feedback problems is to use Vaseline or putty around the probe tube next to the outer edge of the earmold or ITE to seal off the source of the leak. If this does not allow the VCW to be rotated to the desired position, a third procedure can be performed, involving the following steps:

1. obtain the desired aided response (REAR or REIR, whichever is being used) at a VCW setting that does not produce feedback,
2. without changing the VCW, remove the hearing aid and measure the gain in a 2-cm³ coupler,
3. rotate the VCW to the desired higher position and measure the gain again in the 2-cm³ coupler, and
4. subtract the two 2-cm³ gain values and add the differences to the probe-measured gain. This derived probe-microphone gain should be equal to what would have been measured in the real ear at the desired VCW position.

Effect of Cerumen in the Probe Tube

When substantial cerumen is observed in the ear canal on the initial otoscopic evaluation, it is necessary to determine if probe-microphone testing should even be attempted. In extreme cases, the entire ear canal is occluded, and testing is not possible. In many instances, however, probe-microphone measurements can be conducted with cerumen present. For example, regular hearing aid users often have a dried rim of cerumen located at the point where the tip of their hearing aid or earmold terminates in their ears. This ridge is usually thin and only occludes one fourth to one third of the ear canal. It is possible to slide the probe past this ridge and obtain an appropriate placement depth. On a limited number of pre- and post-cerumenectomy cases, we have found that this minimal amount of dried cerumen in the ear canal does not significantly affect probe-microphone results.

When there is excessive wet cerumen in the ear canal, probe-tube blockage is almost certain. If your clinic or office does not engage in cerumen removal, a medical referral is necessary before probe-microphone testing can be accomplished.

If testing is initiated and the probe tube becomes blocked with cerumen, it is easy to observe and identify that blockage has occurred, as there will typically be **negative values on the REUR** (suggesting that sound was attenuated rather than amplified as it moved from the field to the tympanic membrane) or **negative hearing aid gain**. Figure 4–20 shows an REUR when a probe tube was occluded with cerumen. The obvious solution is to remove the cerumen (though not by cutting the tube) or to replace the tube with a clean one.

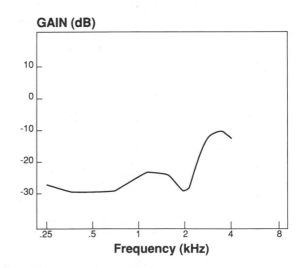

Figure 4–20. REUR obtained when the probe tube was blocked with cerumen.

Probe Tube Crimped or Against Ear Canal Wall

An almost identical result will occur as with the cerumen-blocked tube if the probe tube is crimped or the tip is directly against the wall of the ear canal. Negative values will again appear. Reinsertion or removal of the crimp will solve the problem.

Middle-Ear Pathology

Hearing aids are occasionally selected for persons with various types of middle-ear pathologies. The condition of the middle ear can have a substantial effect on both the unaided and aided response. Perhaps the most significant effect is observed for people with tympanic membrane perforations. The enlarged cavity and resultant change in the ear canal and middle-ear resonance can rather dramatically change the appearance of the REUR. While considerable variability is present, the REUR typically has two peaks when a perforation is present, especially if the perforation is relatively large (Moryl, Danhauer, & DiBartolomeo, 1992). The primary peak is often located between 750 and 1500 Hz and can have an amplitude of greater than 20 dB. This same type of REUR pattern has been reported for patients with mastoidectomies (Civantos & Meyer, 1990).

An example of a REUR from a patient with a large tympanic membrane perforation is shown in Figure 4–21A from Moryl et al. (1992). A normal amplitude peak is observed not at 2700 Hz, but at 1500 Hz. After a large drop in the REUR just above 2000 Hz, a large and rather broad peak occurs at 3000 Hz and above. After a tympanoplasty in which the perforation was closed, the normal REUR shown in Figure 4–21B was obtained for the same patient. Findings such as these raise the issue of **whether insertion gain measures are valid when a perforation is present**. No research data are available at this time, and until more information is available, we recommend that FG be used as an additional measure.

Children and adults with ventilating tubes in place also have unusual REURs (Talbott & Matsumoto, 1990). The results are not as dramatic as observed with perforations, as the large peak around 1000 Hz is not typically present.

Simple changes in **middle-ear pressure** and compliance can also have significant effects on probe-microphone measurements. Such effects can be easily demonstrated by conducting pre- and post-Toynbee test REURs. Figure 4–22 shows the effects of mild negative middle-ear pressure (−150 daPa) on an individual's REUR. Notice that when negative middle-ear pressure and slightly reduced compliance were

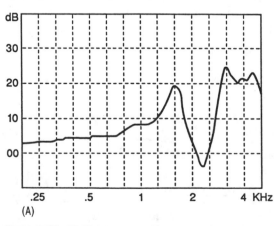

(A)

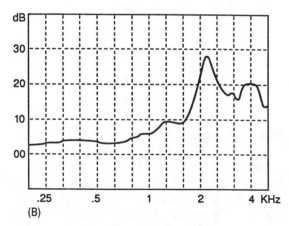

(B)

Figure 4–21. REUR (A) obtained on a patient with a large tympanic membrane perforation. REUR (B) obtained on the same patient after a tympanoplasty had closed the perforation. (Reprinted from Moryl, C., Danhauer, J., & DiBartolomeo, J. 1992. Real ear unaided responses in ears with tympanic membrane perforations. *Journal of the American Academy of Audiology, 3,* 60–65, with permission.)

present, the peak of the REUR shifted downward in frequency. Unless the REAR changed in a similar manner, this minor alteration in middle ear pressure could cause REIR values to appear better or worse when compared to desired target gain.

Larson, Egolf, and Cooper (1991) reported that **abnormal eardrum impedance** can cause pronounced changes in the real-ear performance of a hearing aid. It seems reasonable, therefore, that if a patient has transient middle-ear pathology at the time of the hearing aid fitting, such as negative middle-ear pressure caused by allergies, it would be useful to repeat the probe-microphone measurements when the condition has resolved to insure that the hearing aid fitting is satisfactory.

CONCLUSIONS

It should be clear that a wide variety of variables can affect probe-microphone measurements. At the same time, the reader should recognize that the problems and variables in these measurements can be dealt with easily. The first step is awareness of the major problem areas and knowledge of the many simple strategies to deal with them. Listed below are some of our recommendations, which should lead to reliable and useful probe-microphone measurements:

■ perform the measurements in a sound booth if possible; if not, minimize reflective surfaces near the test position
■ inspect the ear first and avoid cerumen
■ position the loudspeaker at a 0° or 45° azimuth
■ instruct the patient to look at the loudspeaker and not to move his or her head
■ use the modified pressure method of sound-field equalization
■ insert the probe tube 25–30 mm past the tragus and maintain the same position for all measurements
■ use a broad-band signal (such as speech-shaped noise) for all REAR and REIR measurements with hearing aids that are not simple linear instruments
■ use a signal level that is representative of a typical input (70 dB SPL with speech-shaped noise and 60 dB SPL with warble tones) for REAR and REIR measurements and one that will saturate the hearing aid (90 dB SPL with pure tones) for RESR measurements
■ as the measurements are obtained, be vigilant for artifacts and invalid results.

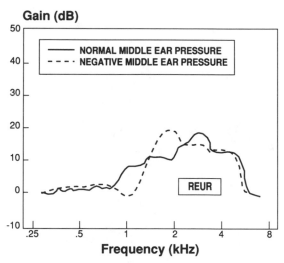

Figure 4–22. REURs obtained before and after a Toynbee test, which creates negative middle-ear pressure.

CHAPTER 5

Prescriptive Approaches to Selection of Gain and Frequency Response

■ DAVID B. HAWKINS, Ph.D. ■

The two most important decisions made when choosing the electroacoustic characteristics of a hearing aid concern selection of maximum power output, or SSPL90, and the gain/frequency response. This chapter discusses some of the currently popular procedures for specifying the gain and frequency response of hearing aids. Selection options for SSPL90 are covered in Chapter 7.

Guidelines in the literature on selection of gain and frequency response were sparse until the mid 1970s. While some of the current procedures have their roots in a method first described in 1940 (Watson & Knudsen, 1940), it was not until the 1980s that practicing clinicians became interested in specifying the precise gain of the hearing aid at different frequencies. Although hearing aid gain and frequency response specification is now more sophisticated, logical, and defensible, it is doubtful that present procedures could be claimed to be major breakthroughs.

Approaches to specification of the gain and frequency response can be categorized in several ways. Some approaches are based on theoretical constructs. For instance, researchers decide systematically what they want the hearing aid to do and why. Then specific formulas are developed to achieve the stated goal. An example is a procedure in which the average levels of speech are to be amplified to most comfortable levels (MCLs) across frequency. Alternatively, other procedures can be characterized as pragmatic in approach. Researchers observe what current hearing aid wearers prefer in terms of gain and then develop a scheme to replicate these characteristics for others.

Another way of categorizing frequency-response selection schemes is by the data necessary to implement the procedure. For instance, some procedures require only auditory thresholds at certain frequencies, as in a pure-tone audiogram. Other approaches require certain suprathreshold measures, such as MCLs or upper level of comfortable loudness (ULCL). The choice of approach may well relate to the population being evaluated. For instance, if a clinician deals mostly with children, then an approach that requires MCLs will clearly not be appropriate.

USE GAIN AS A FUNCTION OF DEGREE OF HEARING LOSS

An initial question often asked by those interested in selecting gain and frequency response is "How much gain does the hearing aid wearer desire for everyday listening?" More specifically, the issue typically becomes whether the desired **use gain** tends to be some percentage of the degree of hearing loss. Many studies over recent years have investigated this issue by gathering groups of people who wear hearing aids and determining where their volume control wheels (VCWs) are set for everyday listening. This use gain is then compared with the degree of hearing loss. If a group acts in a reasonably homogeneous way, then predictions as to the amount of gain required can be made for other potential wearers of hearing aids.

The first person to examine this issue scientifically was Samuel Lybarger in the 1940s. He proposed that gain should be equal to one half of the hearing loss. Gain at that time was expressed in a 2-cm³ coupler, and hearing thresholds were measured by a different standard (ASA 1951 instead of our current ANSI S3.6–1989). The first database published on what is now known as **Lybarger's Half-Gain Rule** was provided by Brooks (1973). He showed that gain at 1000 Hz for experienced hearing aid users was best fit by the following equation:

Gain at 1000 Hz = (0.49 × Hearing Loss at 1000 Hz) + 1

For example, if the hearing loss was 50 dB HL, then the predicted use gain would be (0.49 × 50) + 1, or 25.5 dB. While there was substan-

tial intersubject variability, Brook's study (1973) provided the first empirical data confirming the half-gain rule.

Numerous researchers since Brooks (1973) have reported similar results. Perhaps the largest study came from Berger et al. (1980); results for functional gain (FG) were reported at 500, 1000, and 2000 Hz as a function of degree of hearing loss for 486 wearers of hearing aids. While the half-gain rule described the mean data rather well, there was **substantial intersubject variability**, suggesting that some people desire more gain and others less gain. It should be noted that these use-gain data reflect the philosophy of the audiologist fitting the hearing aid in terms of the amount of gain and the specific frequency response that was made available to the wearers of the hearing aids. If different frequency response shapes had been provided, the desired gain might have been different. In addition, these half-gain values are use gain, not full-on gain, which is seen on hearing aid specification sheets. To convert from FG at a use VCW setting to full-on 2-cm³ coupler gain, appropriate correction values must be applied (see Chapter 12 on CORFIGs), as well as 10–15 dB of reserve gain.

Data are also available that suggest that the half-gain rule may not be valid for mild hearing losses (Leijon, Eriksson-Mangold, & Bech-Karlsen, 1984), and gain equal to approximately one third of the degree of hearing loss has been proposed. For instance, Libby (1985) has suggested that gain should be approximately one third of the hearing loss for mild and moderate losses, one half for moderate and severe losses, and two thirds for more severe losses. This concept is discussed later in more detail.

Many of the pragmatically based selection procedures discussed in this chapter are based on gain equal to one third or one half of the hearing loss. While the theoretically based schemes do not start with such a rule, it is interesting that the gain prescribed by these procedures typically falls within this same general gain range. While many of the schemes do recommend different gain and frequency responses, reasonably similar values are often obtained when the issue is approached from different perspectives.

The remainder of this chapter describes the major selection or prescription procedures and compares and contrasts them.

GAIN AND FREQUENCY RESPONSE SELECTION SCHEMES

THE BERGER PROCEDURE

The procedure advocated by Berger was first described in 1977 (Berger, Hagberg, & Rane, 1977) and has undergone several subsequent revisions, with the latest version being Berger, Hagberg, and Rane (1988). The Berger procedure was the first comprehensive procedure dealing with both gain and frequency response and SSPL90. It has corrections for whether the hearing aid fitting is monaural or binaural and takes into account the presence of air-bone gaps.

Because Berger et al. felt that MCL measurements were too variable, the procedure was developed to require only pure-tone thresholds. It is based on the following assumptions:

■ The intensity of speech is between 55 and 75 dB SPL. (Further specifics are not given as to what levels are assumed in the different frequency regions.)
■ Desired gain is slightly greater than one half of the hearing loss.
■ Amplification of low-frequency ambient noise is detrimental.
■ Less gain is needed at 500 Hz and below than in higher frequencies.
■ In general, information above 4000 Hz is not too useful, but one may want to include 6000 Hz in selection decisions.
■ The frequency response should be smooth and not have prominent resonant peaks.

Gain values are determined through a series of equations that are different for behind-the-

ear (BTE), in-the-ear (ITE), and body hearing aids. The equations assume a sensorineural hearing loss and yield full-on 2-cm^3 coupler gain values. This approach is appropriate as the hearing aid must be selected from full-on 2-cm^3 coupler values on a specification sheet in the case of a BTE or body hearing aid, or ordered from a manufacturer in the case of an ITE. The specific equations are shown in Table 5–1.

These formulas assume sensorineural hearing loss. If conductive or mixed hearing loss is present, additional gain is added equal to the size of the air-bone gap divided by five, up to a maximum additional gain of 8 dB.

The values in Table 5–1 only apply to a monaural hearing aid fitting. If binaural hearing aids are being used, 3 dB is subtracted from the gain at each frequency to account for binaural loudness summation. The 10 dB addition to the end of each equation is for reserve gain so that the formula will be for full-on gain.

The Berger procedure prescribes gain equal to one half of the hearing loss at 500 Hz (note that the denominator in the 500-Hz equations in Table 5–1 is 2 for both BTEs and ITEs), yielding values that are higher than most other procedures. The gain at 500 Hz is reduced, however, if the hearing loss is less than 50 dB HL. Berger et al. (1988) do not mention 250 Hz, but we can assume that the frequency-response slope continues to decline at the same rate present from 1000 to 500 Hz. With a denominator of less than 2 at 1000, 2000, and 3000 Hz, the Berger procedure gain at these frequencies is also **higher than the gain in other procedures** and is also greater than the results of the half-gain rule.

Although the Berger procedure provides an approach to determine if the prescription is a success, it actually only verifies if the target gain values are reached. For instance, predicted aided thresholds are determined from the prescribed 2-cm^3 coupler gain, and the actual aided thresholds should be within 9 dB at all frequencies except 500 and 2000 Hz. (Interestingly, FG and 2-cm^3 coupler gain are assumed to be equal for ITEs and only 2 dB and 3 dB different at 2000 and 3000 Hz, respectively, for

TABLE 5–1. BERGER PROCEDURE FORMULAS FOR FULL-ON 2-CM^3 GAIN FOR BTE AND ITE HEARING AIDS

Frequency (Hz)	BTE	ITE
500	$\dfrac{\text{HL at 500 Hz}}{2} + 10^*$	$\dfrac{\text{HL at 500 Hz}}{2} + 10^*$
1000	$\dfrac{\text{HL at 1000 Hz}}{1.6} + 10$	$\dfrac{\text{HL at 1000 Hz}}{1.6} + 10$
2000	$\dfrac{\text{HL at 2000 Hz}}{1.5} + 12$	$\dfrac{\text{HL at 2000 Hz}}{1.5} + 10$
3000	$\dfrac{\text{HL at 3000 Hz}}{1.7} + 13$	$\dfrac{\text{HL at 3000 Hz}}{1.7} + 10$
4000	$\dfrac{\text{HL at 4000 Hz}}{1.9} + 10$	$\dfrac{\text{HL at 4000 Hz}}{1.9} + 10$
6000	$\dfrac{\text{HL at 6000 Hz}}{2} + 10$	$\dfrac{\text{HL at 6000 Hz}}{2} + 10$

*When hearing loss at 500 Hz is below 50 dB HL, gain at 500 is reduced.

BTEs.) At 500 Hz, the gain cannot be more than 5 dB above the predicted gain, and at 2000 Hz it cannot be more than 5 dB worse than the predicted gain.

THE NATIONAL ACOUSTIC LABORATORIES PROCEDURE

In 1976, Byrne and Tonisson introduced the first version of a procedure developed at the National Acoustic Laboratories (NAL) in Australia. It is a pure-tone threshold based procedure and does not require suprathreshold loudness judgments. The rationale behind the procedure is to amplify the long-term spectrum of speech so that it is comfortably and equally loud across frequency. The speech signal is shaped so that each frequency band contributes equally to its loudness. To determine the desired gain, Byrne and Tonisson originally examined preferred sensation level (PSL) data, as represented by the MCL values minus thresholds. They found that for each 10-dB increase in hearing loss, the PSL decreased 5.6 dB. To compensate for an overall decrease of 5.4 dB Sensation Level (SL) (i.e., 10 − 5.6) for each 10-dB increase in hearing loss, the gain in their formula is increased by 4.6 dB for each 10 dB of hearing loss, thus producing a value quite close to the half-gain rule. Two sets of corrections are then made, one for loudness differences across frequency (the 60-phon line is the reference) and one for the shape of the long-term speech spectrum. For the final values, differences between 2-cm^3 coupler and FG are added, and a reserve gain of 15 dB is added, thus yielding a recommended full-on 2-cm^3 coupler gain curve.

In 1986, Byrne and Dillon published a **revised version of the NAL procedure** based on data collected on the efficacy of the 1976 procedure. The revised NAL formulas for desired real ear insertion gain (REIG) at each of nine frequencies are shown in Table 5–2 for both BTE and ITE hearing aids. These formulas yield the target insertion gain values for probe-microphone measurements.

Since BTEs must be selected from 2-cm³ coupler specification sheets and ITEs are ordered from the manufacturer by providing desired full-on 2-cm³ coupler gain values, the NAL procedure also yields the predicted full-on 2-cm³ coupler gain that should produce the desired REIG for the average person when 15 dB of reserve gain is left on the VCW. The formulas for

the desired full-on 2-cm³ coupler gain values are shown in Table 5–3 for BTEs and ITEs.

It should be noted that **the desired REIG is the same for BTE and ITE hearing aids, but different 2-cm³ coupler gain values are needed to produce the same REIG.** This is due to the different hearing aid microphone locations for the two types of hearing aids and the resulting different field-to-hearing-aid-microphone transfer functions (see Chapter 12 for more details).

It should be emphasized that these formulas assume average REIG/2-cm³ coupler differences (CORFIGs), no venting, and, with BTEs, earmolds with #13 tubing extended to the end of the canal portion. See Chapter 9 for information on how conversions from desired REIG to 2-cm³ gain can be customized for the individual.

The NAL procedure is a careful approach with some validation data. Byrne and Cotton (1988) compared the NAL procedure to a variety of frequency responses that represented deviations from the desired responses. In nearly all cases, individuals with impaired hearing preferred the NAL response in terms of speech intelligibility and pleasantness of sound quality.

Byrne, Parkinson, and Newall (1990, 1991) recommended that the **formulas be changed for persons with severe sensorineural hearing losses.** Two specific modifications to the origi-

TABLE 5–2. NAL PROCEDURE REAL EAR INSERTION GAIN FORMULAS FOR BTEs AND ITEs AT USE VCW POSITION

Frequency (Hz)	Formulas
250	$X + 0.31\ HL_{250} - 17$
500	$X + 0.31\ HL_{500} - 8$
750	$X + 0.31\ HL_{750} - 3$
1000	$X + 0.31\ HL_{1000} + 1$
1500	$X + 0.31\ HL_{1500} + 1$
2000	$X + 0.31\ HL_{2000} - 1$
3000	$X + 0.31\ HL_{3000} - 2$
4000	$X + 0.31\ HL_{4000} - 2$
6000	$X + 0.31\ HL_{6000} - 2$

$$X = .05\ (HL_{500} + HL_{1000} + HL_{2000})$$

TABLE 5–3. NAL PROCEDURE FULL-ON 2-CM³ GAIN FORMULAS

Frequency (Hz)	Formulas	Hearing Aid Style BTE	Hearing Aid Style ITE
250	$X + .31\ HL_{250}$	+ 1	− 1
500	$X + .31\ HL_{500}$	+ 9	+ 9
750	$X + .31\ HL_{750}$	+12	+13
1000	$X + .31\ HL_{1000}$	+16	+16
1500	$X + .31\ HL_{1500}$	+13	+14
2000	$X + .31\ HL_{2000}$	+15	+14
3000	$X + .31\ HL_{3000}$	+22	+15
4000	$X + .31\ HL_{4000}$	+18	+13
6000	$X + .31\ HL_{6000}$	+12	+ 4

$$X = .05\ (HL_{500} + HL_{1000} + HL_{2000})$$

TABLE 5–4. NAL FORMULA MODIFICATION DATA WHEN HEARING LOSS EXCEEDS 90 dB HL AT 2000 Hz

Hearing Loss (in dB HL) at 2000 Hz	Frequency (KHz)								
	0.25	0.5	0.75	1	1.5	2	3	4	6
95	4	3	1	0	−1	−2	−2	−2	−2
100	6	4	2	0	−2	−3	−3	−3	−3
105	8	5	2	0	−3	−5	−5	−5	−5
110	11	7	3	0	−3	−6	−6	−6	−6
115	13	8	4	0	−4	−8	−8	−8	−8
120	15	9	4	0	−5	−9	−9	−9	−9

nal NAL formulas were suggested. First, the X factor in the equations is increased if the three-frequency average exceeds 60 dB; then the following is added to the X portion of the NAL equations if the sum of the thresholds at 500, 1000, and 2000 Hz exceeds 180:

$$0.116 \ (X - 180)$$
$$(X = \text{combined total of HL}$$
$$\text{at } 500, 1000, \text{ and } 2000)$$

As an example, if the thresholds at 500, 1000, and 2000 Hz were 80 dB HL, then the sum of the thresholds (240) exceeds 180 by 60, therefore 7 dB (0.116 × 60) is added to the X factor in the gain equation.

A second modification changes the gain in the low and high frequencies if the degree of hearing loss at 2000 Hz exceeds 90 dB HL (Table 5–4).

THE PRESCRIPTION OF GAIN AND OUTPUT PROCEDURE

McCandless and Lyregaard (1983) described a procedure for specifying the gain and SSPL90 of a hearing aid for a person with a sensorineural hearing loss of less than 80 dB HL. There were three objectives in formulating the prescription of gain and output (POGO) approach: (1) the procedure must be simple, (2) it

must be practical, and (3) it must have some basis in what is known about users of hearing aids and their gain preferences.

The POGO procedure specifies desired REIG target values at use VCW position according to the formulas provided in Table 5–5. In essence, POGO is simply **a half gain rule using REIG,** but with a reduction at 500 Hz and below. Such an approach is indeed quite simple to conceptualize and lends itself well to verification with probe-microphone measurements.

POGO full-on 2-cm³ coupler gain (assuming 10 dB of reserve gain) values are determined with the formulas in Table 5–6. The numbers that are added to the basic formulas are combinations of the REIG/2-cm³ difference and 10 dB of reserve gain.

A recent modification was made to POGO by Schwartz, Lyregaard, and Lundh (1988) to make the procedure applicable to those with severe hearing losses. The formulas were altered to change gain when the hearing loss was greater than 65 dB HL. This procedure, called **POGO II,** changes the formulas to those in Table 5–7. The modification simply **increases the gain by one half the amount that the hearing loss exceeds 65 dB HL.** For example, if the hearing loss is 95 dB HL at 1000 Hz, then the gain will be increased by 15 dB (95 − 65 = 30/2 = 15) over the regular half-gain formula. To convert these POGO II values to full-on 2-cm³ coupler gain, the same corrections as in Table 5–6 are added to these values.

TABLE 5–5. POGO PROCEDURE REAL EAR INSERTION GAIN FORMULAS FOR USE VCW POSITION

Frequency (Hz)	Formulas
250	½ HL − 10
500	½ HL − 5
1000	½ HL
2000	½ HL
3000	½ HL
4000	½ HL

TABLE 5–6. POGO PROCEDURE FULL-ON 2-CM^3 GAIN FORMULAS

Frequency (Hz)	Formulas	Hearing Aid Style		
		ITE	BTE	Body
250	½ HL − 10 +	7	7	3
500	½ HL − 5 +	9	9	3
1000	½ HL +	8	10	0
2000	½ HL +	16	12	21
3000	½ HL +	16	21	23
4000	½ HL +	15	19	23

TABLE 5–7. POGO II PROCEDURE REAL EAR INSERTION GAIN FORMULAS FOR USE VCW POSITION

Frequency (Hz)	Formulas
250	½ HL + ½ (HL − 65) − 10
500	½ HL + ½ (HL − 65) − 5
1000	½ HL + ½ (HL − 65)
2000	½ HL + ½ (HL − 65)
3000	½ HL + ½ (HL − 65)
4000	½ HL + ½ (HL − 65)

The articles describing POGO provide little explanation or rationale for the formulas or how they were developed. No data have been published on the accuracy or validity of the procedure. As with the Berger procedure, validation involves measuring REIG and determining how close the obtained values come to the desired target values.

THE LIBBY PROCEDURE

Articles in 1985 and 1986 by Libby described a modification to the POGO procedure that varies the amount of REIG depending on the degree of hearing loss. Libby stated that his experience indicated that persons with **mild and moderate hearing losses preferred REIG equal to one third** of their hearing loss rather than one half. Libby's formulas for REIG for mild and moderate sensorineural hearing losses are provided in Table 5–8.

The formulas in Table 5–9 are used for full-on 2-cm^3 gain values for ITE, BTE, and body hearing aids. Notice that these formulas are very close to those of POGO with the following exceptions: (a) one third instead of one half is used, and (b) there is less gain reduction in the low frequencies (5 and 3 dB at 250 and 500 Hz, respectively, instead of 10 and 5 dB).

Libby stated that as the hearing loss exceeded the mild-to-moderate category, the gain should be increased to one half and then to two thirds of the hearing loss. He did not, however, clearly specify when the formula changes from one third to one half to two thirds. One would guess that the half-gain rule is applied to severe losses, and two-thirds gain rule is applied to severe-to-profound losses. For binaural fittings, 3 dB of gain is subtracted. When an air-bone gap is present, gain is added equal to one fourth of the air-bone gap up to a maximum of 8 dB.

As with POGO, there are no research data to support the procedure. Studies have not been done in which alterations to the formulas have been made and comparisons to the original formulas have been evaluated.

THE MEMPHIS STATE UNIVERSITY PROCEDURE

The Memphis State University (MSU) procedure was developed by Cox and described in publications in 1983, 1985, and 1988. The basic premise of the procedure is that the hearing aid should amplify the long-term speech spectrum to a point halfway between the auditory threshold and the Upper Limit of Comfortable Loudness (ULCL). Cox (1989) suggested that ULCL be changed to Highest Comfortable Loudness (HCL) to avoid confusion with Uncomfortable Loudness Level (UCL).

The difference in decibels between auditory threshold and HCL is the **long-term listening range**, similar in concept to the dynamic range. Speech levels in the various frequency regions are amplified so that they bisect the long-term listening range.

In the original MSU procedure, it was necessary to obtain the person's thresholds and HCLs to define the long-term listening range. In MSU version #3 (Cox, 1988), it is possible to have the HCLs predicted based on the auditory thresholds. Also, in the original procedure it was necessary to obtain the thresholds and HCLs via an insert receiver that was calibrated in a 2-cm^3 coupler. In MSU-3, however, standard audiometric earphones may be substituted. In either case, the auditory thresholds and HCLs are expressed in dB SPL rather than dB HL. (See Chapter 12 for conversion values from dB HL to dB SPL for a variety of earphones.)

If audiometric data are gathered with a standard supra-aural earphone and a BTE hearing aid is being selected, the formulas in Table 5–10 can be employed to determine the full-on 2-cm^3 coupler gain, assuming 10 dB of reserve gain. These formulas assume the use of an HA-2 earmold (3-mm bore that is 18-mm long) or measurement of 2-cm^3 coupler gain with the person's actual earmold attached to an HA-1 2-cm^3 coupler. For an ITE instrument, the values in Table 5–11 are subtracted from the BTE gain values from the formulas in Table 5–10.

If HCL values cannot be obtained on a person due to his or her inability to make reliable

TABLE 5–8. LIBBY PROCEDURE REAL EAR INSERTION GAIN FORMULAS FOR USE VCW POSITION FOR MILD AND MODERATE HEARING LOSSES

Frequency (Hz)	Formulas
250	⅓ HL − 5
500	⅓ HL − 3
1000	⅓ HL
2000	⅓ HL
3000	⅓ HL
4000	⅓ HL
6000	⅓ HL − 5

TABLE 5–9. LIBBY PROCEDURE FULL-ON 2-CM^3 GAIN FORMULAS

Frequency (Hz)	Formulas	Hearing Aid Style		
		ITE	BTE	Body
250	⅓ HL +	6	6	3
500	⅓ HL +	8	8	5
1000	⅓ HL +	11	12	5
2000	⅓ HL +	16	21	26
3000	⅓ HL +	18	25	28
4000	⅓ HL +	12	20	28
6000	⅓ HL +	2	13	10

TABLE 5-10. COX MSU PROCEDURE FULL-ON 2-CM^3 GAIN FORMULAS FOR BTE HEARING AID

Frequency (Hz)	Formula 1[1]	Formula 2[1]
250	½ HCL (dB SPL) + ½ HL (dB SPL) − 62	HCL (dB SPL) − 77
500	½ HCL (dB SPL) + ½ HL (dB SPL) − 55	HCL (dB SPL) − 70
800	½ HCL (dB SPL) + ½ HL (dB SPL) − 49	HCL (dB SPL) − 64
1000	½ HCL (dB SPL) + ½ HL (dB SPL) − 47	HCL (dB SPL) − 62
1600	½ HCL (dB SPL) + ½ HL (dB SPL) − 47	HCL (dB SPL) − 62
2500	½ HCL (dB SPL) + ½ HL (dB SPL) − 42	HCL (dB SPL) − 57
4000	½ HCL (dB SPL) + ½ HL (dB SPL) − 46	HCL (dB SPL) − 61
6300	½ HCL (dB SPL) + ½ HL (dB SPL) − 47	HCL (dB SPL) − 62

[1]Choose the formula that yields the lowest gain value at each frequency. HCL is Highest Comfortable Loudness.

suprathreshold loudness judgments, then these values are predicted with the equations in Table 5–12. The predicted HCLs are then used in the formulas in Table 5–10 to determine full-on 2-cm³ coupler gain.

Since the rationale for the MSU procedure is to amplify the speech spectrum into the long-term listening range, the procedure is **not an insertion-gain based approach**. It is best visualized as utilizing a speech spectrum input and creating target Real Ear Aided Response (REAR)

TABLE 5–11. COX MSU PROCEDURE CORRECTIONS TO TABLE 5–10 VALUES FOR FULL-ON 2-CM³ GAIN FOR ITE HEARING AID

Frequency (Hz)	Corrections
250	−1.0
500	−1.0
800	−1.5
1000	−1.0
1600	−1.0
2500	−4.5
4000	−6.0
6300	−3.0

TABLE 5–12. COX MSU PROCEDURE FORMULAS TO PREDICT HCL FROM AUDITORY THRESHOLDS

Frequency (Hz)	Formulas
250	0.37 (HL in dB SPL) + 85
500	0.25 (HL in dB SPL) + 83
800	0.45 (HL in dB SPL) + 73
1000	0.44 (HL in dB SPL) + 71
1600	0.41 (HL in dB SPL) + 69
2500	0.37 (HL in dB SPL) + 69
4000	0.39 (HL in dB SPL) + 68
6300	0.39 (HL in dB SPL) + 68

values. With a speech-spectrum input, the hearing aid is adjusted until the output levels in the ear canal match target values and thus bisect the long-term listening range. Such a procedure was described by Cox and Alexander (1990).[1]

THE DESIRED SENSATION LEVEL APPROACH

In a series of articles, Seewald, Ross, and Spiro (1985); Seewald, Ross, and Stelmachowicz (1987); Seewald (1988); Seewald and Ross (1988); Seewald, Zelisko, Ramji, and Jamieson (1991); and Seewald (1992) describe a different approach to selecting characteristics of hearing aids. In this procedure, desired sensation levels (DSLs) for the amplified speech spectrum are determined at each frequency for all degrees of sensorineural hearing loss. Table 5–13 shows the DSLs at nine frequencies as a function of auditory thresholds (Seewald et al., 1991).

In this approach, hearing aid gain characteristics are chosen such that the **long-term spectrum of speech is amplified to the DSLs**. Figure 5–1 from Seewald et al. (1987) shows the basic approach. The auditory thresholds are expressed in dB SPL and target levels for the amplified speech spectrum are determined by adding the DSLs to the thresholds. With a speech-spectrum input, the hearing aid settings are adjusted to best match the target values. Table 5–14 shows the amplified target levels in the ear canal for a long-term speech-spectrum input to the hearing aid microphone (Seewald et al., 1991). Using these values, an example of an ideal fitting is shown in Figure 5–2. This **procedure can be implemented totally with probe-microphone measurements** and has appeal as a tool in fitting children with hearing impairment.

Although the DSL procedure is not an insertion-gain based approach, Seewald et al.

---

[1]Since many audiologists use the Real Ear Insertion Gain (REIG) approach and the calculations discussed here can be tedious if done manually, Cox will provide interested persons with an IBM-compatible program that calculates all of these values, including REIG, and allows for audiometric data gathered with either an insert receiver or standard earphone. Write to Robyn Cox, Ph.D., Memphis Speech and Hearing Center, 807 Jefferson Avenue, Memphis, TN 38105.

TABLE 5–13. DESIRED SENSATION LEVELS (IN dB) FOR THE AMPLIFIED SPEECH SPECTRUM

Threshold (dB HL)	Frequency (Hz)								
	250	500	750	1000	1500	2000	3000	4000	6000
0	47	53	53	48	46	46	43	40	30
5	41	48	49	44	42	43	40	38	27
10	36	44	44	41	39	40	37	35	24
15	32	40	41	38	37	38	35	33	22
20	28	36	37	35	34	35	33	31	20
25	25	33	34	33	32	33	31	29	19
30	23	30	32	31	30	31	30	27	17
35	20	28	30	29	29	30	28	26	16
40	18	26	28	28	27	28	27	25	15
45	17	24	26	26	26	27	25	23	14
50	16	22	24	25	25	25	24	22	13
55	14	21	23	25	24	25	22	21	15
60	13	19	22	22	22	23	22	19	11
65	13	18	20	21	21	21	21	18	10
70	12	17	19	20	20	20	19	17	9
75	11	16	18	18	19	18	18	15	8
80	10	14	17	17	17	16	16	14	7
85	8	13	15	15	16	15	15	12	5
90	7	12	14	13	14	13	13	11	3
95	5	10	12	11	12	11	11	9	0
100	3	8	10	9	10	8	8	7	—
105	—	6	7	6	7	5	5	5	—
110	—	4	5	4	4	2	2	3	—

Source: Reprinted from Seewald, R., Zelisko, D., Ramji, K., & Jamieson, D. 1991. *DSL 3.0 user's manual*. London, Ontario, Canada: University of Western Ontario, with permission.

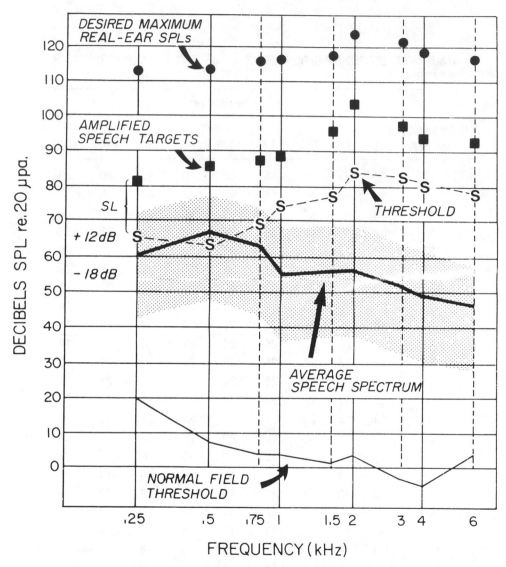

Figure 5–1. Schematic approach of the desired sensation level (DSL) approach. First, target desired maximum real-ear output (real-ear SSPL90; circles) and amplified speech targets (boxes) are determined. Then the amplified speech targets are determined by adding the DSLs from Table 5–13 to the auditory thresholds. The required hearing aid gain is the difference between the average speech spectrum and the amplified speech targets. (Reprinted from Seewald, R., Ross, M., & Stelmachowicz, P. 1987. Selecting and verifying hearing aid performance characteristics for children. *Journal of the Academy of Rehabilitative Audiology, 20,* 25–37, with permission.)

TABLE 5–14. DESIRED TARGET LEVELS FOR THE AMPLIFIED SPEECH SPECTRUM (IN dB SPL) FOR THE DSL PROCEDURE

Threshold (dB HL)	Frequency (Hz)								
	250	500	750	1000	1500	2000	3000	4000	6000
0	64	67	64	57	56	62	60	55	48
5	64	67	64	59	58	63	62	57	50
10	64	67	65	61	60	66	64	60	52
15	65	68	66	63	62	68	67	63	55
20	66	69	68	65	65	71	70	66	58
25	68	71	70	68	68	74	73	69	61
30	70	73	72	71	71	77	76	72	65
35	73	76	75	74	74	80	80	76	69
40	76	79	78	78	78	83	83	79	73
45	80	82	81	81	81	87	87	83	77
50	83	85	85	85	85	91	91	86	81
55	87	89	88	88	89	94	95	90	85
60	91	93	92	92	92	98	99	94	89
65	95	96	96	96	96	101	102	98	93
70	99	100	99	100	100	105	106	101	97
75	103	104	103	103	104	108	110	105	101
80	107	108	107	107	107	112	113	109	104
85	111	111	110	110	111	115	116	112	108
90	115	115	114	113	114	118	119	115	111
95	118	118	117	116	117	121	122	119	113
100	121	121	120	119	120	123	125	122	115
105	—	124	123	121	122	126	127	125	—
110	—	127	125	123	124	128	129	127	—

Source: Reprinted from Seewald, R., Zelisko, D., Ramji, K., & Jamieson, D. 1991. *DSL 3.0 user's manual*. London, Ontario, Canada: University of Western Ontario, with permission.

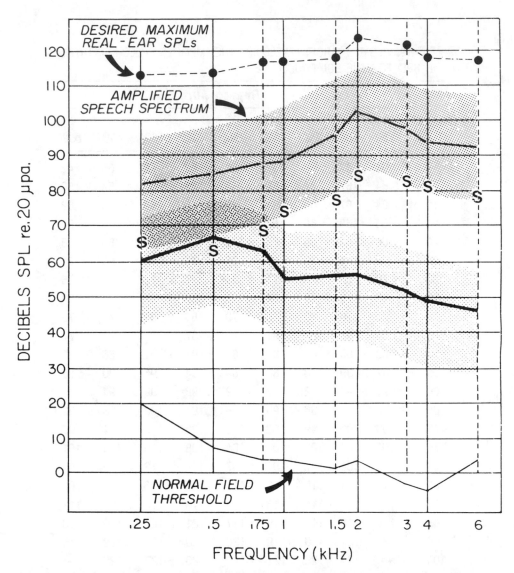

Figure 5–2. The desired result with the DSL approach for the case shown in Figure 5–1. The amplified speech spectrum is audible across frequency and has been placed at the appropriate desired sensation levels. An adequate residual dynamic range (the distance between the threshold and SSPL90) has been created, and the peaks of the amplified speech spectrum do not saturate the hearing aid. (Reprinted from Seewald, R., Ross, M., & Stelmachowicz, P. 1987. Selecting and verifying hearing aid performance characteristics for children. *Journal of the Academy of Rehabilitative Audiology, 20,* 25–37, with permission.)

(1991) have calculated the REIGs necessary for different hearing thresholds to accomplish the goals of the procedure. These values are shown in Table 5-15.

The DSL procedure is easily computerized, and as with the Cox (MSU) procedure, a computer program that makes the approach easily implemented on an IBM-compatible system is available from Seewald.[2] The DSL procedure and its implementation with probe measurements and children is presented in more detail in Chapter 8.

THE PASCOE PROCEDURE

The Pascoe procedure was developed at the Central Institute for the Deaf and has been described by Pascoe (1978); Skinner, Pascoe, Miller, and Popelka (1982); and Skinner (1988). The procedure is similar to that described by Cox (1988), in that suprathreshold loudness judgments are obtained and a residual auditory area is defined. The Pascoe procedure also shares similarities with the Seewald and Ross (1988) DSL procedure in that desired aided speech levels are determined. The long-term speech-spectrum is amplified to a point that represents a certain percentage of the difference between auditory threshold and the MCL for the frequency range 500–4000 Hz. At 250 and 6000 Hz, amplified speech is placed at one half of the distance between the threshold and the MCL. The goals are to make speech audible over the range of 250–6000 Hz and close to the MCLs and to provide a normal balance of loudness across frequency.

This approach is complicated to compute manually and is greatly assisted by a computer program. Sample values are provided in Table 5–16 for one frequency (1000 Hz) for a hypothetical person having a threshold of 45 dB HL and an MCL of 85 dB HL. For more complete details on the Pascoe procedure, the reader is referred to Skinner (1988).

COMPARISON OF THE VARIOUS PRESCRIPTIVE PROCEDURES

From the above descriptions, it is obvious that a variety of procedures is available to the audiologist to determine the desired gain and frequency response of a hearing aid. The question is, do significant differences exist among the procedures in speech intelligibility and hearing aid benefit?

This question has not been answered conclusively, but it is clear that **the different procedures do prescribe different REIRs and full-on 2-cm³ coupler values**. Let us consider two different audiograms and examine the REIRs and full-on 2-cm³ coupler values described by six of the prescription procedures: (1) Berger, (2) NAL, (3) POGO, (4) Cox (MSU), (5) Libby, and (6) DSL. The first case represents a common hearing aid candidate with a mild-to-moderate sloping, sensorineural, probably presbycusic, hearing loss. Figure 5–3 shows the audiogram as an inset and the prescribed REIR for a monaural ITE hearing aid. Notice that **all procedures recommend similar REIGs at 250 and 500 Hz**. This is not surprising, as very little hearing loss is present at these frequencies. At 1000 Hz and above, however, some rather large differences emerge in the recommended REIG values. The Libby procedure recommends the least gain with the one third rule, and the Berger procedure prescribes far more than the others, especially at 1000 and 2000 Hz. The DSL procedure also prescribes more gain at 2000 Hz and above, as it attempts to make speech energy audible throughout the frequency range.

Given that the different procedures do not use the same conversions from REIR to 2-cm³ gain and use different values for reserve gain (typically 10 or 15 dB), it is not surprising that the recommended full-on 2-cm³ coupler recommendations are also different. Figure 5–4 shows the full-on 2-cm³ coupler gain curves for

---

[2]For information on the DSL computer program, contact Richard Seewald, Ph.D., Hearing Health Care Research Unit, University of Western Ontario, Department of Communicative Disorders, Elborne College, London, Ontario, Canada N6G 1H1.

TABLE 5–15. REAL EAR INSERTION GAIN VALUES FOR THE DSL PROCEDURE

Threshold (dB HL)	Frequency (Hz)								
	250	500	750	1000	1500	2000	3000	4000	6000
0	0	0	0	0	0	0	0	0	0
5	0	0	0	0	0	0	1	1	1
10	0	1	1	2	2	3	3	3	3
15	1	2	2	4	4	5	6	6	6
20	2	3	4	6	7	8	9	9	9
25	4	5	6	9	10	11	12	12	12
30	6	7	8	12	13	14	15	15	16
35	9	10	11	15	16	17	19	19	19
40	12	13	14	19	20	20	22	22	23
45	16	16	17	22	23	24	26	26	27
50	19	19	21	26	27	28	30	30	32
55	23	23	25	29	31	31	34	34	36
60	27	26	28	33	35	35	37	37	40
65	31	30	32	37	38	38	41	44	44
70	35	34	36	41	42	42	45	45	48
75	40	38	39	44	46	45	48	48	52
80	43	41	43	48	49	49	52	52	55
85	47	45	47	51	53	52	55	55	58
90	51	49	50	54	56	55	58	59	61
95	54	52	53	57	59	58	61	62	64
100	57	55	56	60	62	60	64	65	66
105	—	58	59	62	64	63	66	68	—
110	—	61	61	64	67	65	68	71	—

Source: Reprinted from Seewald, R., Zelisko, D., Ramji, K., & Jamieson, D. 1991. *DSL 3.0 user's manual.* London, Ontario, Canada: University of Western Ontario, with permission.

TABLE 5-16. EXAMPLE OF PASCOE AP-
PROACH INSERTION-GAIN CALCULATION

Auditory threshold	45 dB HL
MCL	85 dB HL
MCL (in dB SL)	40 dB
Percentage multiplier	0.9
Aided-speech SL	36 dB
Add the auditory threshold	45 dB HL
Aided speech (dB HL)	81 dB HL
Unaided speech (dB HL)	49 dB HL
Desired REIG	32 dB

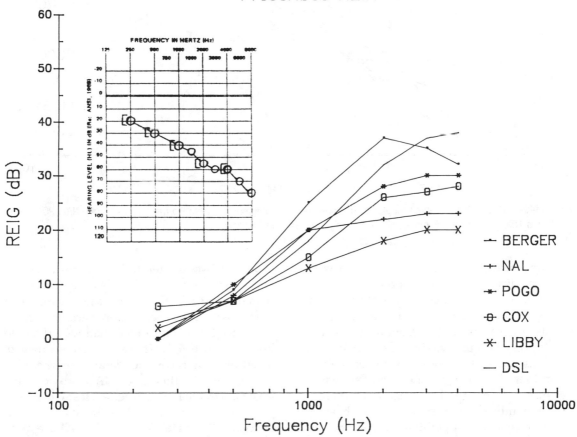

Figure 5-3. Prescribed REIRs for the audiogram shown in the inset using Berger, NAL, POGO, Cox, Libby, and DSL procedures. A monaural ITE hearing aid has been assumed.

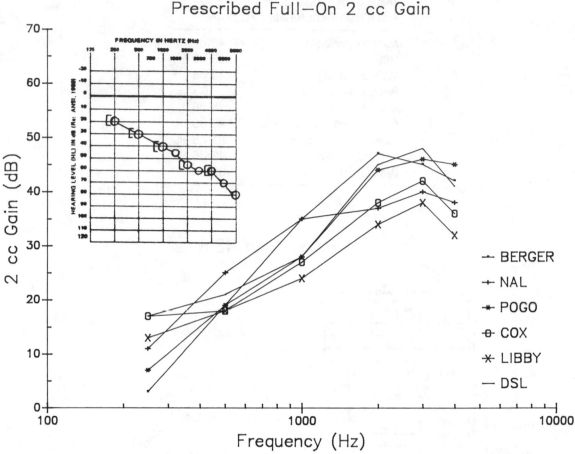

Figure 5–4. Prescribed full-on 2-cm³ coupler gain curves for the audiogram shown in the inset using Berger, NAL, POGO, Cox, Libby, and DSL procedures. A monaural ITE hearing aid has been assumed.

the same hearing loss. Again, there are wide discrepancies across these prescriptive approaches. It is clear that very different BTE hearing aids will be selected, or quite different circuits ordered from ITE manufacturers, depending on which prescriptive procedure is used.

The audiogram for a more severe hearing loss is considered in the second case and shown in the inset of Figure 5–5. This moderate-to-severe, gently sloping, sensorineural hearing loss represents the upper limit of what most of the procedures are able to accommodate. Also shown in Figure 5–5 are the prescribed REIRs for a BTE hearing aid for this hearing loss. Due to the severity of the hearing loss, the Libby

procedure was altered to incorporate insertion gain equal to one half of the hearing loss rather than one third. With the increased hearing loss in the lower frequencies, more variance among the procedures is observed than with the mild loss in Figure 5–3. There is a wide range of insertion-gain recommendations in the high frequencies. In this case, NAL provides the least gain in the higher frequencies. The Berger procedure again prescribes the most gain at 1000 and 2000 Hz. DSL and POGO are quite similar for this hearing loss.

Figure 5–6 shows the full-on 2-cm³ coupler gain recommendations for this severe hearing loss. With the exception of 1000 Hz, where the

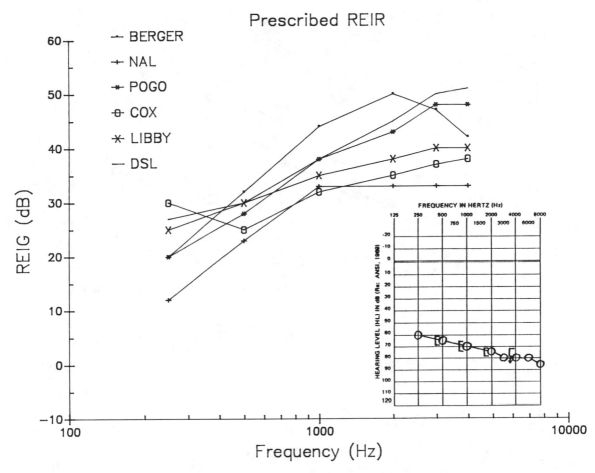

Figure 5–5. Prescribed REIRs for the audiogram shown in the inset using Berger, NAL, POGO, Cox, Libby, and DSL procedures. A monaural BTE hearing aid and occluding earmold have been assumed.

range of recommendations varies only by 7 dB, substantial differences among the procedures are again evident.

Several published studies have compared some of these selection procedures in terms of the prescribed response (Byrne, 1987; Skinner, 1988), predicted performance via the Articulation Index (Humes, 1986), and comparisons of people with impaired hearing on a variety of performance measures (Humes & Hackett, 1990; Sullivan, Levitt, Hwang, & Hennessey, 1988). As shown in Figures 5–3 through 5–6, it is clear that the different procedures do indeed prescribe different REIRs and full-on 2-cm³ coupler gain curves. It has been suggested that when

the user is given control of the VCW, or if the procedures are matched at a given frequency, differences among the prescriptions decrease. For instance, Figure 5–7 shows data from Byrne (1987) in which the responses from six procedures were matched at 1000 Hz in order to show shape differences rather than absolute gain differences. Prescribed frequency responses are shown for a mild flat sensorineural hearing loss and a severe flat hearing loss for six different procedures. The numbers attached to the various curves represent the amount of gain increase or reduction from the absolute prescribed amount in order to match at 1000 Hz. These data show that even when the re-

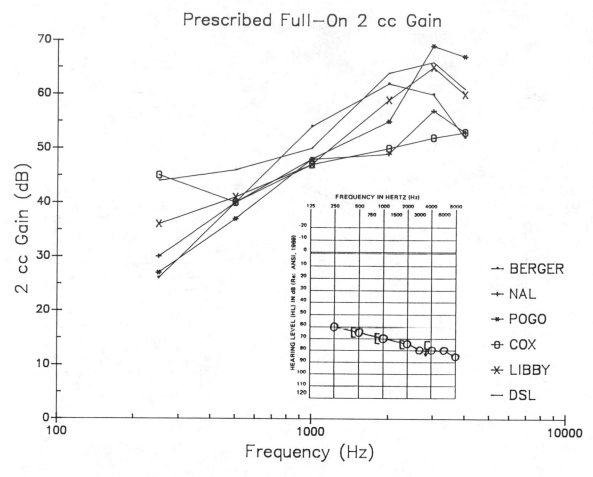

Figure 5–6. Prescribed full-on 2-cm³ coupler gain curves for the audiogram shown in the inset using Berger, NAL, POGO, Cox, Libby, and DSL procedures. A monaural BTE hearing aid and occluding earmold have been assumed.

sponses are matched at a central frequency, differences still remain among the procedures.

Based on her own work and that of Byrne (1987), Skinner (1988) arrived at the following conclusions after comparing the different procedures:

1. The Berger procedure recommends excessive gain at 2000 Hz relative to 500 Hz.
2. The Pascoe procedure may prescribe slightly too much at 500 Hz and the overall gain may need to be reduced.
3. The POGO procedure prescribes excessive gain at 2000 Hz relative to 500 Hz for steeply sloping high-frequency hearing losses.

4. The NAL procedure prescribes less low-frequency gain than the Pascoe and Cox procedures due to the different speech spectra that were used.
5. The Cox procedure may prescribe inadequate gain in order to make the speech spectrum comfortably loud across frequency.
6. The Libby (1985) procedure prescribes the least amount of gain and varies gain as a function of audiogram slope less than the other procedures.
7. The gain prescribed by any of the current prescription procedures may need to be altered for a given hearing-impaired individual.

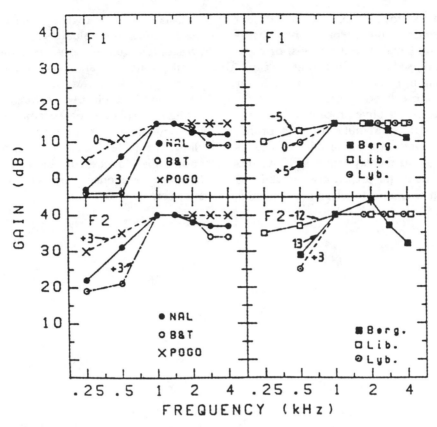

Figure 5–7. Frequency response curves prescribed by six different procedures for a mild flat hearing loss (F1) and a severe flat hearing loss (F2). The procedures are: NAL (Byrne & Dillon, 1986); B & T (Byrne & Tonisson, 1976); POGO (McCandless & Lyregaard, 1983); Berg. (Berger, Hagberg, & Rane, 1977); Lib. (Libby, 1986); Lyb. (Lybarger, 1955). The curves have been matched at 1000 Hz, with the numbers attached to the curves representing the increase or decrease necessary to achieve the absolute recommended gain. (Reprinted from Byrne, D. 1987. Hearing aid selection formulae: Same or different? *Hearing Instruments, 38,* 5–11, with permission.)

CONCLUSIONS

While response differences clearly exist among the various prescriptive procedures, **it is not clear that speech intelligibility is actually different from procedure to procedure** (Humes, 1991b) or if more hearing aid wearers are satisfied as a result of the use of one or another. A realistic, but disconcerting, statement by Sullivan et al. (1988) is pertinent:

A result of important consequence to clinical implementation of these methods is the significant interaction between prescriptive method and subject. This interaction suggests that different methods may be needed for subjects with different hearing loss characteristics. (p. 31)

Perhaps the truth is that one procedure is not best for all persons with impaired hearing. Indeed, there is probably no single optimal frequency response for all situations. A different response might be required for different speakers, background noises, input levels, or combinations of these factors. This complex interaction assumption underlies the rationale for multiple-response hearing aids.

Each of the prescriptive procedures has proponents and critics. Manufacturers of probe-microphone systems include data programs that compute and display target REIG values for many of the major prescriptive procedures discussed in this chapter. Dispensing audiologists must be knowledgeable about each of the procedures, evaluate research studies of prescriptive comparisons, examine their own client population, and reach a decision about which procedure can be best implemented efficiently in their own setting. The use of probe-microphone measurements makes the implementation of prescriptive approaches clinically viable and feasible and allows the audiologist to control the actual gain and frequency response provided to the hearing aid user.

CHAPTER 6

Insertion Gain Measurements

H. GUSTAV MUELLER, Ph.D.

The preceding chapter has provided background information regarding the theoretical and practical application of prescriptive fitting approaches. A critical component of the prescriptive fitting strategy is to assure that prescriptive gain targets have actually been achieved when the hearing aid is worn. Some type of real ear verification process, therefore, is required. Two different probe-microphone measures can be used to accomplish this task: the real ear aided response (REAR) and the real ear insertion response (REIR). Typically, **the prescriptive method chosen dictates whether the REAR or the REIR is used**. While there has been a slight increase in the use of the REAR in recent years, the REIR clearly remains the most commonly used measure for frequency response verification. It is probable that this trend will continue as long as gain-based prescriptive formulae are the preferred method of hearing aid selection.

It is important to emphasize that **REIR measures, in and of themselves, are not a method of fitting hearing aids**. In fact, in the absence of a theoretically based target, REIR findings become rather meaningless. The intent of this chapter, therefore, is to support the notion that, if the audiologist believes in using a prescriptive fitting approach, and, if the prescriptive approach is based on frequency specific gain, then the REIR can serve as a reliable and valid method of target gain verification. An REIR match to prescriptive target gain, however, does not assure that the fitting will be successful, that speech understanding has been maximized, or even that speech has been made audible.

THEORETICAL ISSUES

When an audiologist makes the decision to use insertion gain as a measure of the goodness of the hearing aid fitting, there are several theoretical issues to consider. Some of these issues impact significantly on whether a given hearing aid will be judged as suitable for a patient.

INSERTION GAIN VERSUS FUNCTIONAL GAIN

The frequent clinical use of the REIR for verification of the hearing aid fitting is related directly to the prescriptive methods that presently are popular. Martin and Morris (1989) reported that 71% of audiologists use a prescriptive fitting procedure and that 78% of them use either the Berger method, the Prescription of Gain and Output (POGO) procedure, or the Australian National Acoustic Laboratories (NAL) formula. All three of these prescriptive methods are gain-based and were developed using functional gain (FG) as the verification procedure. When real ear insertion gain (REIG) measurements are used as a substitute for FG to verify a prescriptive target, it is important that the same, or very similar results can be obtained. As summarized in Chapter 4, **research has shown that REIG is, indeed, the equivalent of FG.**

The use of probe-microphone measurements (REIG), rather than the behavioral FG procedure, offers several practical advantages. Some of the most notable include the following:

Information is obtained across frequency range, not just at discrete frequencies.
It is not necessary to mask the non-test ear.
The masking noise of the hearing aid does not prevent determination of real-ear gain for regions of normal, or near-normal hearing.
Real-ear gain can be determined for patients unable to provide behavioral response.
The effects of the input level on real-ear gain can be assessed.
Determination of real-ear gain for individuals with profound hearing loss is not prevented by the upper limits of the soundfield equipment.
There is significantly improved test-retest reliability.

Given the numerous advantages of REIG measures over FG, there is little reason not to routinely use REIG as the method to verify a prescriptive gain target. In fact, when probe-microphone equipment was first introduced, it was the audiologists who had struggled with FG for many years who most eagerly embraced this new technology. Today, most clinics and offices that have purchased probe-microphone equipment rarely conduct FG. There are some instances, however, when FG should still be considered:

■ When the validity of the *unaided thresholds* is in question, such as in difficult to test children or adults, possible vibrotactile responses, etc. FG measures can be used as a cross-check of the unaided thresholds, whereas REIG measurements cannot.
■ When cerumen in the ear canal is sufficient to plug the probe tube but is not completely occluding the ear canal. FG should provide reasonably accurate real-ear gain in this instance when probe-microphone testing would not be possible.
■ When a middle ear pathology is present that could alter significantly the patient's REUR, producing unusual REIG findings. A behavioral FG cross-check is warranted (see Chapter 4).

PRESCRIBED GAIN VERSUS USE GAIN

When REIR measures are conducted for validation of prescriptive targets, the configuration of the response usually is given the most attention. A second important consideration, however, is the relationship between the target prescription gain and an individual patient's use gain. In general, as discussed in Chapter 5, this factor has been carefully studied as part of the development of various prescriptive methods. For example, Byrne and Dillon (1986) reported that their decision to equate the new NAL three-frequency average gain with the three-frequency average gain of the Byrne and Tonisson (1976) procedure was based on the extensive experience showing that these values are a realistic estimate of use gain (except possibly in people with severely impaired hearing). Their recommendation of 15 dB reserve gain was based on the finding that the **standard deviation for use gain is 8 dB for individuals with the same hearing threshold levels** (Byrne & Tonisson, 1976). Hence, 15 dB of reserve gain would accommodate nearly all hearing aid users.

Assuming that the patient's use gain is within the range of the hearing aid's capabilities, a pre-fitting estimate of use gain might not seem very critical, as the patient simply could adjust the volume control wheel (VCW) until a desired gain setting is obtained. There are several reasons, however, why this approach will not always work. First, it usually is desirable to have the patient use the hearing aid at a 1/2 to 2/3 VCW rotation. It is necessary, therefore, to have a reasonably accurate estimate of use gain when the hearing aid is ordered. Secondly, many patients are not comfortable in selecting their own VCW setting, and they rely on guidance from the audiologist. As a result, some audiologists will instruct a patient to use a specific VCW rotation, and will go so far as to place a mark on the hearing aid to assist the patient in obtaining the "correct setting." When this approach is used, the prescriptive gain value becomes more important, and ultimately might determine whether the patient judges the fitting as successful.

Finally, in some cases, an accurate prediction of use gain also is helpful when decisions are made concerning the appropriateness of a custom in-the-ear (ITE) fitting. This is most commonly experienced with new hearing aid users, for whom no use gain history is available. For example, it is normally recommended that a usable gain reserve of approximately 10 dB be available from the hearing aid (Hawkins et al., 1991). If prescriptive target gain for a patient is 20 dB at 2000 and 3000 Hz, and a custom ITE hearing aid begins to produce feedback just as REIG at these frequencies approaches this level, it is possible that this hearing aid could be returned to the manufacturer because of "feedback problems." If, however, this person's use gain was only 10 dB for the 2000–3000 Hz range, and the audiologist

believed that use gain would not increase as the person became experienced with hearing aid use, then there is no feedback problem, and the patient has the desired 10 dB of reserve gain.

When conducting REIG measures, **therefore, there is a need to consider the overall gain as well as the slope of the frequency response**. Factors that might influence these decisions include:

■ Whether the patient is a first-time hearing aid user.
■ The patient's age.
■ The degree of hearing loss.
■ The patient's typical listening environment.

New Users Versus Experienced Users

There appears to be a prevailing belief among dispensers that new hearing aid users prefer less gain than experienced users. This belief also appears to be held by most manufacturers, as many custom ITE hearing aid order forms ask the dispenser to specify whether the hearing aids being ordered are for a new or previous user; while it is not clear what the manufacturers do with this information, presumably the answer to this question will influence how the hearing aids will be built. Recent research using REIR measurements, however, **has not found a difference in preferred gain as a function of experience using hearing aids**.

In an evaluation of the new NAL procedure, Byrne and Cotton (1988) compared use gain to prescribed gain for 44 people (67 ears), 29 of whom were new hearing aid users. Averaged across all subjects, the three-frequency average prescribed gain was 16.2 dB, compared with 15.8 dB for the use gain average. When the patients were divided into four groups according to hearing loss, similar close agreement between use gain and prescribed gain remained. The authors reported that previous hearing aid use did not affect the prescribed gain–use gain relationship.

Leijon, Lindkvist, Ringdahl, and Israelsson (1990) also compared preferred insertion gain for groups of experienced and new hearing aid users. They found no relationship between preferred gain and amount of previous hearing aid use. These findings, in agreement with the work of Byrne and Cotton (1988), suggest that when patients select their preferred gain, experience with hearing aids might not be as important as commonly believed. These studies indicate that there would be little reason to vary a patient's recommended gain setting based solely on whether they had previously used hearing aids.

Elderly Patients

As reviewed by Davies and Mueller (1987) and Gordon-Salant (1991), there are several amplification considerations when fitting hearing aids to the elderly. Researchers have studied the relationship between prescribed and use gain for this population with somewhat differing results.

The study of Byrne and Cotton (1988) cited above, though not specifically a study of the elderly, was conducted using subjects with a median age of 72 years. Their findings showed excellent agreement between preferred gain and that prescribed by the NAL, suggesting that the age of the patient is not a factor when selecting prescriptive gain.

In agreement with the findings of Byrne and Cotton (1988), Ryals and Auther (1990) compared preferred insertion gain for a group of elderly (over 75 years, 12 ears) and younger (under 60 years, 13 ears) experienced hearing aid users. The groups were matched for hearing loss. These researchers reported no significant difference in preferred insertion gain between the two groups. In comparing the preferred gain of both groups to four different prescriptive methods, Ryals and Auther found the closest agreement with the NAL and the Libby 1/3 gain formula methods (see Figure 6–1).

The work of Leijon and colleagues, however, has not shown the close agreement between prescribed and use gain for elderly subjects that was reported by Byrne and Cotton (1988) or Ryals and Auther (1990). Leijon, Eriksson-

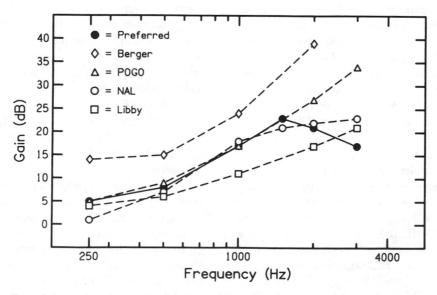

Figure 6–1. Comparison of preferred gain to the prescriptive target gain of four different procedures. (From Gordon-Salant, S. 1991. [Adapted from Ryals & Auther, 1990.] Special amplification considerations for elderly individuals. In G. Studebaker, F. Bess, & L. Beck [Eds.], *The Vanderbilt hearing aid report II* [pp. 245–261]. Parkton, MD: York Press, with permission.)

Mangold, and Bech-Karlson (1984) found that a group of elderly hearing aid users preferred 10–15 dB less gain in the 1000–2000 Hz region than prescribed by the old NAL formula (Byrne & Tonisson, 1976). In a more recent publication, Leijon, Lindkvist, Ringdahl, and Israelsson (1990) discussed the possibility that binaural fittings and a peaked frequency response could have contributed to the reduced use gain measured in the 1984 study. These authors, therefore, conducted a similar study with elderly subjects using monaural fittings that produced relatively smooth REIRs. The mean use-gain results of Leijon et al. (1990) compared with the target gain of three different prescriptive methods are shown in Figure 6–2. Notice that preferred gain (P) falls 5–8 dB below the NAL prescribed gain (N), and more substantially below the gain targets of the Berger method (B) and POGO procedure (PO). Although not plotted on the chart shown in Figure 6–2, the preferred gain values are reasonably close to the 1/3 gain prescriptive fitting approach described by Libby (1986). Leijon et al. (1990) did not study a younger group of subjects; therefore, it cannot be de-

termined if these reduced preferred gain values only apply to the elderly.

In summary, it **does not appear that preferred gain for elderly hearing aid users is much different than that for younger counterparts**. There are data to suggest, however, that the average preferred insertion gain of the elderly may fall below the prescribed gain of some of the popular gain-based prescriptive methods.

Severe-to-Profound Hearing Loss

The agreement between prescribed gain and use gain for individuals with severe-to-profound hearing loss is somewhat dependent on the prescriptive method used. As discussed in Chapter 5, **the same prescriptive method might not be appropriate for all types of hearing loss**. For example, some prescriptive methods call for gain that is as little as one-third of the patient's hearing threshold. While this approach might work quite well for mild-to-moderate hearing losses, normal speech would barely be audible in the high frequencies if these calculations were applied to someone with a hearing loss of 80 dB HL or greater.

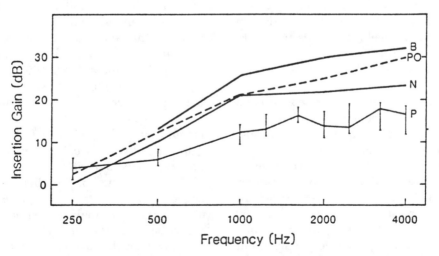

Figure 6–2. Comparison of preferred gain to that prescribed by three different procedures. B = Berger, PO = POGO, and N − NAL. (From Leijon, A., Lindkvist, A., Ringdahl, A., & Israelsson, B. 1990. Preferred hearing aid gain in everyday use after prescriptive fitting. *Ear and Hearing, 11*, 299–305, with permission.)

Some of the threshold gain-based prescriptive formulae, such as the Libby method, POGO, and the NAL procedure have been modified for use with individuals with severe-to-profound hearing losses (e.g., Byrne, Parkinson, & Newall, 1991; Libby, 1986; Schwartz, Lyregaard, & Lundh, 1988 — see Chapter 5 for more details). These modifications provide corrections which result in a prescriptive target gain that is a greater percentage of the hearing loss; Libby (1986), for example, suggests that 2/3 of the hearing loss is appropriate for some patients, although he does not provide specific guidelines concerning when this fitting rule should be used. Byrne et al. (1991) reported that **individuals with severe-to-profound hearing loss prefer about 10 dB more gain than that recommended by the NAL procedure**. When these modifications are employed, closer agreement between prescribed gain and use gain would be expected.

It might be that for people with severe-to-profound hearing loss it is simply better to use a prescriptive method that is not based on insertion gain; such as the Desired Sensation Level (DSL) method of Seewald and Ross (1988). Byrne et al. (1991), however, reported that the corrections they derived for the NAL procedure were in close agreement with the gain required for prescriptions derived from maximum comfort level (MCL) measurements.

High-Frequency Hearing Loss

The relationship between prescribed gain and use gain must also be considered in those individuals with high-frequency hearing loss — in particular, patients with normal hearing through 1500 or even 2000 Hz. Perhaps more so than for other audiometric configurations, the preferred REIG at specific frequencies for this group can be influenced considerably by the hearing aid style that is fitted; this is not a function of the hearing aid style per se, but of the configuration of the REIR that can be obtained with different hearing aid styles.

Figure 6–3, from Mueller et al. (1991) shows the mean REIRs from four different hearing aid styles, all selected for people with normal hearing through 2000 Hz. For this comparison, REIG for the four different instruments was matched at 3000 Hz. The average differences in REIG between hearing aid styles were as much as 15–20 dB at both above and below 3000 Hz. This illustrates how the configuration of the REIR easily can affect the degree that use gain agrees with prescribed gain. For example, if the people who were used to obtain the mean REIRs shown in Figure 6–3 all had normal hearing and little or no prescribed gain at 2000 Hz, and a prescription target gain of 20 dB at 3000 Hz, it is possible that with a style such as the ITE-IROS (see Figure 6–3), the 15 dB REIG in the 1500–2000 Hz range would cause them to use a low VCW setting; as a result, REIG at 3000 Hz might only be 10 dB. This does not mean that the preferred gain would not be 20 dB at 3000 Hz if the REIR configuration resembled the mean results shown in Figure 6–3 obtained from the behind-the-ear (BTE) hearing aid.

Mueller et al. (1991) reported on use gain for twelve individuals with high-frequency hearing loss above 2000 Hz, all fitted binaurally with ITE-IROS hearing aids. The subjects obtained relatively flat mean REIRs for 1500–4000 Hz, similar to the ITE-IROS pattern shown in Figure 6–3. Mueller et al. (1991) reported that average use gain for 1500–4000 Hz was 10 dB; only about 20% of the average hearing threshold at 3000–4000 Hz. This average use gain value decreased by 1–3 dB following a 6-week trial period, and decreased another 1–3 dB when the subjects were using binaural amplification. The final average use gain for individuals using binaural amplification was only 6–7 dB.

These findings of Mueller et al. (1991) suggest that patients with high-frequency loss above 2000 Hz might prefer less gain than prescribed for 3000 and 4000 Hz. It is possible, however, that **if these individuals are fitted with an REIR that meets the configuration of the prescriptive gain targets, REIG and target gain at 3000 and 4000 Hz would be in closer agreement.** Although improved REIRs

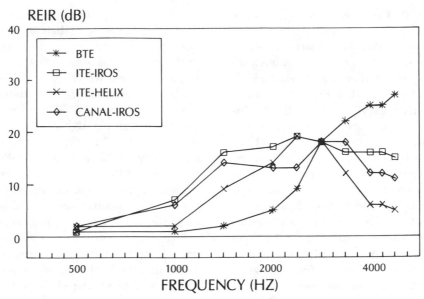

Figure 6–3. Comparison of real ear insertion gain (REIG) for four different hearing aid styles. REIG matched at 3000 Hz. (Reprinted from Mueller, H., Bryant, M., Brown, W., & Budinger, A. 1991. Hearing aid selection for high-frequency hearing loss. In G. Studebaker, F. Bess, & L. Beck [Eds.], *The Vanderbilt hearing aid report II* [pp. 269–287]. Parkton, MD: York Press, with permission.)

were obtained with the BTE instrument, all of the subjects in the Mueller and colleagues study requested the ITE hearing aid style. Since the data were collected for this study, however, new circuitry has been developed for ITE (including in-the-canal) hearing aids using Class D amplifiers and active tone controls. **With this new circuitry, it is possible to obtain REIRs with an IROS-ITE hearing aid that closely resemble the BTE instrument response shown in Figure 6–3.** We predict that use gain in the 3000 – 4000 Hz range will increase when patients with high-frequency hearing loss are fitted with this improved circuitry.

Listening Environment

Another factor to consider when prescriptive gain and use gain are compared is the typical listening environment of the hearing aid user. Anecdotal comments from hearing aid users certainly suggest that preferred gain is reduced for noisy listening situations. This was

recently documented in a study by Cox and Alexander (1991a). These authors compared use gain to that prescribed by the Memphis State University (MSU) prescriptive method for three different listening environments: A, face-to-face conversation in a typical living room or quiet office; B, listening as an audience member to a lecture delivered in an unamplified classroom; and C, face-to-face communication at a social event with numerous people present. The subjects made use gain judgments using three different frequency response slopes, one of which was that prescribed by the MSU procedure.

Cox and Alexander (1991a) reported that for the three response slopes used in this study, **subjects preferred approximately 10–13 dB more gain for environment A than for environments B or C;** there was no significant difference in use gain between environments B and C. When all environments were averaged, use gain was in good agreement with the MSU prescribed gain; however, no single environment resulted in a use gain corresponding to the MSU prescription.

There are two useful clinical applications of the results of the Cox and Alexander study. First, it is important that the **hearing aid is selected and fitted so that the user has the option of altering gain by 10–12 dB for different listening situations**. Second, if it is necessary to instruct the user where to set the gain control, it might be best to offer two settings, one for quiet and one for noisy listening environments. For the MSU fitting procedure, these two settings would be 5–6 dB above (listening in quiet) and 5–6 dB below (listening in noise) the prescribed gain. For individuals using multiple memory digitally programmable hearing aids, it might be **useful to program these gain settings into different user-controlled memory locations**.

INSERTION GAIN VERSUS SPEECH AUDIOMETRY

Another theoretical issue concerns the common practice of using the REIR as the primary validation measure of the hearing aid fitting. There are methods other than the REIR of verifying the appropriateness of the hearing aid's frequency response, the most obvious being the use of speech audiometry. Since patients normally seek amplification because they are unable to understand speech, **it seems reasonable to determine if speech understanding has been maximized, or at least improved, before the fitting is considered appropriate**. In an article advocating the use of a speech-based measure as the ultimate validation of the hearing aid, Jerger (1987) wrote:

Some clinicians eagerly embrace the simplistic concept that the only thing you need to know about a hearing aid's performance is its frequency response. In many respects this view of the world is as obsolete as Carhart's much maligned methodology. Yet it gains new followers daily, seduced by the specious argument that "objective science" is replacing "subjective impression." (p. 50)

Humes (1991b), in agreement with Jerger (1987), commented that audiologists have been preoccupied with real-ear measurements at the expense of other hearing aid evaluation procedures. He wrote that aided-speech audiometry is essential, even if there is a perfect match between the REIR and prescribed target. Humes and Houghton (1992) recommend the use of the 11-subtest version of the City University of New York (CUNY) Nonsense Syllable Test (NST) to obtain an estimate of the improvement in speech understanding after the hearing aid has been fitted and adjusted according to a prescriptive fitting method.

The complex relationship between aided-speech audiometry and prescriptive fitting methods was illustrated in the recent findings of Cox and Alexander (1991b). Using connected speech discourse, these authors studied hearing aid benefit in three different listening environments for three prescriptive gain slopes. They found that one of the three prescriptive responses resulted in a significantly different benefit for 76% of the subjects in at least one listening environment, however, **there was no overall trend for any single frequency response slope to give superior benefit in any listening environment**.

While few audiologists would dispute the merit of using speech-based procedures for validation of the hearing aid fitting, as pointed out by Jerger (1987), **the speech material and test conditions must be carefully selected so that the inherent instability of the measure does not prevent detection of small, but important changes, in hearing aid performance**; Studebaker (1991) has reviewed many issues concerning the reliability of the speech intelligibility and quality measures used in hearing aid assessment.

Few audiologists presently use speech audiometry to select the "best" hearing aid or the most appropriate REIR. This is probably due to the fact that it has not been clearly demonstrated that any clinical speech material has the sensitivity to make this differentiation on an individual basis — at least not within the time frame that normally is allotted for a hearing aid evaluation. Additionally, because of the overwhelming popularity of custom ITE and in-the-canal (ITC) instruments, only one hearing aid usually is available for clinical testing, and comparative testing is not practical. Hence, many audiologists have welcomed the use of probe-microphone measures, and view the REIG as a more reliable measure than speech audiometry to establish if a custom ITE hearing aid fitting is appropriate, since the REIG can be used to assist in determining if the average speech spectrum at least has been made audible. The advantage of the later consideration perhaps is best summarized by Pascoe (1980):

Although it is true that mere detection of a sound does not ensure its recognition, it is even more true that without detection the probabilities of correct identification are greatly diminished. (p. 224)

Pascoe's comment helps emphasize that **both the REIR and speech audiometry play important roles in the validation of the hearing aid fitting, and it is probably best to incorporate both measurements into the hearing aid evaluation.** (This was the recommendation of the 1991 Vanderbilt/VA hearing aid selection consensus statement — see Chapter 1.)

One approach would be to use the REIR to determine if the hearing aid is providing the desired amount of gain at specific frequency regions, based on some prescriptive approach; REIR measurements also would be used at this time to make fine tuning adjustments. Once the desired response was obtained, speech testing could then be conducted. This testing could be used to compare unaided versus aided results (speech audiometry *is* sensitive enough to make this differentiation), and to compare the aided results to a clinic standard of acceptable performance. **Developing a clinic standard for acceptable aided performance for a given speech material is not an easy task. The articulation index, which is discussed next, can be used to provide general guidelines.**

USE OF THE ARTICULATION INDEX

Somewhat related to the above discussion is the combined use of REIR measurements and the articulation index (AI). It is generally believed that the AI is helpful in determining a frequency-gain hearing aid response that will maximize speech understanding. For this reason, the AI has been used to study and compare different prescriptive fitting approaches (e.g., Humes, 1986; Rankovic, 1991).

At one time, calculation of the AI was considered to be too complicated and confusing to be employed routinely in everyday clinical practice. In recent years, however, simplified versions of the AI have been introduced by Mueller and Killion (1990), Humes (1991a), and Pavlovic (1991) which easily can be used by audiologists to predict both unaided and aided speech understanding. All three of these methods employ a series of dots placed on a conventional audiogram, which represent the average speech spectrum. The density of the dots is related to the importance of that particular frequency for understanding speech. An example of the Mueller and Killion (1990) AI audiogram is shown in Figure 6–4.

The unaided AI is calculated by plotting the earphone audiogram on the chart and counting the dots that fall below the unaided thresholds (i.e., the dots that would be audible). The predicted aided thresholds can be obtained by adding the REIG to the unaided thresholds at each frequency. This allows for calculation of the aided AI, a comparison of the unaided AI to the aided AI, and comparison of one aided AI to another.

Humes (1991a) used this procedure to compare both unaided and aided AI calculations to the speech-recognition scores obtained for the CUNY Nonsense Syllable Test (NST). Using his count-the-dot AI method, he found a 0.93 correlation between AI scores and unaided measured speech recognition. The aided correlation coefficient between the two measures was 0.73. Humes (1991a) also reported that, in most instances, the AI scores correlated highly for subjects tested with three different hearing aids; that is, when insertion gain predicted a higher AI for a given hearing aid, higher NST scores were obtained. He concluded that these methods were good *relative* predictors of speech-recognition performance for aided listening in quiet.

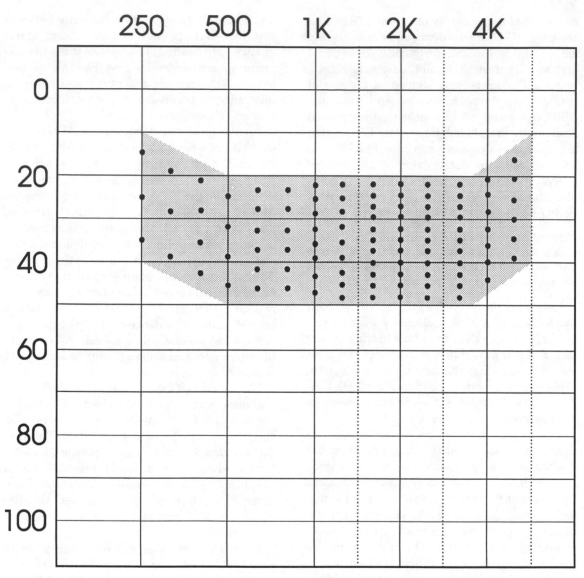

Figure 6–4. Count-the-dot audiogram for use in calculation of the articulation index (AI). (From Mueller, H., & Killion, M. 1990. An easy method for calculating the articulation index. *Hearing Journal, 43,* 14–17, with permission.)

There are some limitations, however, in using the AI for assessing hearing aid performance. These calculations do not take into account hearing aid distortion, internal noise, or patient factors (e.g., reduced loudness discomfort level, central presbycusis) that could result in lower than predicted scores (of course, neither do REIR measurements in general). Byrne (1992) also suggests that the AI

might not be applicable for steep high-frequency hearing losses. As pointed out by Revit (1991b), raising the hearing aid gain and increasing the high frequencies to improve the AI often results in patient dissatisfaction and acoustic feedback. It is also possible that the increased high frequencies could cause increased sound power and loudness, and the patient would lower the gain of the hearing aid as a result — a reaction that would *lower* the AI (Studebaker, 1992).

A final caution concerns the combined use of earphone thresholds and REIG measurements, that is, the procedure of subtracting REIG values from unaided thresholds to obtain predicted soundfield aided thresholds. While this procedure is usually easier than conducting aided soundfield thresholds, and it is reasonably accurate for the average person, it is possible that significant errors could be present for patients with unusual REURs.

PRACTICAL CONSIDERATIONS

When using the REIR to validate a hearing aid fitting, it often is necessary to make a pass/fail decision, and a later section of this chapter discusses this topic in detail. There are several practical considerations, however, that can assist the audiologist in obtaining closer agreement between the REIR and the prescriptive gain target.

ORDERING METHOD FOR ITE HEARING AIDS

A simple, yet critical principle is that **custom ITE hearing aids must be ordered according to the prescriptive method that will be used for validation**. Examining the underlying math of the popular prescriptive fitting methods will reveal that a hearing aid ordered according to the POGO method would probably appear to have too much gain if the Libby 1/3 rule were used when REIR measurements were conducted. While this would seem to be an easy principle to adhere to, implementation is compromised by the fact that **80–95% of custom hearing aids are ordered without any specification regarding gain or frequency response** (Bratt & Sammeth, 1991; Valente, Valente, & Vass, 1990). This means that the manufacturer must make the gain, frequency response, and SSPL90 selection based pure-tone audiogram. In other words, **manufacturers have been forced to develop their own prescriptive fitting method**.

When custom hearing aids that are ordered simply by mailing in an audiogram are fitted, the manufacturer's prescriptive method should be used to determine if REIG values are appropriate. For example, if a given manufacturer believes that insertion gain at 4000 Hz is unnecessary, and the audiologist allowed the manufacturer to choose the prescription, then the custom product should not be returned due to the absence of REIG at 4000 Hz.

In most cases, however, manufacturers have their own modifications of the published prescriptive methods, and little or no data are available that would allow the audiologist to calculate specific target gain values. As a result, validation is usually difficult, sometimes impossible, and at best haphazard. This clearly points out why the **best approach simply is to order custom products either by matrix or by full-on 2-cm^3 coupler gain**, as discussed in Chapter 9.

CIRCUITRY LIMITATION

When making decisions regarding the acceptability of REIR measurements, **it is important to consider the limitations of the hearing aid circuitry**. This is most commonly an issue of concern when custom ITE products are returned for credit or frequency-response change because the REIR does not meet the prescriptive target gain. It is counterproductive to return an ITE hearing aid for 10 dB more gain at 4000 Hz if the present instrument already has the greatest high-frequency gain offered by that manufacturer. Most manufacturers offer a matrix book which displays 2-cm^3 coupler responses for their different circuitry and circuitry combinations. It is helpful to become very familiar with the product line of two or three manufacturers, as this approach provides a frame of reference for making REIR value judgments for ITE instruments. While 2-cm^3 coupler curves might not accurately predict the REIR (see Chapter 12), they can be used effectively to determine whether other circuitry is available that would be better suited for a given patient. This will become less of an issue in a few years, as each audiologist will have the majority of the manufacturers' gain and output responses available at the time of the hearing aid fitting through the use of digital programmers.

MAKING SPEECH AUDIBLE

The goal of most prescriptive fitting procedures, whether stated explicitly or not, is to place amplified speech at the hearing aid user's MCL. As hearing loss becomes greater, this task becomes more difficult, and sometimes it is difficult to even make speech audible. In some cases, **when it appears impossible to make average speech (or even the peaks of speech) audible, it is best to ignore these frequencies when REIR results are analyzed**. For example, consider a patient with a precipitous high-frequency hearing loss of 20 dB at 1000 Hz, 60 dB at 2000 Hz, and 90 dB at 3000 and 4000 Hz. On occasion, audiologists will return a custom instrument for patients with hearing loss similar to this because the REIG did not meet the prescriptive target gain at 3000 and 4000 Hz. However, even if the REIG *did* reach the prescriptive gain target (e.g., per the POGO or NAL method) loud speech in the 3000–4000 Hz range would barely be audible, and average speech would still be inaudible. Inaudible is inaudible. Hence, for this type of hearing loss, it probably is best to focus on obtaining appropriate REIGs for 2000 Hz and below. This could mean ordering a hearing aid with a 2-cm³ coupler gain that peaked in the 2000 Hz range, rather than at 3000 Hz. The AI audiogram shown in Figure 6–4 can be used in conjunction with earphone thresholds and prescribed target gain to help determine when it is not feasible to make speech audible for a specific frequency region.

THE PATIENT'S REUR

As discussed in Chapter 3, **the patient's REUR often determines whether the REIR meets the** **prescriptive gain target**. The primary reason that a prescriptive target gain is difficult to obtain at 3000 Hz is because this is the frequency region where the primary peak of many patient's REUR is located. Theoretically, therefore, people with small REURs in the 3000–4000 Hz range should be receiving the most benefit from their hearing aids because it is almost always possible to obtain target prescriptive gain for these individuals. Because of this direct relationship between the REUR and the REIR, a hearing aid should not be rejected because of a bad REIR without first considering the patient's REUR. Some individual's REUR has a peak intensity as high as 25 or 30 dB. When the peak intensity of the REUR is 25 dB or greater, and the peak is located at 3000 Hz or above, a dip in the REIR at the peak frequency is almost inevitable given the current limitations of hearing aid circuitry. On the other hand, if the REUR peak is no more than 15 dB, an upward-sloping REIR curve, the desired outcome for most patients, should be easily attainable.

ACOUSTIC FEEDBACK

It is not unusual that **two of the most important aspects of the hearing aid fitting, achieving target gain and avoiding acoustic feedback, work in direct opposition**. When a REIR slope is obtained that places the peak of the response in the 3000 to 4000 Hz range, acoustic feedback might occur when the patient adjusts the hearing aid gain to a comfortable listening level. Elimination of feedback must then take priority. In some cases, this can be accomplished through making a vent smaller, extending the canal length, or other shell modifications. Sometimes, however, the only solution is to reduce the high frequency gain. Most manufacturers offer the option of a high-frequency gain reduction potentiometer, often referred to as a feedback control circuit — a more desirable marketing term than a "speech intelligibility reduction potentiometer."

While the goal of many hearing aid fittings is to maximize the audibility of high frequency speech sounds, in some cases, reducing the high frequency gain seems to be the only method of eliminating a feedback problem. Figure 6–5 shows the range of REIG variation that can be obtained using this type of circuitry. While prescriptive target gain for the person in Figure 6–5 closely resembled the solid-line REIR, it was necessary to fit the hearing aid with high-frequency REIG closer to the dashed REIR.

USE OF NONLINEAR CIRCUITRY

Prescriptive fitting rationales have been designed and verified using linear hearing aid circuitry. When REIR measurements are conducted for nonlinear hearing aids, therefore, there are two issues to be considered. First, the prescriptive target gain used for linear hearing aids is sometimes difficult to apply to these instruments. Gain might vary as a function of input, and whether the REIR meets target gain depends on the input that is selected for testing. Second, in some models using input-controlled gain, the configuration of the REIR can vary significantly as a function of the input intensity used to conduct the measure. Figure 6–6 shows the REIRs obtained at 50, 60, and 70 dB for an input automatic gain control (AGC) ITE instrument. Depending on whether the audiologist considered the 50 dB-input REIR or the 70 dB-input REIR, agreement with the target gain configuration could be viewed as either very good or very bad. The reduction of REIG for only the higher frequencies for an input AGC hearing aid, as shown in Figure 6–6, is probably partially due to a measurement artifact (referred to as *blooming*), as these measurements were obtained using a swept puretone signal (Preves, Beck, Burnett, & Teder 1989 — see Chapter 10 for further description). **When evaluating nonlinear instruments, it is best to use speech-shaped noise as the**

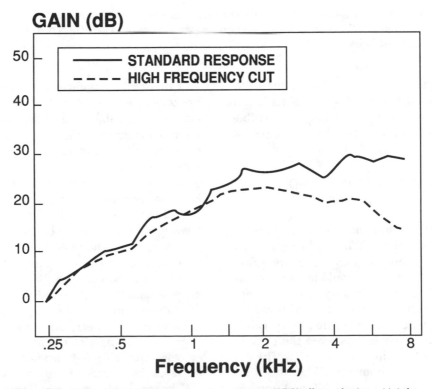

Figure 6–5. Illustration of the real ear insertion response (REIR) effects of using a high frequency gain-reduction potentiometer.

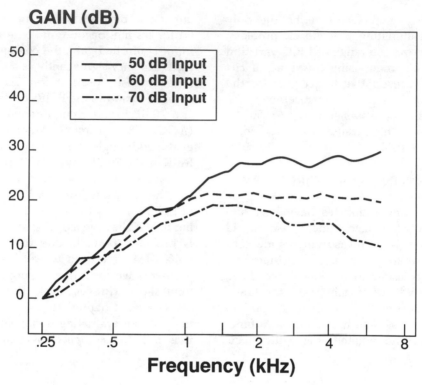

Figure 6–6. Variation in real ear insertion response (REIR) for three different inputs (warbletones) for an AGC-I hearing aid. The alteration in the configuration of the REIR is due to the blooming artifact.

input signal and to conduct at least one REIR measurement of the hearing aid in its linear mode, although this might not be possible with some hearing aids that have a compression knee as low as 45 dB.

MODIFICATIONS AND ADJUSTMENTS

Before the final judgment is made concerning the acceptability of the REIR of a hearing aid, it is important to consider all possible modifications or adjustments that could be made other than changing the circuitry itself. Potentiometers offer the ability to increase or reduce the low-frequency and high-frequency gains; in some newer instruments, even the peak in the frequency response can be varied. The degree that the potentiometer affects the REIR varies considerably among different models

and different manufacturers. Given that this option is present on nearly all BTE hearing aids, and available from most ITE instrument manufacturers for little or no cost, potentiometers provide a convenient method of fine-tuning the REIR.

Another common method of altering the REIR is through venting. Select-a-vents can provide the option of altering vent size at the hearing aid fitting. Much of the research literature concerning the effects of venting is based on BTE hearing aids and earmolds coupled to 2-cm³ couplers, with a tight seal between the earmold and the coupler. REIR measures with ITE hearing aids, which usually have a slit leak around the periphery, do not show the same degree of venting effect as shown in this earlier research. Table 6–1, from Tecca (1991), illustrates the effects of different vent sizes of ITE hearing aids, measured using the REIR.

TABLE 6–1. COMPARISON OF THE EFFECTS OF THREE DIFFERENT VENT SIZES ON HEARING AID GAIN

	Frequency (Hz)				
	200 Hz	*500 Hz*	*1000 Hz*	*1500 Hz*	*2000 Hz*
1.0/1.3 mm Vent					
Tecca (sealed)	− 6.8	2.8	0.8	0.3	−0.2
Lybarger	2.0	2.0	0.0	0.0	—
Kates	−13.0	2.0	4.0	0.0	—
Tecca (slit vent)	− 7.1	0.3	1.5	0.5	0.1
2.0 mm Vent					
Tecca (sealed)	−12.1	2.2	1.7	0.6	0.3
Lybarger	−14.0	9.0	2.0	1.0	—
Kates	−17.0	−12.0	0.0	1.0	—
Tecca (slit vent)	−11.1	− 0.9	1.9	0.7	0.2
3.0 mm Vent					
Tecca (sealed)	−25.0	− 9.8	5.1	2.9	2.0
Lybarger	−22.0	− 2.0	2.0	2.0	—
Kates	—	—	—	—	—
Tecca (slit vent)	−21.9	−10.5	3.1	2.6	1.9

Source: From Tecca, J. 1991b. Real ear vent effects in ITE hearing instrument fittings. *Hearing Instruments, 42*, 10–12, with permission.

For comparison Table 6–1 also displays data from BTE hearing aids and ear molds on an ear simulator (Lybarger, 1985) and KEMAR (Knowles Electronics Manikin for Acoustic Research) measurements and computer simulation of ITE venting effects (Kates, 1988).

The data from Tecca shown in Table 6–1, offer some practical guidelines for use when venting is applied to alter the REIR of an ITE fitting. For ITC hearing aids, a vent style referred to as a "D" vent often is employed. Stuart et al. (1992) compared the real-ear effects of pressure vents (1 mm), standard D vents (1.4 mm × 2.8 mm), and IROS D vents (1.7 mm × 3.4 mm) for ITC instruments. The mean results of their comparisons are shown in Figure 6–7. Notice that the **different venting can be used to significantly alter real-ear gain, but only for the frequencies below 600–800 Hz**.

A final application to alter the REIR that can be applied to both earmolds and ITE hearing aids is extending the canal length. This approach is known to help reduce the occlusion effect, but it also causes a slight increase in high-frequency gain. Figure 6–8, for example, shows the effect of extending the canal of an earmold an additional 8–10 mm into the ear canal. Observe that **when the canal is longer, the REIR becomes smoother, and additional gain is achieved for the higher frequencies**. Simply extending the receiver tubing of an ITE hearing aid can cause a slight increase in high-frequency gain, although not as significant as the increase shown for the long canal in Figure 6–8.

There are some other modifications, such as the use of dampers and horn acoustics, which can be used easily with earmolds and tone hooks when BTE hearing aids are fitted. These techniques also have some limited applications with ITE instruments. In general, the REIR offers a useful and rapid method to measure the effects of these modifications; and likewise,

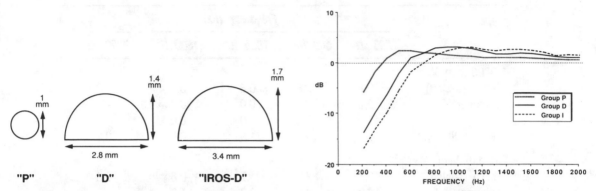

Figure 6–7. Left panel: Illustration of the different vent sizes for in-the-canal (ITC) hearing aids used in this study. Right panel: The real-ear effects of three different types of ITC vents. (Reprinted from Stuart, A., Stenstrom, R., MacDonald, O., Schmidt, M., & Maclean, G. 1992. Probe-tube microphone measures of vent effects with in-the-canal hearing aid shells. *American Journal of Audiology, 1*(2), 58–62, with permission.)

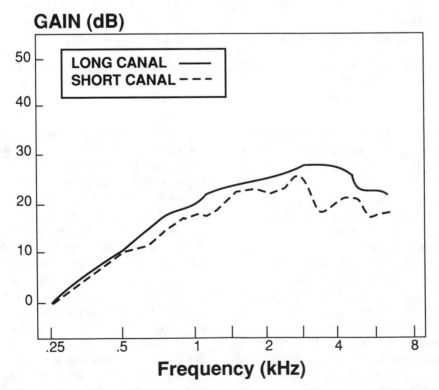

Figure 6–8. The effects of two different hearing aid ear canal lengths (10 mm and 20 mm) on the real ear insertion response (REIR).

the modifications often provide the necessary alteration in the REIR so that an acceptable rating of the fitting can be rendered.

PATIENT'S SUBJECTIVE JUDGMENTS

What if REIG values are a perfect match to prescriptive gain targets and the patient says that he or she does not like the way the hearing aid sounds? Does it matter if the patient is a new or experienced hearing aid user? Does it matter if these comments are made at the time of the hearing aid fitting or after the patient has used the hearing aid for a few weeks? Does it matter if the comment is from a patient who is not motivated to use hearing aids?

The degree that the REIG of a hearing aid should be altered because of patient comments is not an easy decision. Consider, for example, the typical new hearing aid user who has had at least a mild downward-sloping high-frequency hearing loss for the past 10 or more years. If target REIG is achieved, the *expected* response from the patient would be that things sound "tinny." Removing high-frequency gain probably would make things "normal" for this patient. But what about the goal of maximizing audibility of high-frequency speech signals? Who is the best judge of what is best for the patient?

The solution usually involves compromise and is facilitated through frequent follow-up visits and the use of programmable hearing aids or hearing aids with active tone-control potentiometers. Small deviations from prescriptive gain target usually do not alter speech understanding significantly, and if a small change in the REIR causes the patient to judge the fitting as more satisfactory, then changing the response is probably the best decision. On the other hand, the benefit of a specific REIR might not be realized by the patient until after extended listening in a variety of everyday environments. **Relying too heavily on the patient's opinion at the time of the fitting could prevent the user from experiencing the REIR**

that ultimately would be optimal for him or her. For example, previous users of hearing aids with little high-frequency gain often want the new hearing aids to sound like their old ones. An approach that works quite well for these patients is to gradually adjust the REIR toward the desired high-frequency gain on follow-up visits. It might take 3–6 months to bring the high-frequency REIG to the desired level, but ultimately, both the audiologist and the patient will be happy.

ESTABLISHING PASS/FAIL CRITERIA

During the 1980s, there were several changes regarding the way that audiologists routinely select and evaluate hearing aids. These changes primarily were driven by four factors:

■ The larger number of audiologists involved in direct dispensing.
■ The popularity of custom ITE hearing aids.
■ The increased use of prescriptive fitting methods.
■ The emergence of computerized probe-microphone systems.

Today, nearly 80% of all hearing aid sales in the United States are custom ITE instruments (Kirkwood, 1991). Because it is not practical to order multiple ITE hearing aids for the same patient, the once-common **comparative evaluation of different hearing aids is now seldom conducted**. Rather, at the time of the evaluation, patients typically are tested with only one hearing aid — the custom-made ITE with which they will be fitted.

Because most popular prescriptive methods are gain-based, REIG values usually are used to determine if the *gold standard* (prescriptive gain targets) for the fitting has been met. Unfortunately, even after the audiologist has made all possible in-house modifications, it is unusual for the REIG to meet the target for all frequencies of interest. The clinician, therefore, must establish what is an acceptable decibel deviation from target and what is not — that is, pass/fail criteria must be developed for the verification process. Presumably the hearing aids that pass are fitted to the patient and the ones that fail are returned to the manufacturer for alteration of the frequency response or a different model is selected. Obviously, criteria that are too lax could result in an unacceptable number of patients being fitted with hearing aids that, at least theoretically, are not maximizing their speech understanding. On the other hand, a pass/fail standard that is too rigid could result in an extremely large number of hearing aids being returned to the manufacturer — a situation that is not desirable for the patient, audiologist, or manufacturer.

Because the **pass/fail rules are ambiguous, audiologists often are not in agreement concerning what REIG–prescriptive target gain match constitutes an acceptable fitting**. We recently surveyed 100 experienced audiologists who were using prescriptive fitting methods and probe-microphone measurements for fitting ITE hearing aids. We asked them to judge whether they would consider the four REIRs shown in Figure 6–9 acceptable based on the agreement with the prescriptive target gain — that is, would they sell a hearing aid to someone if the best frequency response obtainable had this degree of deviation from target gain. As displayed in Figure 6–9, even the REIR with the greatest deviations from prescriptive target was judged as acceptable by nearly one-half of the audiologists, yet a number of audiologists did not consider the "best" REIR to be acceptable.

Mueller et al. (1991) discussed two different approaches to establishing reasonable decibel cut-off values for the REIG — target gain differences. The ideal, but perhaps least practical, approach would be to fail the hearing aid if the deviation from target gain was great enough to cause a significant decrease in the patient's speech-understanding ability. For example, if target gain for a given patient at 3000 Hz was 24 dB, and the REIG was 18 dB, and if it was known that 6 dB below target at 3000 Hz would cause a significant decrease in speech

understanding, then the hearing aid would fail and it would not be fitted to the patient. While in theory this approach seems sound, implementation is difficult as the precise decibel deviations that begin to cause a reduction in speech understanding are not known (not to mention other variables, such as the patient's use gain). The use of an AI procedure, such as discussed earlier in this chapter, could possibly help solve this problem. But, again, one would have to determine what is the maximum AI possible for a given patient, and then determine what variation below this value would warrant a hearing aid rejection.

A second approach for establishing an insertion gain pass/fail protocol is to compare the REIG–target gain differences for a given patient to similar measures obtained from a large pool of hearing aid fittings. The hearing aid would be judged as good or bad, therefore, based on how similar the deviations from target are to previous findings. This procedure takes into account the present day limitations in hearing aid circuitry. For example, as in the previous illustrative case, if REIG at 3000 Hz was 6 dB below target, but in 70% of similar fittings the deviation from target was greater than 6 dB, then the hearing aid likely would pass the verification process for that frequency.

Until the data or clinical test procedures are available to allow for the implementation of the first-mentioned pass/fail procedure, the second alternative approach would seem to provide a reasonable method of establishing clinical standards. Each fitting could be compared to these standards to assure that the patient left the clinic using a hearing aid with target gain–REIG agreement that at least was close to "the best possible." With this approach, it is important that the data used to establish clinical standards are obtained in such a way that the REIG–prescriptive target comparisons truly represent the "best case" scenario. This means that the hearing aids must be ordered by individualized prescriptions, only manufacturers capable of producing a wide range of responses are used, and the manufacturer is aware of the priorities of the audiolo-

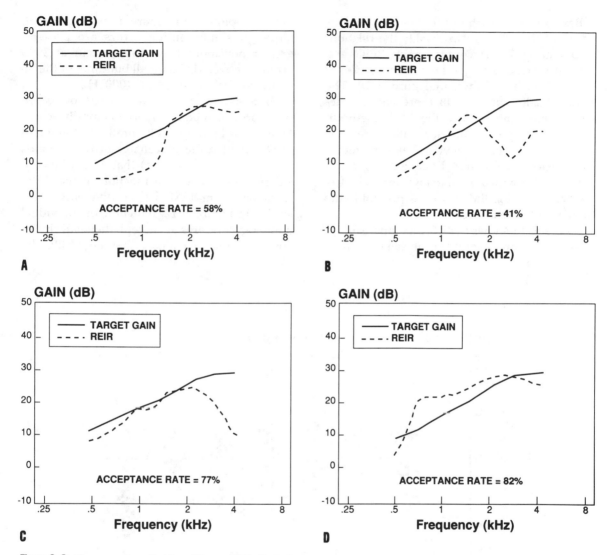

Figure 6–9. The percentage that four different REIRs (A, B, C, and D) were rated as acceptable by 100 dispensing audiologists.

gist when the hearing aids are built (e.g., If there is only room for one potentiometer, which one do you want?). There have been two large studies at government agencies that have used this approach to establish some baseline clinical guidelines for pass/fail decisions regarding custom ITE fittings.

NASHVILLE VA MEDICAL CENTER STUDY

As part of a long-term study on hearing aid selection and fitting, audiologists at the Nash-

ville VA compared 2-cm³ coupler values and REIG to prescriptive target gain for 90 ears fitted with analog custom ITEs (Bratt & Sammeth, 1991). The hearing aids were ordered using the NAL procedure. The manufacturer was provided the desired full-on gain 2-cm³ coupler values, based on average real-ear-to-coupler correction factors. All possible potentiometer and/or venting adjustments were made prior to recording final REIG values to obtain the closest match to the NAL prescriptive gain target.

Bratt and Sammeth (1991) randomly select- ed 35 of the 90 cases to display the relation- ship among 2-cm³ coupler gain, REIG and NAL prescriptive target. Data from the 2-cm³ comparison are shown in Figure 6–10. The horizontal line at zero dB represents the de- sired 2-cm³ values (per the NAL method); each datum point, therefore, illustrates the measured difference above or below target for each custom hearing aid. In general, too much gain was provided in the low and mid fre- quencies, and too little gain was present in the high frequencies.

Figure 6–11 shows the REIG comparisons to NAL prescriptive target for the same 35 hear-

ing aids plotted in Figure 6–10. Note that, although similar fitting errors are present, greater deviations from target occur at 3000 Hz and above. REIGs for all but three of the 35 cases fell below target at 4000 Hz.

To assist in determining what deviation from target can be considered clinically accep- table, or at least tolerable, Bratt and Sammeth (1991) plotted the percentage of hearing aids (using the 90 ear sample) that would be con- sidered acceptable as a function of the REIG deviation from NAL prescriptive target. As shown in Figure 6–12, if a clinic or individual audiologist desires to accept the majority of custom ITE hearing aids, rather large REIG de-

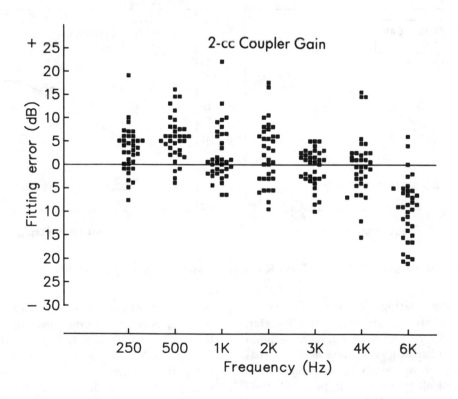

Figure 6–10. Scatterplot illustrating magnitude and distribution of fitting error based on 2-cm³ coupler gain. (From Bratt, G., & Sammeth, C. 1991. Clinical implications of pre- scriptive formulas for hearing aid selection. In G. Studebaker, F. Bess, and L. Beck [Eds.], *The Vanderbilt hearing aid report II* [pp. 23–35]. Parkton, MD: York Press, with permission.)

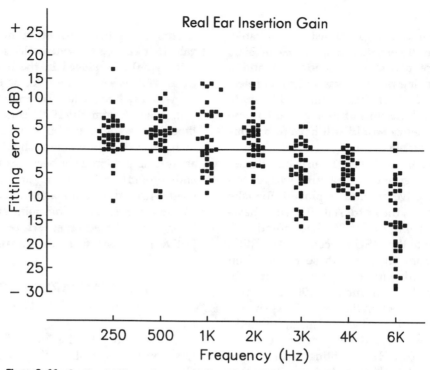

Figure 6–11. Scatterplot illustrating magnitude and distribution of fitting error based on real ear insertion gain. (From Bratt, G., & Sammeth, C. 1991. Clinical implications of prescriptive formulas for hearing aid selection. In G. Studebaker, F. Bess, & L. Beck [Eds.], *The Vanderbilt hearing aid report II* [pp. 23–35]. Parkton, MD: York Press, with permission.)

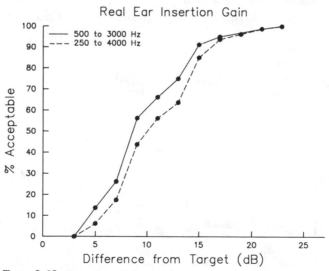

Figure 6–12. Illustration of the relation between fitting error and the acceptance rate based on real ear insertion gain measurements. (From Bratt, G., & Sammeth, C. 1991. Clinical implications of prescriptive formulas for hearing aid selection. In G. Studebaker, F. Bess, & L. Beck [Eds.], *The Vanderbilt hearing aid report II* [pp. 23–35]. Parkton, MD: York Press, with permission.)

viations from target gain must be tolerated. For example, if only the frequencies of 500–3000 Hz are considered (solid line) and a given dispensing practice was willing to reject as many as 20% of their fittings, this study suggests that **deviations of nearly 15 dB at one or more frequency would still have to be considered acceptable**.

Bratt and Sammeth (1991) also questioned whether the degree of fitting error was related to the prescriptive method employed. To make this comparison, they ordered 20 custom hearing aids according to the POGO method, and 20 according to the MSU procedure. The REIG deviations from target for these fittings then were compared with the previous data obtained using the NAL method (90 ears). This comparison is shown in Figure 6–13. As shown, the fitting error is similar for the three methods in the low and mid frequencies; however, at 3000 and 4000 Hz the fitting error for the POGO method is about 5 dB larger than that obtained using the NAL. This finding most likely is a reflection of the fact that POGO gain targets are higher than the NAL targets at 3000 and 4000 Hz when a downward-sloping hearing loss is present. Because the **manufacturer is limited in the amount of high-frequency gain that can be provided, the same circuitry often would be placed in the hearing aid regardless of whether the NAL or POGO method was used to order the instrument**.

Bratt and Sammeth (1991) concluded that although these deviations from target are greater than desired, improvement should be possible as hearing aid circuitry becomes more flexible and programmable units are more widely used. Also, they emphasized that the **target values are only a starting point and may need to be altered based on speech testing and subjective responses from the hearing aid user**.

LETTERMAN ARMY MEDICAL CENTER STUDY

A similar study to the Nashville VA project was conducted at Letterman Army Medical Center in San Francisco (with some data collected at Walter Reed Army Medical Center in Washington, DC). Preliminary reports of these findings have been made by Mueller and Jons (1989), Mueller (1990), and Bryant, Mueller, and Reidel (1990).

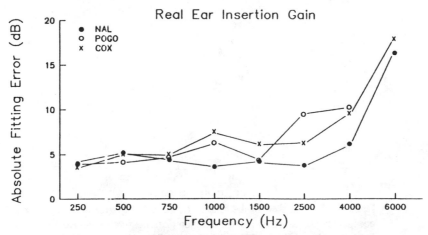

Figure 6–13. Comparison of the fitting error for three different prescriptive procedures. (Reprinted from Bratt, G., & Sammeth, C. 1991. Clinical implications of prescriptive formulas for hearing aid selection. In G. Studebaker, F. Bess, & L. Beck [Eds.], *The Vanderbilt hearing aid report II* [pp. 23–35]. Parkton, MD: York Press, with permission.)

Custom ITE hearing aids were ordered from two major manufacturers using the NAL prescriptive method. The desired frequency response was expressed to the manufacturers in full-on gain 2-cm³ coupler values using the 2-cm³ coupler ITE corrections recommended by Byrne and Dillon (1986). The manufacturers were not furnished audiograms. Two modifications to the Byrne and Dillon NAL procedure were employed when the hearing aids were ordered. First, using the REUR correction procedure described by Mueller (1989), the requested 2-cm³ coupler gain was altered when the patient's REUR deviated significantly from average. Second, only 10 dB reserve gain was requested, rather than the 15 dB incorporated by Byrne and Dillon (1986).

The insertion gain data reported here were taken from over 500 consecutive fittings that occurred over a 4–6 month period. Patients were eliminated from the data base if:

■ The audiometric configuration was not downward sloping.
■ A conductive hearing loss was present.
■ Hearing loss at 500 Hz was greater than 60 dB.

For some patients, specific frequencies were eliminated from the analysis if the hearing loss at that frequency was greater than 80 dB. Using these criteria, the resulting number of patients in the database ranged from 416 to 466, depending on the frequency of interest.

Given that pass/fail criteria might vary as a function of the slope of the hearing loss, the subjects were divided into five groups based on the frequency at which their hearing loss began (threshold, >20 dB HL) and the degree of hearing loss at 500 Hz. The group divisions were as follows:

Group 1: Hearing loss beginning at 2000 Hz
Group 2: Hearing loss beginning at 1500 Hz
Group 3: Hearing loss beginning at 1000 Hz
Group 4: Hearing loss of 25-40 dB at 500 Hz
Group 5: Hearing loss of 45-60 dB at 500 Hz

The mean audiograms of the five different groups are shown in Figure 6–14.

To allow for meaningful comparisons of deviations from NAL prescriptive target gain among patients and groups, REIG was matched to NAL target gain at 2000 Hz for all patients. The frequency of 2000 Hz was chosen for three reasons:

■ This frequency is recognized as important for speech intelligibility.
■ All subjects had a hearing loss at this frequency.
■ It was almost always possible to obtain NAL prescribed REIG at 2000 Hz.

Figures 6–15 through 6–19 show the REIG findings, plotted as a function of frequency, audiometric configuration, deviation from desired gain, and the degree of desired gain. Only data for 3000 and 4000 Hz are shown as these are the two frequencies that usually determine whether the fitting is judged as acceptable. Using these data, it is possible to formulate reasonable REIG expectations for a given patient. For example, if (a) an individual's audiogram revealed normal hearing through 1000 Hz (Group 2), (b) NAL target gain at 4000 Hz was 25 dB, and (c) the measured REIG fell 5 dB below target, the data in Figure 6–16 show that this outcome actually is *better* than typically observed in this sample.

When examining the target gain–REIG difference, many audiologists prefer to use a fixed decibel difference value in order to rate the hearing aid as good or bad — for instance, deviations less than 10 dB are acceptable, while at greater than 10 dB the hearing aid is returned to the manufacturer. Figure 6–20 organizes the data from Figures 6–15 through 6–19 so that pass/fail percentages can be observed for two different decibel tolerance windows at either 3000 or 4000 Hz. **A rigid cut-off value such as 5 dB would result in a large number of hearing aid rejections.** For 3000 Hz, 10 dB might be considered a reasonable value. **For 4000 Hz, however, even a 10 dB deviation tolerance causes 13–44% (depending on audiogram type) of the fittings to fail the verification procedure.**

A final way to view these data is to establish REIG deviation values for various percentiles,

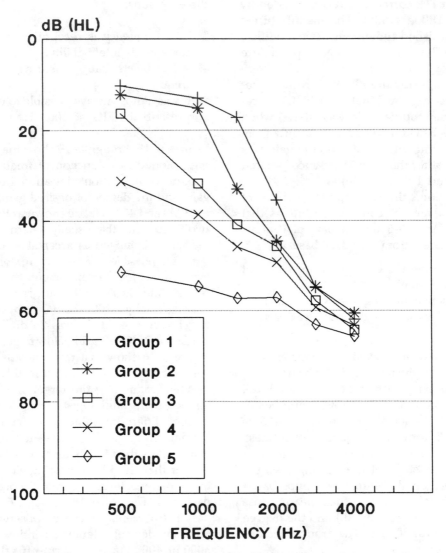

Figure 6–14. Mean audiograms for the five different subject groups used in the Letterman Army Medical Center Study.

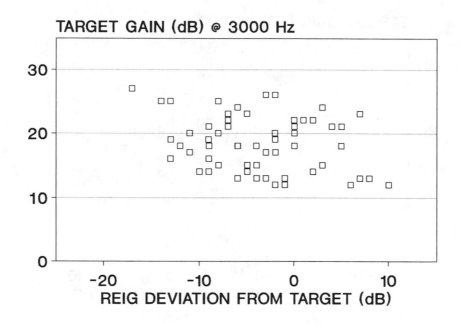

TARGET GAIN (dB) @ 3000 Hz

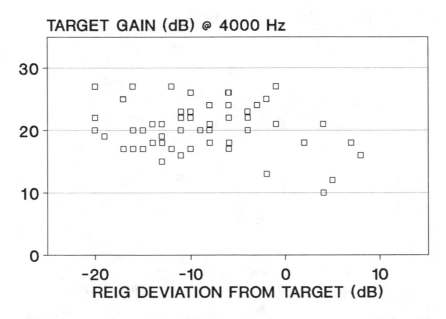

TARGET GAIN (dB) @ 4000 Hz

Figure 6–15. Deviation of real ear insertion gain (REIG) from prescriptive target gain as a function of desired gain for 3000 and 4000 Hz. Subjects are from hearing loss Group 1 (see Figure 6–14).

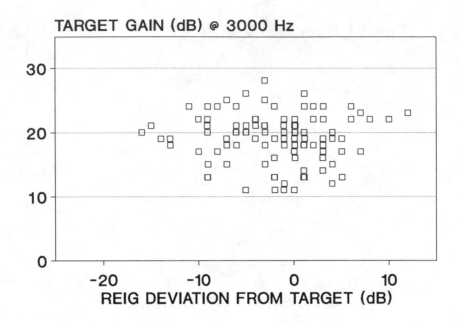

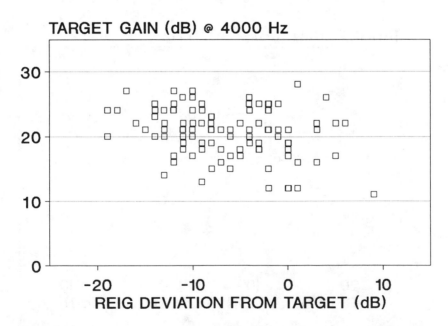

Figure 6-16. Deviation of real ear insertion gain (REIG) from prescriptive target gain as a function of desired gain for 3000 and 4000 Hz. Subjects are from hearing loss Group 2 (see Figure 6-14).

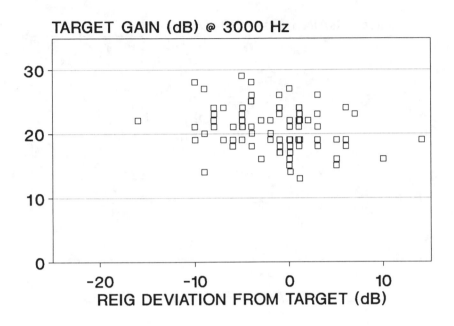

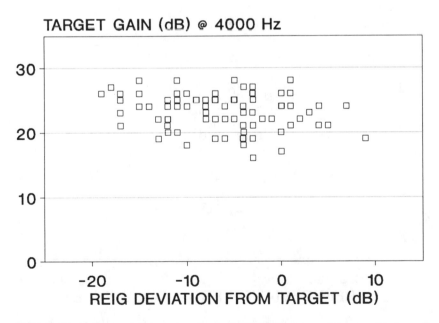

Figure 6–17. Deviation of real ear insertion gain (REIG) from prescriptive target gain as a function of desired gain for 3000 and 4000 Hz. Subjects are from hearing loss Group 3 (see Figure 6–14).

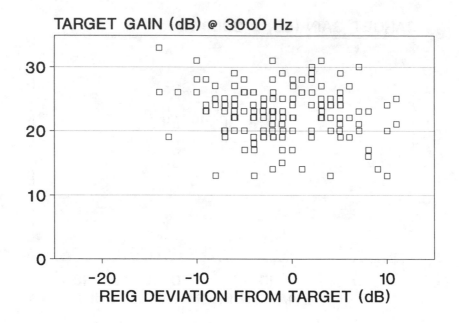

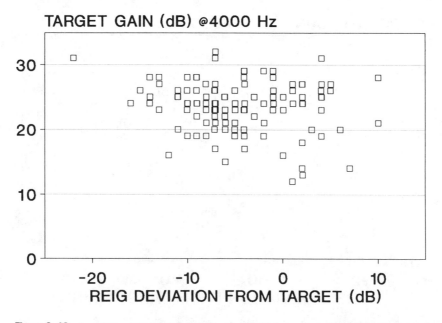

Figure 6–18. Deviation of real ear insertion gain (REIG) from prescriptive target gain as a function of desired gain for 3000 and 4000 Hz. Subjects are from hearing loss Group 4 (see Figure 6–14).

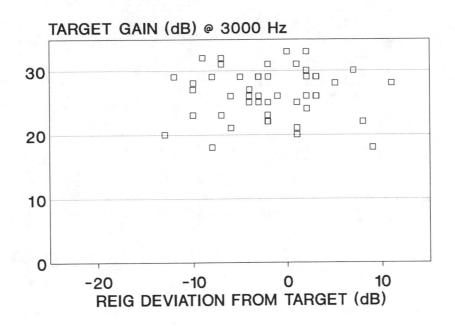

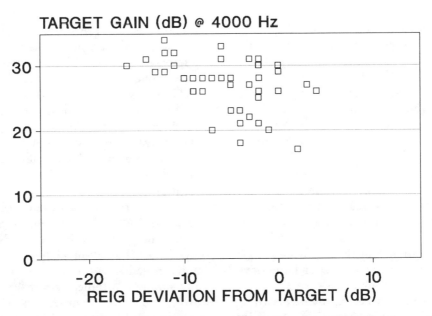

Figure 6–19. Deviation of real ear insertion gain (REIG) from prescriptive target gain as a function of desired gain for 3000 and 4000 Hz. Subjects are from hearing loss Group 5 (see Figure 6–14).

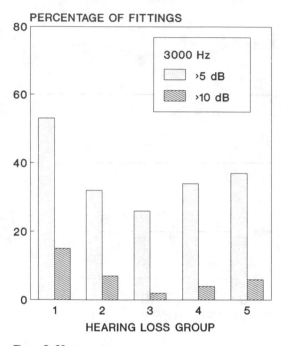

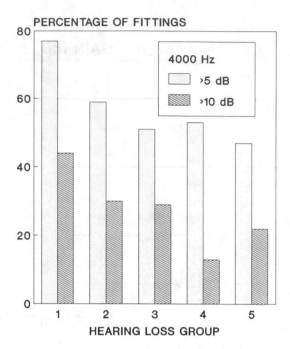

Figure 6–20. Percentage of fittings that exceeded target gain by more than 5 or 10 dB for 3000 and 4000 Hz for five different hearing loss groups (see Figure 6–14).

much like those shown earlier from the Nashville VA study. Table 6–2 presents the REIG decibel cut-off values for four different percentile levels. For this analysis, the data were collapsed across groups, and the results for 1500 Hz were added (recall that REIG was arbitrarily matched to NAL target at 2000 Hz). Table 6–2 provides a general indication of the number of fittings that would fail the verification procedure relative to the decibel deviation value that is selected. These results suggest that **it may be necessary to use different decibel windows of acceptance relative to the frequency of interest**. Unless one is willing to reject a great number of their hearing aids, it appears to be necessary to accept a large deviation from target at 4000 Hz.

These data can be used to provide a starting point for establishing a pass/fail protocol for ITE hearing aid verification. Factors such as the ordering procedure, the custom hearing aid manufacturer, and the specific prescriptive method utilized will influence the applicability

of these results. Adjustments, however, could be made to account for some of the expected differences that would be obtained when other prescriptive methods are used. In this study, REIG and NAL target were matched at 2000 Hz; therefore, deviations at 3000 and 4000 Hz are directly related to the slope of the prescriptive gain target for the higher frequencies. If one used a prescriptive method that called for a steeper slope than the NAL above 2000 Hz, REIG deviations from target gain probably would be greater, as in the results of the Nashville VA study (see Figure 6–13).

The data presented here could be helpful in day-to-day decision-making or in clinical quality-improvement efforts. It would be reasonably simple to predict custom hearing aid returns for different hearing loss configurations and decibel deviation values simply by reviewing the data shown in Figures 6–15 to 6–19. The results in Table 6–2 ignore the direction of the deviation from prescriptive target gain. It may be that the tolerance window should

TABLE 6–2. RELATIONSHIP BETWEEN THE REAL EAR INSERTION GAIN (REIG) FITTING ERROR AND THE PERCENTAGE OF HEARING AIDS THAT WOULD BE ACCEPTED AT THAT FREQUENCY

	Percentile			
	70th	**80th**	**90th**	**95th**
1500 Hz	4 dB	6 dB	8 dB	10 dB
3000 Hz	6 dB	7 dB	9 dB	11 dB
4000 Hz	9 dB	11 dB	13 dB	16 dB

be greater for deviations that are larger than target, based on the logic that *too much audibility* is better than *no audibility*. This would be an issue only for the lower and mid frequencies, however, since deviations of 10 dB or greater almost always are below, rather than above, target gain for 3000 and 4000 Hz.

CONCLUSION

REIR measurements provide a useful method to validate prescriptive gain targets. These measures, in and of themselves, however, are not sufficient for fitting hearing aids. Using REIG deviation values as pass/fail criteria for custom hearing aid fittings, therefore, is only as good as the underlying theory behind the prescriptive method(s) to which the REIG values are compared. This again leads to the issue that, even when REIR measurements are in good agreement with the prescriptive gain target, there is no guarantee that the optimal fitting has been obtained. As outlined by Bratt and Sammeth (1991), prescriptive targets should only be preliminary goals, with the final REIR determined through the use of speech measures, assessment of individual needs, and the subjective reports of the hearing aid user.

CHAPTER 7

Selecting SSPL90 Using Probe-Microphone Measurements

■ DAVID B. HAWKINS, PH.D. ■

In the last 15 years, attention has focused on the selection of hearing aid gain and frequency response. As discussed in the previous chapter, the development of probe-microphone measurements has made rapid assessment and verification of two important electroacoustic characteristics possible through direct measurement of insertion gain. In contrast, the maximum output, or saturation sound pressure level (SSPL90, ANSI S3.22–1987), an equally important electroacoustic characteristic, has received little attention. Several investigators (Hawkins, 1984; Libby, 1985; Walker, Dillon, Byrne, & Christen, 1984) have speculated that an appropriate maximum output may be **the characteristic most related to user acceptance of the hearing aid**.

This chapter describes several methods of selecting and verifying SSPL90 and the role of probe-microphone measurements in determining this important electroacoustic parameter.

CRITERIA FOR AN APPROPRIATE MAXIMUM OUTPUT (SSPL90)

LOUDNESS DISCOMFORT SHOULD NOT BE EXPERIENCED

The hearing aid user should not experience loudness discomfort while wearing a hearing aid. This is a commonly held tenet of hearing aid fitting and has significant clinical importance. When the SSPL90 is too high and exceeds the hearing aid user's loudness discomfort level (LDL), or uncomfortable loudness level (UCL), or threshold of discomfort (TD),

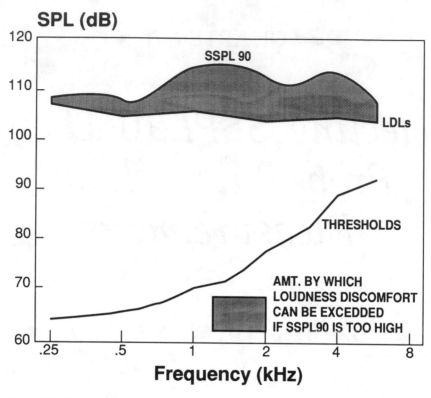

Figure 7–1. The relationship that exists when the SSPL90 of a hearing aid exceeds LDLs.

as shown in Figure 7–1, then one of several unfortunate consequences may occur (Hawkins, 1984).

■ The hearing aid user may **constantly change the volume control wheel** (VCW) to adjust for different input levels. For instance, if a low-level input arrives, the VCW is turned up to make the low-intensity sound audible. However, if a higher level input is encountered that causes the hearing aid output to exceed the LDL, the user turns the VCW down. As a result, the user is constantly adjusting the VCW to assure audibility for lower level inputs and to avoid discomfort for higher level inputs.

■ To avoid this constant adjustment, the user may simply leave the hearing aid VCW at a lower than optimal position to minimize the number of times that the output produces loudness discomfort. In other words, the user utilizes a VCW setting that reduces the gain so that the input plus the gain will not exceed the LDL. In this case, audibility of lower level inputs is sacrificed to avoid discomfort.

■ The hearing aid is worn only in relatively quiet environments where input levels are low. These lower input levels, when combined with the gain of the hearing aid, are not likely to exceed the LDL. The user avoids large noisy gatherings or takes the hearing aid off in these situations to avoid loudness discomfort.

■ The user **may reject the hearing aid**, as the discomfort experienced outweighs the communication benefits received.

Given these four possible negative outcomes when the SSPL90 is too high, it becomes clear that attention must be directed in the selection process toward assuring that the hearing aid's maximum output does not exceed the user's LDLs.

WIDE DYNAMIC RANGE SHOULD BE PRESENT

The second criterion for appropriate output is that the SSPL90 be adjusted to assure maximum dynamic range for the hearing aid user. That is, if the only criterion for selecting SSPL90 is avoidance of loudness discomfort, then selection is simple: the SSPL90 for all hearing aid users would be 85–90 dB SPL. At this limiting level, virtually no one would experience loudness discomfort. However, if this limiting level were selected for everyone, the residual dynamic range (i.e., the range from the auditory threshold to the maximum output of

the hearing aid) would be severely restricted for many users who have higher LDLs. This reduction in dynamic range is shown in Figure 7–2.

A reduced dynamic range leads to fewer amplitude cues and a hearing aid that could be in constant saturation, a situation leading to increased distortion, especially if a peak-clipping circuit is employed. Therefore, the SSPL90 should be adjusted so that the hearing aid **limits output just below the LDLs** (preventing discomfort) and **yet leaves the widest possible dynamic range** (preventing frequent saturation of the instrument).

AVOIDANCE OF DISTORTED OUTPUT

The third criterion for appropriate output is that the limiting level of the hearing aid be adjusted to avoid distorted output. This crite-

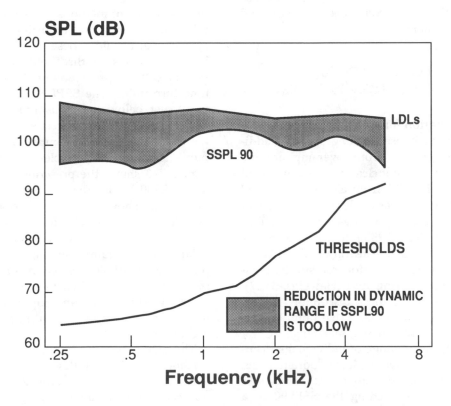

Figure 7–2. The relationship that exists when the SSPL90 of a hearing aid is well below the LDLs.

rion involves the concept of headroom, which is the distance from the amplified signal to the limiting level of the hearing aid. If the amplified signal is constantly saturating the hearing aid (i.e., the input plus the gain equals or exceeds the SSPL90), then the resulting output signal contains significant distortion if the output limiting is accomplished with peak clipping. When low-distortion output limiting, such as automatic gain control (AGC) or compression, is employed by the hearing aid, then this criterion loses much of its importance. In cases of relatively narrow dynamic ranges, which especially occur with moderate and severe hearing losses, the situation of frequent saturation is often present. In the cases of milder losses, frequent saturation occurs in higher input level environments, such as noisy situations. This higher distortion for peak clipping has led some authors (Hawkins & Naidoo, 1992; Mueller, Hawkins, & Sedge, 1984) to advocate **routine use of compression** as a method of output limitation.

POSSIBILITY OF OVERAMPLIFICATION IS MINIMIZED

The final criterion for selecting maximum output is that the chosen setting prevents additional hearing loss from overamplification. Unfortunately, it is not clear what output sound pressure level (SPL) from a hearing aid will cause additional hearing loss. (An excellent summary on this topic can be found in Rintelmann and Bess, 1988.) It has been established, however, that a hearing aid that is not causing loudness discomfort can still be causing additional hearing loss (Hawkins, 1982). The absence of loudness discomfort per se, cannot be taken to indicate that output levels are necessarily within the safe range.

Due to the large range of individual susceptibility to acoustic trauma, it is important to **set output limiting at what are thought to be safe levels.** This means setting the SSPL90 to a point well below the LDLs in some cases. For instance, suppose a person with a mild-to-

moderate sensorineural hearing loss provided reliable LDLs of 125–130 dB SPL. Providing for adequate headroom (as mentioned earlier), there would be no justification for setting the SSPL90 above 110–115 dB SPL. The additional dynamic range width is not necessary given the expected gain requirements for such a hearing loss, and allowing an SSPL90 of 130 dB SPL in this case simply increases the chances of overamplification.

If the potential hearing aid user cannot provide valid LDLs or the LDLs are very high, a decision must be made regarding an output setting that provides adequate headroom and reduces any chances for overamplification. Such an approach is discussed in the next section.

METHODS FOR SELECTION OF THE DESIRED SSPL90

Several types of methods are employed clinically for selecting and adjusting the SSPL90 of the hearing aid. These methods typically involve either suprathreshold measurements such as LDLs or prediction of LDLs from pure-tone thresholds. The SSPL90 is adjusted to a point just below the measured or predicted LDLs. A recent study by Hawkins, Ball, Beasley, and Cooper (1992) compared a number of published methods for selecting the SSPL90. Figure 7–3 shows the prescribed SSPL90 values at 2000 Hz for the procedures evaluated. These data show that the prescribed SSPL90 will depend on the selection procedure used. Given that none of the procedures has proven validity, one suprathreshold approach and one pure-tone threshold prediction approach were selected to be described in this chapter. The ways in which probe-microphone measurements are integrated with each approach are outlined.

The LDL procedure had its initial roots in a method described by Pascoe (1978) in which loudness category judgments are made to define the entire dynamic range. This category scaling approach was then employed in an LDL procedure published by Hawkins, Wal-

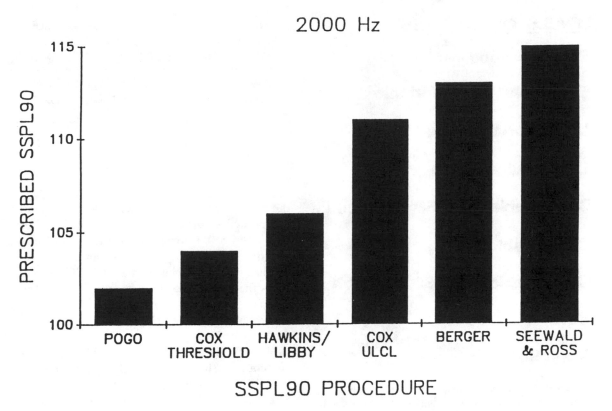

Figure 7–3. Prescribed SSPL90 values at 2000 Hz from different SSPL90 selection procedures. (From Hawkins et al. 1992. A comparison of SSPL90 selection procedures. *Journal of the American Academy of Audiology, 3,* 46–50, with permission.)

den, Montgomery, and Prosek (1987), and further modified by Hawkins, Ball, Beasley, and Cooper (1992). It can be adapted to include probe-microphone measurements with suggestions from Seewald (1990a), Stelmachowicz (1991), and Stuart, Durieux-Smith, and Stenstrom (1991).

In this procedure, pure tones or narrow bands of noise centered at 500, 1000, and 2000 Hz (other frequencies may be added at the audiologist's discretion) are produced by a standard audiometer and **delivered through Etymotic ER-3A insert earphones** coupled to the ear with a foam earplug. The potential hearing aid user is given a sheet with the **loudness categories** shown in Figure 7–4 along with the following instructions:

We need to do a test to determine where to set the amplifier on your hearing aid. We want to set it such that sounds do not become uncomfortably loud. You will hear some sounds, and after each one I want you to tell me which of the loudness categories on this sheet best describes the sound to you. So after each sound tell me if it was "Comfortable," "Comfortable, But Slightly Loud," or "Loud, But OK," or "Uncomfortably Loud," etc. I will be zeroing in on the uncomfortably loud category because that is where we want the hearing aid to stop and not get any louder. So after each sound, tell me which category best describes the sound to you. (p. 163)

Starting at approximately 90 dB SPL, an ascending approach using 2.5- or 5-dB steps is employed and the category judgment uncomfortably loud is crossed several times. The in-

LEVELS OF LOUDNESS

Painfully Loud

Extremely Uncomfortable

Uncomfortably Loud

Loud, But O.K.

Comfortable, But Slightly Loud

Comfortable

Comfortable, But Slightly Soft

Soft

Very Soft

Figure 7–4. Loudness categories for LDL measurements. (From Hawkins et al. 1987b. Description and validation of an LDL procedure designed to select SSPL90. *Ear and Hearing, 8,* 162–169, with permission.)

tensity at which a consistent judgment of uncomfortably loud is obtained is considered to be the LDL.

The integration of probe-microphone measurements is accomplished by inserting the probe tube through the foam earplug and into the ear canal. Although the probe tube can be placed along the outside edge of the foam plug, a large needle may be used to thread the probe tube through the foam plug, thus eliminating any compression of the tube against the ear canal wall or unwanted slit leaks. After the LDL has been determined, the signal is turned on at the point of loudness discomfort, and the SPL in the ear canal is measured by

TABLE 7–1. EXAMPLE OF VALUES AVAILABLE WHEN LDLS ARE OBTAINED VIA INSERT EARPHONES WITH A PROBE TUBE IN THE EAR CANAL

Frequency (Hz)	LDL in dB HL	2-cm³ Coupler SPL at LDL	Target RESR
500	100	109	110
1000	105	109	112
2000	100	107	113

the probe-microphone system. Depending on the particular probe system, the loudspeaker may need to be turned off to make this measurement; the probe system is essentially acting like a sound-level meter. This SPL represents the **target maximum output level in the ear canal** for the hearing aid, or the Real Ear Saturation Response (RESR), which will be described shortly.

Since the insert earphone is calibrated in 2-cm³ coupler, the LDL is directly converted from dB HL on the audiometer dial reading to dB SPL in a 2-cm³ coupler.[1] With the probe tube in the ear canal, the target RESR is also now available. The audiologist now has three values at each frequency from the measurement, as shown in Table 7–1.

The LDL in dB HL is not of interest in hearing aid selection; rather, the 2-cm³ coupler SPL is necessary for specifying the SSPL90 or appropriate matrix for an in-the-ear (ITE) order or for selecting a behind-the-ear (BTE) hearing aid from specification sheets. In the example in Table 7–1, a hearing aid would be selected or ordered that had a 2-cm³ coupler SSPL90 range of approximately 100–115 dB SPL. (The lower limit of 100 dB SPL allows for error in the LDL measurements and SSPL90 reduction if loudness discomfort is experienced.) The output control, an essential option for setting the SSPL90 accurately, would be adjusted initially at a mid-point position and then it could be

---

[1]To calibrate the insert earphone, the foam plug is placed on a HA-1 2-cm³ coupler (the type used for ITE hearing aids). The audiometer is set to 70 dB HL, the output is measured in the 2-cm³ coupler, and conversion factors at each frequency from dB HL to dB SPL in the 2-cm³ coupler are determined. It is important to check linearity of the audiometer dial to determine the highest attenuator dial setting that can be used for accurate results.

turned, lowered, or raised as necessary based on client reactions. The SPLs in the ear canal at the point of loudness discomfort serve as targets for adjustment of the maximum output during the hearing aid fitting via RESR (discussed below).

This LDL procedure, combined with probe-microphone measurements, can be completed in approximately 5 min for each ear with a cooperative adult. The procedure can be accomplished in a sound-treated room or in a reverberant room, depending on where the probe-microphone system is located. In either setting a portable audiometer can be located next to the probe-microphone system to generate the signals for LDL measurement.

An SSPL90 selection procedure that utilizes pure-tone thresholds to determine maximum output is described by Seewald, Ross, and Stelmachowicz (1987) and Stelmachowicz and Seewald (1991). Based on known relationships between pure-tone thresholds and LDLs, the need for adequate headroom, and overamplification concerns, hearing aid real-ear maximum output levels (RESRs) have been recommended by Seewald, Zelisco, Ramji, and Jamieson (1991) for all typical test frequencies for hearing thresholds up to 110 dB HL. These recommended values are shown in Table 7–2 and serve as targets for the RESR.

RESR MEASUREMENT AND SETTING THE SSPL90

The RESR of a hearing aid is the maximum output in dB SPL that the hearing aid is capable of producing in the user's ear canal. There are two methods of measuring the RESR of a hearing aid. One method directly measures the RESR (Hawkins, 1987b), while the other derives the RESR from other measurements (Sullivan, 1987).

DIRECT RESR MEASUREMENT METHOD

In the direct RESR measurement method, the hearing aid is fitted to the ear with the probe tube in the ear canal. The hearing aid VCW is rotated to a point just below feedback. A sweep-frequency pure tone or warble tone is delivered from the loudspeaker at 90 dB SPL, and an output-SPL curve in the ear canal is obtained. This output-SPL curve with the hearing aid saturated is the RESR. The high VCW position in combination with the high loudspeaker output is designed to assure that the hearing aid has been saturated and that the maximum output of the hearing aid has been reached.[2] A different VCW setting is necessary if the hearing aid has input compression, as the SSPL90 is tied to the VCW setting with this type of output-limiting circuit. In other words, as the VCW is turned up, the SSPL90 will increase. With an input-compression hearing aid, the VCW is adjusted to a location that is thought to represent the highest use VCW setting; that is, a setting that might be chosen for low-intensity speech inputs.

It is important to emphasize that the SSPL90 control on the hearing aid should be set to the minimum-output position (or a position known not to cause loudness discomfort) before the first RESR measurement is obtained. This is important for two reasons. First, **the user should not experience excessive loudness discomfort during the measurement**. This is especially true for children, who may reject any further participation in the measurement procedure if discomfort is experienced (see Chapter 8 for further discussion about children and RESR measurements). Second, **high SPLs in the ear canal must be avoided** to minimize any possibility of acoustic trauma from the measurement. If the hearing aid has been preselected in a reasonable way based on LDLs or estimated LDLs, and the hearing aid has an output control that can bracket the estimated LDL (an essential condition in many cases), this initial adjustment of the output control is easy to achieve. For example, suppose a prospective hearing aid client with a moderate sensorineural hearing loss provided the LDLs in Table 7–3, measured

---

[2]The input of 90 dB SPL with the VCW just below feedback should saturate the hearing aid. It is possible, however, that the hearing aid would not reach its maximum output using this procedure in a few cases, such as with a relatively high SSPL90 and a nonoccluding earmold.

TABLE 7–2. RECOMMENDED RESR VALUES BASED ON PURE-TONE THRESHOLDS

Threshold (dB HL)	Frequency (Hz)								
	250	500	750	1000	1500	2000	3000	4000	6000
0	94	102	101	99	99	100	100	98	97
5	94	102	101	99	99	101	100	99	97
10	94	102	101	100	100	102	101	100	98
15	95	103	102	101	100	103	102	101	98
20	95	103	102	101	101	104	103	102	99
25	96	104	103	103	102	105	105	103	100
30	97	105	104	104	104	106	106	104	101
35	99	106	106	105	105	108	108	106	103
40	100	107	107	107	107	110	110	108	105
45	102	109	109	109	109	112	112	109	106
50	104	111	110	110	111	114	114	111	108
55	106	113	112	112	113	116	116	113	111
60	109	115	114	114	115	118	118	115	113
65	111	117	117	117	117	120	120	118	115
70	114	119	119	119	119	122	123	120	117
75	117	121	121	121	121	124	125	122	120
80	120	123	123	123	123	126	127	124	122
85	123	126	125	125	125	128	129	126	124
90	126	128	127	127	127	130	130	128	125
95	129	130	129	129	129	131	132	130	127
100	132	131	131	130	131	133	133	132	128
105	—	133	132	131	132	134	135	133	—
110	—	134	134	133	133	135	136	135	—

Source: Reprinted from Seewald, R., Zelisko, D., Ramji, K., & Jamieson, D. 1991. *DSL 3.0 user's manual*. London, Ontario, Canada: The University of Western Ontario, with permission.

TABLE 7–3. HYPOTHETICAL LDLs DEFINED IN A 2-CM³ COUPLER AND REAL EAR

Frequency (Hz)	2-cm³ Coupler SPL at LDL	Target RESR
500	100	112
1000	113	117
2000	114	120

using insert earphones calibrated in a 2-cm³ coupler and a probe tube in the ear canal to measure the real-ear SPL at the point of loudness discomfort.

A hearing aid would be chosen with an SSPL90 control that can vary the maximum output from approximately 100 to 120 dB SPL in a 2-cm³ coupler. The first RESR measurement would be made with the SSPL90 control at its minimum position, which should not produce loudness discomfort. The control would be slowly adjusted upward in several small steps until the RESR was just below the target values or until the user experienced loudness discomfort during the measurement.

An example of RESRs obtained at three different SSPL90 control settings is shown in Figure 7–5. These curves were obtained on a Knowles Electronics Manikin for Acoustic Re-

search (KEMAR), with a high-gain BTE hearing aid with a 1000 ohm damper in the earhook. These curves demonstrate the RESR with different SSPL90 control settings. At the lowest output control setting, the 2-cm³ coupler SSPL90 was measured. Figure 7–6 shows the RESR and the 2-cm³ coupler SSPL90 curve. The difference between the two curves is the real ear coupler difference (RECD). Notice that the output is greater in the real ear, especially in the higher frequencies, a finding that has been verified in many studies (see Chapters 8 and 12 for more information about the magnitude of the RECD in children and adults).

A variation of this procedure involves obtaining only aided suprathreshold loudness judgments. This variation is justified only if the hearing aid has an output-control adjustment with a sufficiently wide range of settings. In this

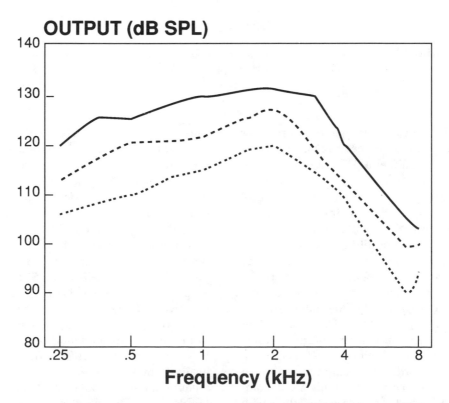

Figure 7–5. RESR curves for a high-gain BTE hearing aid on a KEMAR with three different output-control settings.

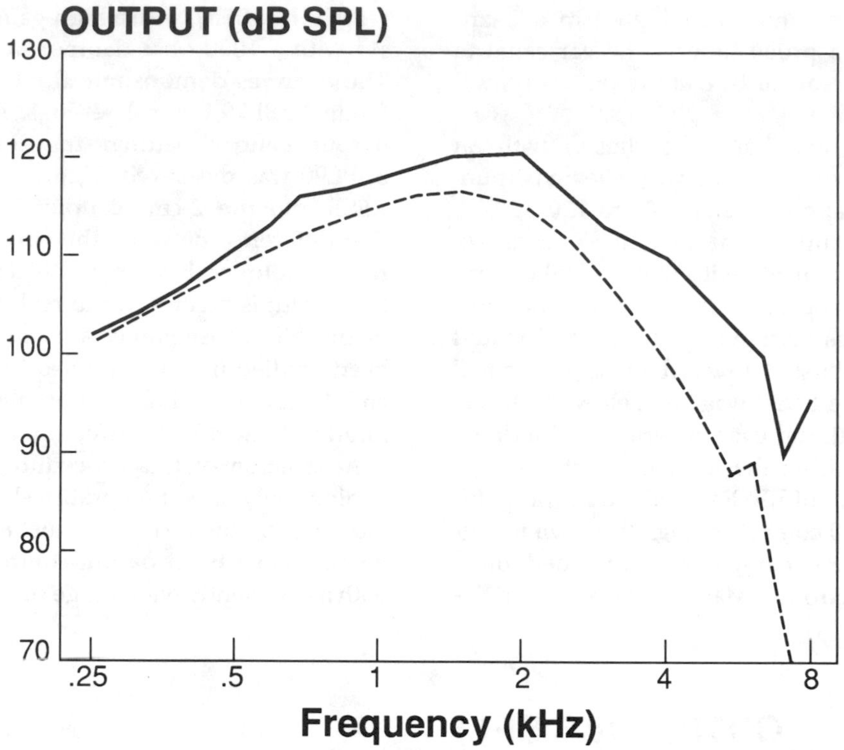

Figure 7–6. RESR curve (solid line) for a BTE hearing aid on KEMAR and the 2-cm³ coupler SSPL90 curve (dashed line) for the same hearing aid. The difference between the two curves is the RECD.

approach, it is not necessary to measure LDLs prior to the fitting of the hearing aid (Hawkins & Schum, 1992). Either a BTE hearing aid with a wide range of SSPL90 settings is chosen, or an ITE hearing aid with an output control capable of a 15–20 dB adjustment is ordered with the maximum SSPL90 slightly above the predicted LDLs. At the fitting and orientation, the hearing aid is placed on the ear with the output control at the minimum, and the probe tube is placed in the ear canal. A 90 dB SPL swept pure tone or warble tone is delivered by the loudspeaker, and the client is asked to raise his or her hand if any of the sounds reach the uncomfortably loud level. The probe microphone records the maximum output in the ear canal. If any of the sounds are uncomfortable, the SSPL90 is increased slightly with the output screw and the swept signal repeated.

This procedure is repeated until an uncomfortably loud judgment is obtained, at which point the output screw is reduced slightly. If the recorded RESR is deemed excessive at this point of loudness discomfort, then the output can be reduced to a safer level, regardless of the LDL, as described above.

In the above approaches, the probe-microphone system measures the RESR and allows the audiologist **to adjust the SSPL90 until the output in the real ear is acceptable and does not exceed the LDLs.** In some cases, the potential hearing aid user may not be able to perform a suprathreshold loudness judgment task. In such cases, the SSPL90 control can be adjusted to match a target RESR curve based on recommendations such as those of Seewald (Table 7–2). The client can be questioned at follow-up visits concerning any loudness discomfort. If discomfort has occurred, then the output control can be reduced slightly and follow-up questions continued.

INDIRECT RESR MEASUREMENT METHOD

The indirect RESR measurement method uses probe-microphone and 2-cm^3 coupler measurements. This method was advocated by Sullivan (1987), who wrote that "emotional and acoustic trauma" may occur as part of the RESR procedure. (This author believes that if an appropriate SSPL90 is preselected and the output control is set to minimum output before the first measurement, as described above, then there is virtually no possibility of any type of trauma, especially for such a short-duration signal.) Sullivan's procedure determines the RECD and adds it to the 2-cm^3 coupler SSPL90 curve. That is, the hearing aid VCW is set to a predicted use setting and the output in a 2-cm^3 coupler is measured with a 60 dB SPL input. Without changing the VCW, the hearing aid is then placed on the ear and the output in the ear canal, the real ear aided response (REAR) is also measured with a 60 dB SPL input. The difference between the 2-cm^3 coupler output and the REAR is the RECD, which typically indicates that more output is being developed in the ear canal than in the coupler. The RECD is then added to the 2-cm^3 coupler SSPL90 to yield the derived, or predicted, RESR.

STIMULUS TYPE FOR RESR MEASUREMENTS

The choice of stimulus type for the RESR measurement is important. The two options that are typically available include discrete-frequency signals (pure tones or warble tones) or a broad-band noise (such as white noise or a speech-shaped noise). When the RESR is measured with a tonal signal, then the curve will show the maximum output for any single input frequency. This RESR curve represents the maximum output capability for the hearing aid for narrow-band signals. When a broad-band

signal, such as a speech-shaped multitone complex, is used, the output curve will be reduced. This finding is demonstrated in Figure 7–7 from Stelmachowicz, Lewis, Seewald, and Hawkins (1990), which shows the maximum output from one hearing aid with a pure-tone signal and a complex signal at different input levels. If the pure-tone curve is compared with the complex-signal curve at saturation, a difference of 15–20 dB is observed between the apparent maximum outputs.

Explaining this pure-tone/complex-signal difference, Stelmachowicz et al. (1990) wrote that:

When a complex signal is processed . . . the power-handling capabilities of the system must be shared by all of the frequency components simultaneously. As such, the maximum output at each frequency will be less than that observed when only a single tone is processed independently. (p. 384)

The output curve for the complex signal represents the maximum output at a given frequency when a broad-band signal is applied. The output levels for narrower band signals will be much higher. Given that many signals that send a hearing aid into saturation have narrow-band spectra (Stelmachowicz, 1991), it is **important that the RESR be determined with frequency-specific signals** and that loudness discomfort not occur during measurement. Stelmachowicz et al. (1990) concluded that:

The most conservative approach would be to obtain LDLs using pure-tone stimuli and set the maximum output using the same signals. Under these circumstances, any broader frequency environmental signals encountered while wearing the hearing aid would cause the hearing aid to saturate at or below the levels designated. (p. 384)

Revit (1991a) agreed with this position and wrote that:

The broadband tests . . . are excellent for checking how the frequency response of an instrument changes for changing speech-like inputs. But for checking the maximum output of an instrument, the pure-tone SSPL90 saturation test is still the best. The reason is that narrow-band inputs (such as whistles,

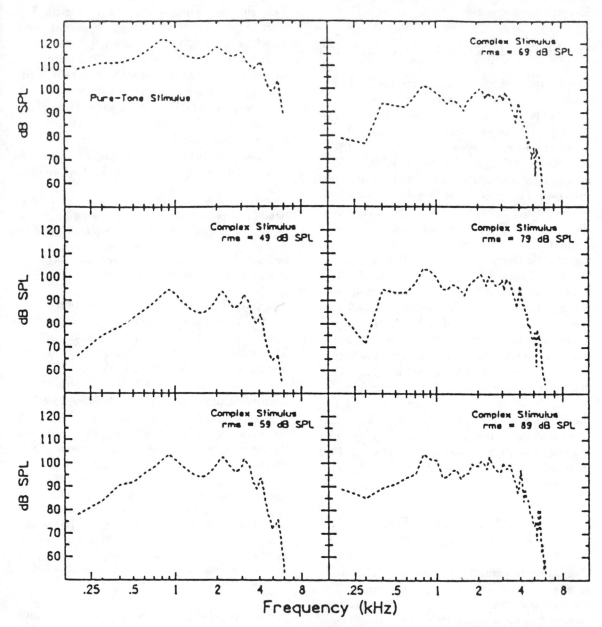

Figure 7–7. Maximum output curves for a hearing aid with a 90 dB SPL pure-tone input (top left). Other curves show the output from the same hearing aid with a complex noise input at 49, 59, 69, 79, and 89 dB SPL. The hearing aid is saturated at inputs of 59 dB SPL and above. (From Stelmachowicz, P., Lewis, D., Seewald, R., & Hawkins, D., 1990. Complex and pure-tone signals in the evaluation of hearing-aid characteristics. *Journal of Speech and Hearing Research, 33,* 612–615, with permission.)

beeps, sirens, musical notes, and pure tones) are likely to cause higher outputs per frequency than a broadband signal would indicate. (p. 23)

Revit demonstrated this effect through the curves shown in Figure 7–8. The top curve shows the pure-tone maximum output and the lower dashed curve represents the broad-band maximum output. The narrow-band curve centered around 800 Hz is the output of the hearing aid resulting from a loud beeping sound of a FAX machine, demonstrating that a narrow-band signal can exceed the SSPL90, as represented by the complex noise.

These data and considerations lead to the recommendation that **RESR measurements be made with frequency-specific signals** such as pure tones or warble tones.

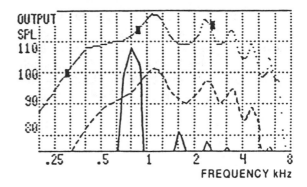

Figure 7–8. Maximum output of a hearing aid with a 90 dB SPL pure-tone input (top curve) and a complex-noise input (dashed line). The output that is centered around 800 Hz represents the output of the hearing aid for a loud beeping sound from a FAX machine. (From Revit, L. 1991a. New tests for signal-processing and multichannel hearing instruments. *The Hearing Journal, 44*(5), 20–23, with permission.)

VERIFICATION OF SSPL90 SETTINGS

Regardless of what measurements are made involving SSPL90, it is essential that the audiologist **verify that loudness discomfort is not being experienced** before the user is released for the first exposure to hearing aids in everyday life. This verification can be implemented in a variety of ways, ranging from informal to formal assessments. Informally, a variety of environmental sounds can be produced and the client asked if any produce loudness discomfort. For instance, as a final verification after it has been demonstrated that a high-level pure-tone sweep does not cause discomfort, this author exposes the person to three signals: (a) loud speech into the hearing aid microphone, (b) hand clapping next to the head, and (c) a stapler banging on a metal table. If the SSPL90 has been set appropriately, each of these sounds should be loud, but not uncomfortable.

If a more formal procedure is preferred, the probe-microphone system can be utilized to present both frequency-specific signals and a broad-band signal at high intensities to saturate the hearing aid. Similar to the procedure outlined earlier, the SSPL90 setting can receive final approval by presenting a 90 dB SPL sweep-frequency pure-tone or warble-tone signal and verifying that no uncomfortable loudness is present. A broad-band noise, such as the speech-weighted noise present on many probe-microphone systems, should also be presented. This is necessary, since it is possible that, due to loudness summation with increasing bandwidth, some people may find pure-tone signals acceptable yet experience loudness discomfort for a broad-band signal. If discomfort is experienced with the wider band signals, the output control can be reduced slightly and the procedure repeated until discomfort is eliminated.

CONCLUSIONS

The careful selection of the maximum output capabilities of a hearing aid is important to the successful adaptation and adjustment of the wearer to amplification. For maximum benefit from a hearing aid, it is critical that the user does not experience discomfort during its use. Further, it is essential that caution is taken to prevent any additional hearing loss as a result of excessive output levels. It is well-established through RECDs that more SPL arrives at the cochlea than is indicated in 2-cm^3 coupler measurements. Given the large intersubject variability in the RECD (Feigin, Kopun, Stelmachowicz, & Gorga, 1989; Hawkins, Cooper, & Thompson, 1990), it is important that an **RESR be measured for each individual hearing aid user to verify that safe maximum-output levels are present**. This is important both for the welfare of the client and to avoid professional liability for the audiologist.

CHAPTER 8

Probe-Microphone Measurements with Children

■ DAVID B. HAWKINS, Ph.D. ■

■ JERRY L. NORTHERN, Ph.D. ■

Although more has been written concerning probe-microphone measurements with adults, the application of this technology to children is one of the most useful new developments in pediatric hearing aid selection. As hearing loss can be identified in infancy, it is possible to begin amplification immediately. The use of probe-microphone measurements offers a reliable method to verify hearing aid selection decisions. Gabbard and Northern (1987) presented several pediatric case studies in which probe-microphone measurements revealed information that otherwise was unavailable with traditional comparative hearing aid evaluation techniques.

The assessment of hearing aids on children, especially infants, has always been somewhat limited due to the inability to utilize standard behavioral tests. Measures of speech intelligibility and sound-quality judgments are typically not appropriate with younger children. As a result, the traditional hearing aid assessment procedure has consisted of measuring functional gain or aided soundfield thresholds. Several hearing aids, or different settings of the same hearing aid, are tested in the soundfield. With each hearing aid change, the audiologist must repeat a set of soundfield thresholds, each time hoping that the child will not lose interest in the task. Cooperation from the child is required for these measurements, testing time can be extensive, and test-retest reliability can be poor. With the variability typically seen in young children, the differences between two sets of thresholds can easily exceed the differences between two hearing aids. For instance, Stuart, Durieux-Smith, and Stenstrom (1990) recently reported that even when the volume control wheel (VCW) was taped, repeated aided soundfield thresholds for children aged 5–14 years had to differ by greater than 10 dB to be considered significant at the .05 level of confidence. One can only assume that with younger children and infants these differences would be even larger. Aided soundfield thresholds assess performance only at octave intervals, leaving the audiologist unaware of possible peaks and valleys in the response between the frequencies tested. Such difficulties and problems have led some to conclude that fitting hearing aids on children is more an art than a science (Martin, 1989). The use of probe-microphone measurements, however, allows a **level of certainty** that has not been possible in the past as to the acoustic signal that the child is receiving.

Probe-microphone measurements offer many advantages over the traditional approach with children. Seewald (1990) summarized four basic advantages of probe-microphone measurements in children: (a) better frequency resolution, (b) enhanced reliability, (c) efficiency, and (d) lower level of cooperation required. Other important probe-microphone advantages include verification of the maximum output in the ear canal (real ear saturation response, or

RESR) for safety and comfort, adjustment and knowledge of the sensation level of the long-term speech spectrum to maximize speech intelligibility potential, and determination of appropriate hearing aid responses for each ear separately for children with asymmetrical hearing losses (Northern & Downs, 1991).

This chapter describes some of the knowledge learned about children and hearing aids from probe-microphone measurements and provides suggestions for using this technology with the pediatric population.

THE REAL EAR UNAIDED RESPONSE (REUR) IN INFANTS AND CHILDREN

Many audiologists select hearing aids by determining a desired target real ear insertion response (REIR) and adjusting the hearing aid until it best matches the target values (see Chapters 6 and 9). Since the REIR is determined by subtracting the REUR from the real ear aided response (REAR), knowledge of how the unaided response differs in children and how it changes as a function of age is important.

Several studies have provided basic normative data on the REUR of infants, children, and adults. Kruger and Ruben (1987) measured the REURs of two adults and 13 children under the age of 40 months. Figure 8–1 shows a typical

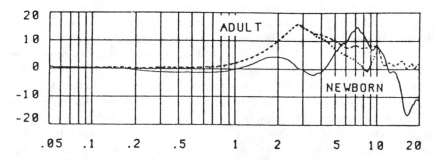

Figure 8–1. A comparison of the typical REUR curves obtained from an adult and a newborn. (From Kruger, B., & Ruben, R. 1987. The acoustic properties of the infant ear. *Acta Otolaryngologica, 103*, 578–585, with permission.)

REUR for an adult and a newborn child. Notice that the adult REUR resonant peak is at approximately 2700 Hz, while the REUR peak for the newborn is at 7200 Hz. The higher peak resonant frequency in the infant is due to a smaller concha and shorter ear-canal length.

Examples of REURs from children of different ages are shown in Figure 8–2 from Kruger (1987), who measured REURs on 26 children ranging from birth to 3 years of age. The REUR resonant peak frequency is indicated by the arrow in each curve. As an infant's age increases, the REUR resonance frequency decreases rapidly and **reaches the typical adult value of 2700 Hz by 12–24 months of age.**

Bentler (1989) extended the REUR database by providing information on 78 children ages 3–13. Figure 8–3 shows the peak resonant fre-

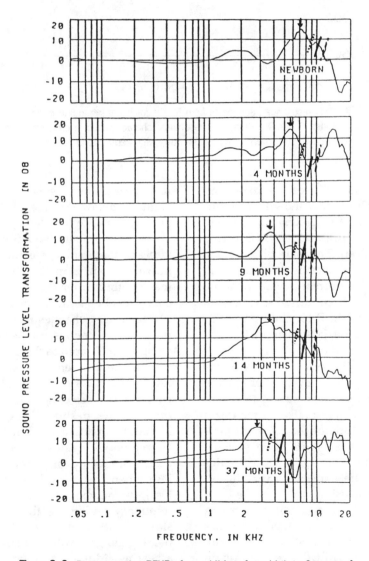

Figure 8–2. Representative REURs from children from birth to 3 years of age. (From Kruger, B. 1987. An update on the external ear canal response in infants and young children. *Ear and Hearing, 8,* 333–336, with permission.)

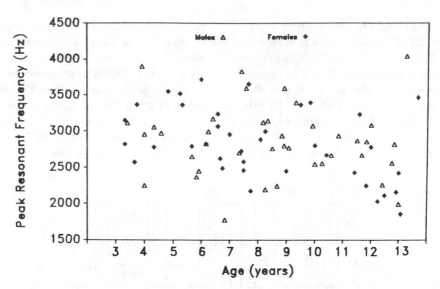

Figure 8–3. Peak resonance frequencies from REURs for children ranging in age from 3 to 13. (From Bentler, R. 1989. External ear resonance characteristics in children. *Journal of Speech and Hearing Disorders, 54*(2), 264–268, with permission.)

quency as a function of age for male and female children. These data show two important trends. First, wide variability can be seen in the location of the peak in the REUR across this group of children. This variability makes probe-microphone measurements attractive in that they allow these normal deviations to be taken into account. Second, consistent with the Kruger data, the REUR for children in this age range (3–13 years) is similar to that expected for adults.

The amplitude of the resonant peak in the REUR was also measured by Bentler (1989). Figure 8–4 shows the amplitude of the resonant peak for 78 children. For comparison purposes, the amplitude of the resonant peak in the average adult is 17 dB. Note that the data for the children are quite close to this value, again with the expected variability.

A different conclusion was reached by Dempster and Mackenzie (1990) concerning the age at which the resonant peak reaches adult values. Their results, shown in Figure 8–5, suggest that the REUR does not attain adult form until the age of 7 years. However, the actual amount of shift in the REUR reso-

nant peak is quite small. Their sample of 15 children below the age of 4 had an average peak resonance of 3002 Hz, only 250 Hz above the comparative adult values. It would appear that small, clinically insignificant downward shifts in the REUR resonant peak may continue after the age of 2, but the REUR curve reaches adult form in early childhood.

Age-related changes in the REUR have important implications for hearing aid selection using a REIR approach. Since the REIR represents the difference between the REAR and the REUR, the REUR must be taken into account when selecting hearing aids that will produce the desired REIR (see Chapter 9). That is, in an infant, the REIR in the 2500–3000 Hz region will gradually decrease as the child ages. Without a peak in the 2700-Hz region to lose when the earmold is in place (insertion loss), the newborn REIR will be higher in this frequency region. As the resonant frequency slowly changes downward in frequency, the hearing aid gain will decrease. In other words, a hearing aid fit on an infant that has 40 dB of real ear insertion gain (REIG) at 2500 Hz may have only 25 dB of REIG by the time the child

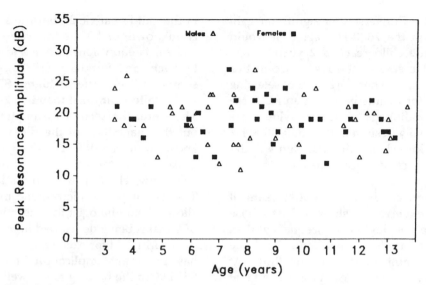

Figure 8–4. Peak resonance amplitudes from REURs for children ranging in age from 3 to 13. (From Bentler, R. 1989. External ear resonance characteristics in children. *Journal of Speech and Hearing Disorders, 54*(2), 264–268, with permission.)

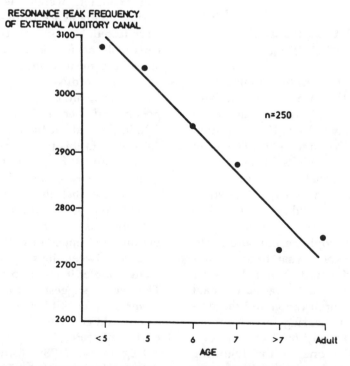

Figure 8–5. Peak resonant frequency as a function of age. (From Dempster, J., & Mackenzie, K. 1990. The resonance frequency of the external auditory canal in children. *Ear and Hearing, 11*(4), 296–298, with permission.)

is 2 years old. Conversely, if significant gain was present in the 7000-Hz region, it would increase as the child reached 2 years of age due to the decrease of the resonance in this frequency region. Therefore, when selecting hearing aids for infants based on an REIR approach, the audiologist should provide more gain than initially desired in the 2500–3000 Hz region, with knowledge that the gain will decrease as the child approaches the age of 2 years.

In summary, children below 1–2 years of age may be expected to show REURs whose resonant peak is higher in frequency than older children or adults. This factor should be taken into account when assessing REIG. At ages older than 2 years, it can be expected that the REUR will be similar to adult values. As with adults, **rather large variability will be observed** in the amplitude and frequency location of the peak in the REUR.

DIFFERENCES IN OUTPUT IN THE 2-CM³ COUPLER AND THE REAL EAR

It is well known that the residual volume of air between the tip of the earmold and the tympanic membrane is greatly reduced in a child compared with an adult. Bratt (1980) reported the average residual volume to be 0.66 cm³ in children and 1.26 cm³ in adults. This reduction in volume, plus potential middle ear impedance differences, can cause large differences in the output of a hearing aid as measured in a 2-cm³ coupler and in the ear canal.

Prior to probe-microphone measurements, there was no way to know what the actual output of a hearing aid would be in a child's ear canal. This lack of knowledge raised constant **concern about overamplification** and the possibility of additional hearing loss. Audiologists were forced to rely on 2-cm³ coupler measures and make one of the following assumptions: (a) 2-cm³ coupler values represent the actual sound pressure level (SPL) in the child's ear; (b) greater SPLs are developed

in the child's ear canal, but the actual amount is unknown; or (c) the increase in SPL in the real ear is equivalent to that shown for adults by Sachs and Burkhard (1972a). The first assumption is not true, as **higher SPL is present in the child's ear canal than in a 2-cm³ coupler**. Therefore, the second assumption is correct, but the magnitude of the difference was not known until recently. The third assumption is a reasonable starting point, but as data below will show, children and adults are different. The use of probe-microphone measurements allows the audiologist to determine the actual SPL that is being developed in the ear canal by the hearing aid for each child. This knowledge has important implications for setting the SSPL90 of the hearing aid as well as determining the gain and frequency response.

A study by Feigin, Kopun, Stelmachowicz, and Gorga (1989) used probe-microphone measurements to compare the SPLs in the ear canals of children and adults to those in a 2-cm³ coupler. Twenty-one adults and 31 children (ranging in age from 4 weeks to 5 years) were tested. Measurements were made in the ear canal and in a 2-cm³ coupler. Figure 8–6 shows the mean results for the children and adults. The ordinate is plotted as real-ear output minus 2-cm³ coupler output, meaning that positive numbers indicate that there is more SPL in the real ear than in the 2-cm³ coupler. All values in this figure are positive except at the very lowest frequencies. In general, as frequency increases, the difference becomes larger. Notice that the real-ear/2-cm³ coupler difference is larger for the children, consistent with the smaller ear canal volumes and possibly different impedance. For example, the difference between the output in a real ear and a 2-cm³ coupler in children at 1000 Hz is 10 dB. This would suggest that a hearing aid with a 2-cm³ coupler SSPL90 at 1000 Hz of 120 dB SPL would generate a real-ear SSPL90 (RESR) of 130 dB SPL.

Feigin et al. (1989) further analyzed these data as a function of age. Figure 8–7 shows the real-ear/2-cm³ coupler differences at four frequencies for adults and five age groups of chil-

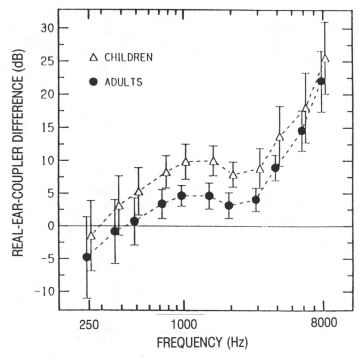

Figure 8–6. Real-ear/2-cm³ coupler differences for children and adults. (From Feigin, J., Kopun, J., Stelmachowicz, P., & Gorga, M. 1989. Probe-tube microphone measures of ear-canal sound pressure levels in infants and children, *Ear and Hearing, 11*, 321–326, with permission.)

dren. There is a clear trend for the **magnitude of the real-ear/2-cm³ coupler difference to decrease with age**. The values for the highest age group (49–60 months), however, are still greater than those for adults.

Feigin et al. (1989) concluded that:

In cases where real ear measures are not feasible, the magnitude of this difference should be considered when limiting the output of hearing aids for infants and young children (p. 258).

These data are interesting and useful for several reasons:

■ They demonstrate the large differences that can be observed between the output in the ear canal of a child and a 2-cm³ coupler, with the output being greater in the real ear.
■ The real-ear/2-cm³ coupler difference is shown to be larger in younger children.

■ These data can be helpful in estimating the 2-cm³ coupler SSPL90 for a desired real-ear SSPL90 (RESR) for the average child of a certain age.
■ These data demonstrate the need for probe-microphone measurements to measure and verify the actual SPL developed by a hearing aid in a child's ear canal.

The standard deviations of the real-ear/2-cm³ coupler differences shown in Figure 8–6 make it clear that actual probe-microphone **measurements of the RESR are preferable to using mean correction factors**. The availability of probe-microphone measurements allows the audiologist to determine the output in the ear canal for each child. Coupler output levels are important for initial hearing aid selection decisions and ordering purposes. Fitting and

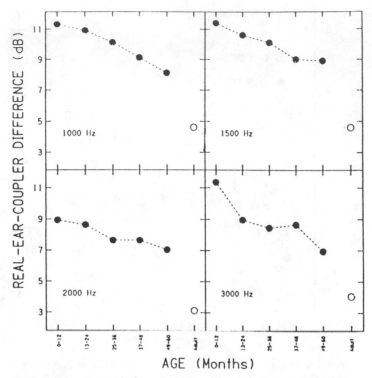

Figure 8–7. Real-ear/2-cm³ coupler differences at four frequencies as a function of age. (From Feigin, J., Kopun, J., Stelmachowicz, P., & Gorga, M. 1989. Probe-tube microphone measures of ear-canal sound pressure levels in infants and children, *Ear and Hearing, 11,* 321–326, with permission.)

adjustment decisions can be made based on the SPLs in the ear canal of each individual child.

CLINICAL APPLICATION

Although less cooperation is required from a child for probe measurements than aided soundfield thresholds, the procedure still presents a challenge. With an infant, the ideal situation for testing is similar to that used in obtaining evoked potentials. The procedure is easiest when the infant is either very drowsy or asleep. However, measurements can be made with the infant awake. Figure 8–8 shows an awake infant with the probe assembly, probe tube, and hearing aid in place. Note that the mother is distracting the infant while ad-

justments are being made to the hearing aid by the audiologist. Measurements with older children are shown in Figures 8–9 and 8–10. If the child is awake, it is necessary that he or she be quiet and remain passive while the signal is being presented. In between signal presentations and measurements, the child may talk and play quietly in the chair, but the probe tube should not be allowed to move.

Stelmachowicz and Seewald (1991) offer several useful suggestions when testing children. They suggest that a loaner hearing aid be used by the child for 2–4 weeks prior to probe-microphone measurements. This will allow the child to become accustomed to having a hearing aid on the ear, and the challenging task will be limited to acceptance of the probe tube. The use of a **visual distractor**, such as a puppet, toy, or picture, **is recommended**

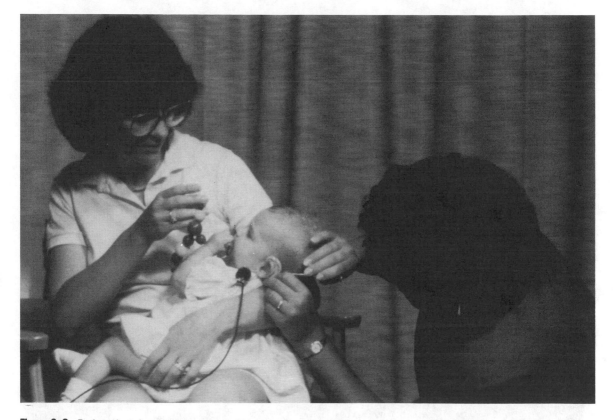

Figure 8–8. Probe-microphone measurements being made on an infant.

during testing. Similar to the traditional protocol with visual reinforcement audiometry (VRA), the visual stimulus can serve to keep the child looking in the correct direction. It is not necessary to keep the child in an alert state ready to respond to a stimulus. In fact, it can be advantageous to have the child quietly involved in the toy or object while the probe-microphone measurements are conducted. To save time, Stelmachowicz and Seewald suggest that the audiologist carefully preselect the hearing aid(s) based on appropriate 2-cm³ coupler electroacoustic characteristics before actually trying instruments on the child.

Because of the shortened ear canal length in children, the insertion depth of the probe is slightly different than for adults (see Chapter 4 for details concerning the effect of probe-tube insertion depth on measured SPL in the ear canal and recommended insertion depths for adults). Stelmachowicz and Seewald recommend that, for children less than 5 years old, the probe tube should be inserted **10 mm past the ear canal entrance**. If the child is over 5 years, the insertion depth beyond the ear canal entrance should be 15 mm. Based on data from Gilman and Dirks (1986), these insertion depths will provide measurement accuracy within ±2 dB through 4000 Hz.

When conducting measurements with high-gain hearing aids, the presence of the probe tube can sometimes create sufficient leakage to cause feedback at the desired VCW position. Stelmachowicz and Seewald recommend placement of a sealing substance, such as putty, around the earmold and probe tube to mini-

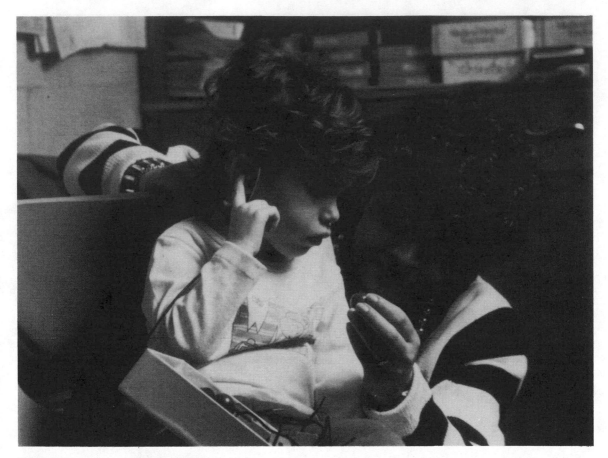

Figure 8–9. Probe-microphone measurements being made on a child.

mize acoustic feedback due to leakage (see Chapter 4 for another alternative employing both coupler and probe measurements in cases with feedback).

SELECTION OF SSPL90

Given the difference described previously between the hearing aid output in a 2-cm³ coupler and the real ear of a child, it becomes clear that the optimal method for fitting a hearing aid should include determination of the SSPL90 and careful setting of the RESR. Given this premise, there are two issues that must be addressed: how to determine an appropriate RESR and how to verify the RESR with probe-microphone measurements.

An appropriate SSPL90 should meet the following four criteria:

- Low enough to prevent loudness discomfort.
- Low enough to prevent additional hearing loss from overamplification.
- High enough to leave an adequately wide dynamic range (distance between the auditory threshold and the SSPL90 of the hearing aid).
- High enough such that normal conversational speech does not constantly saturate the hearing aid.

While it is simple to propose these criteria, it is virtually impossible to know for sure if each premise has been satisfied with the selected

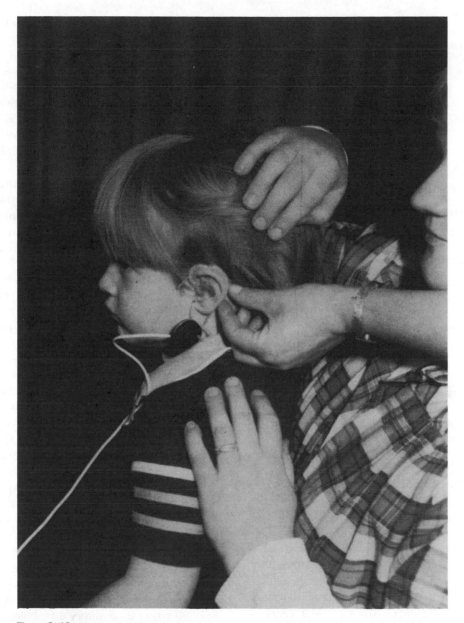

Figure 8–10. Probe-microphone measurements being made on a child.

SSPL90. For instance, it is not clear what SPLs may cause additional hearing loss or how wide a dynamic range should be for optimal speech intelligibility.

One approach often used with adults is to measure the loudness discomfort level (LDL) and set the SSPL90 to a point just below the LDL, attempting to satisfy the first criterion listed above. With children, this technique can present problems as the approach requires subjective loudness judgments. Kawell, Kopun, and Stelmachowicz (1988) developed an LDL procedure specifically for children and evaluated its reliability on a group of 20 children

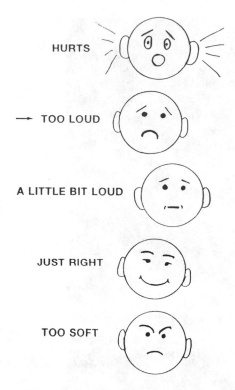

HURTS

TOO LOUD

A LITTLE BIT LOUD

JUST RIGHT

TOO SOFT

Figure 8–11. Loudness category sheet used to obtain loudness discomfort levels with children. (From Kawell, M., Kopun, J., & Stelmachowicz, P. 1988. Loudness discomfort levels in children. *Ear and Hearing, 9,* 133–136, with permission.)

ages 7–14 who were hearing-impaired. The procedure is a variation on an adult LDL method proposed by Hawkins, Walden, Montgomery, & Prosek (1987b), which utilizes loudness categories such as comfortable, comfortable but slightly loud, loud but ok, uncomfortably loud, and so on. Kawell and colleagues altered the instructions and the categories so that they were appropriate for children above 7 years of age. Figure 8–11 shows the loudness category form that is given to the child. The instructions are as follows:

We are going to see how loud this hearing aid makes sounds. You will hear some whistles and I want you to tell me how loud the whistle is. (Go over the descriptor list, explaining each choice, starting with "Too Soft.") When the sounds are "Too Loud," this is where you want the hearing aid to stop and you do not want the sounds to get any

louder. Now, for every whistle, tell me how loud it sounds. (p. 136)

Reliability using this procedure was equivalent to that obtained using the Hawkins et al. (1987) procedure with a group of 20 hearing-impaired adults. Figure 8–12 shows the auditory thresholds and LDLs for the children and adults studied. Similar mean LDLs were obtained for the two groups, indicating that the procedure holds promise as a method of determining LDLs for older children.

Stuart, Durieux-Smith, and Stenstrom (1991) reported measuring LDLs using the Kawell et al. procedure with children ages 7–14 years. However, instead of using a standard earphone to present the signals for LDL judgments, they used an insert earphone attached to the child's personal earmold. A probe tube connected to a probe-microphone system was placed in the ear canal to measure the SPL at the point of loudness discomfort. If the LDLs can be considered valid for the child tested, then the probe-measured SPL in the ear canal at the point of loudness discomfort becomes the target RESR for the hearing aid.

Since loudness judgments are obviously not possible with young children, the audiologist must make decisions as to the appropriate SSPL90, considering the above four criteria. Surprisingly, very little has been written regarding such decisions. Since the only audiometric data typically available to the audiologist are pure-tone or warble-tone thresholds (or minimum response levels), one option would be to examine the literature on selecting SSPL90 based on auditory thresholds for adults. Using regression equations relating LDLs to degree of hearing loss, Cox (1985) proposed that the LDL could be predicted by the simple equation: LDL = 100 + 1/4 Hearing Loss (dB HL). Assuming that the SSPL90 would be set to the LDLs, the same equation applies to SSPL90. For example, if the auditory threshold is 60 dB HL, the SSPL90 would be set to 115 dB SPL (100 + 60/4 = 115). It must be remembered, however, that these are values measured in a

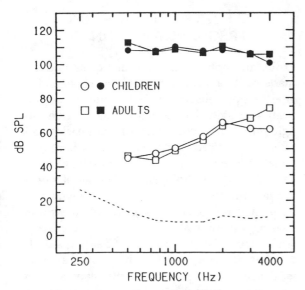

Figure 8-12. Mean auditory thresholds (open symbols) and loudness discomfort levels (black symbols) for a group of children (circles) and adults (squares). (From Kawell, M., Kopun, J., & Stelmachowicz, P. 1988. Loudness discomfort levels in children. *Ear and Hearing, 9,* 133–136, with permission).

2-cm³ coupler, not the ear canal. From the earlier discussion of real ear coupler differences (RECDs), it is clear that 2-cm³ coupler SSPL90 curves will not be representative of the RESR in a child's ear. An SSPL90 of 115 dB SPL in a 2-cm³ coupler might yield 120 dB SPL in the ear canal of an adult and 125 dB SPL in the ear canal of the child. Further, the individual variability mentioned earlier makes it **difficult to predict what the RESR will be for a particular child** given a recommended 2-cm³ coupler SSPL90.

An attempt to define the desired RESR for children was made by Seewald and Ross (1988). Figure 8–13 shows the desired relationship between the level of the amplified speech spectrum and the amount of distance between amplified speech and the RESR. For instance, if the projected level of the amplified-speech spectrum was 100 dB SPL, the desired RESR would be 100 + 20 or 120 dB SPL. Using this approach, Seewald, Zelisko, Ramji, and Jamieson (1991) constructed a revised table showing the de-

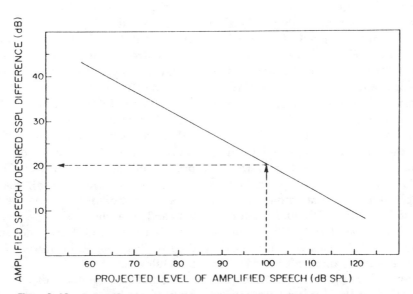

Figure 8-13. The desired amplified-speech/SSPL90 difference as a function of the level of the amplified-speech spectrum. (From Seewald, R., & Ross, M. 1988. Amplification for young hearing-impaired children. In M. Pollack [Ed.], *Amplification for the hearing impaired* [pp. 213–271]. Orlando, FL: Grune & Stratton, with permission.)

sired RESR at nine frequencies as a function of degree of hearing loss. These desired RESR values are shown in Table 8–1. Using these numbers, the audiologist can set RESR targets for the hearing aid as measured in the child's ear canal. It is not clear that these values will satisfy the above four criteria, but they represent the most systematic approach to date with respect to this difficult issue.

Once appropriate RESR values have been determined, probe-microphone measurements can be utilized to adjust the hearing aid to the appropriate output control setting to match the desired values. As discussed in detail in Chapter 7, the probe tube is inserted into the ear canal (10 or 15 mm past the ear canal opening) and the hearing aid and earmold are positioned on the child. The output control is set initially to a point well below the estimated desired setting to yield an appropriate RESR. The purpose of the low initial setting is to minimize the possibility of the child experiencing any loudness discomfort during the measurement procedure. If the initial setting is too high, the child may become agitated, attempt to remove the hearing aid and/or probe tube, and refuse to cooperate further. The VCW is set to a point just below audible feedback and a soundfield signal of 85 or 90 dB SPL is introduced. The high VCW setting in combination with the intense input should saturate the hearing aid and produce the maximum possible SPL in the ear canal as measured by the probe microphone (RESR). The **output control on the hearing aid is then increased and the procedure repeated until the best match is obtained with the desired real-ear SSPL90 values**. The entire procedure can be accomplished in several minutes.

Regardless of how the SSPL90 is determined and set, it is imperative that the audiologist **monitor the child closely** for possible evidence of loudness discomfort and/or overamplification. Our recommendation is that a brief hearing evaluation and hearing aid check be performed **every 3 months** during the first year of hearing aid use with all children.

SELECTION OF GAIN AND FREQUENCY RESPONSE

Probe-microphone measurements should be made with a predetermined purpose and a goal. Simply observing the amount of amplification provided by a hearing aid can be enlightening, but adjustment of the hearing aid to some desired performance is where the benefits of probe measurements are realized. Therefore, the audiologist needs a set of working hypotheses as to the appropriate gain and frequency response for a given child who is hearing impaired.

Unfortunately, the science of hearing aid fitting has not progressed to the point that clear guidance is available. As a result, many audiologists use frequency-response selection schemes (reviewed in Chapter 5) that were developed for adults and apply them to children. While this approach might be appropriate, research is needed to verify this assumption. One could argue that the amplified signal needs to be at a greater sensation level for the child who is learning speech and language than for the adult with a slowly progressive hearing loss.

It should be noted that most of the procedures were developed for adult hearing losses of less than 80 dB HL and are not appropriate for children with severe and severe-to-profound hearing impairment. Suggestions were made by Byrne, Parkinson, and Newall (1990, 1991) for modification of the National Acoustics Laboratories (NAL) procedure for individuals with severe and profound hearing loss. A revision of the Prescription of Gain and Output procedure, known as POGO II (Schwartz, Lyregaard, & Lundh, 1988), changes the formulas for persons having severe hearing losses. The authors of these two procedures, NAL-R and POGO II, have not stated whether they believe their procedures are appropriate for children.

A gain and frequency response selection approach that has received some recent interest with children is the desired sensation level (DSL) procedure described by Seewald and colleagues (see Chapter 5), which lends itself

TABLE 8–1. DESIRED RESR VALUES

Threshold (dB HL)	Frequency (Hz)								
	250	500	750	1000	1500	2000	3000	4000	6000
0	94	102	101	99	99	100	100	98	97
5	94	102	101	99	99	101	100	99	97
10	94	102	101	100	100	102	101	100	98
15	95	103	102	101	100	103	102	101	98
20	95	103	102	101	101	104	103	102	99
25	96	104	103	103	102	105	105	103	100
30	97	105	104	104	104	106	106	104	101
35	99	106	106	105	105	108	108	106	103
40	100	107	107	107	107	110	110	108	105
45	102	109	109	109	109	112	112	109	106
50	104	111	110	110	111	114	114	111	108
55	106	113	112	112	113	116	116	113	111
60	109	115	114	114	115	118	118	115	113
65	111	117	117	117	117	120	120	118	115
70	114	119	119	119	119	122	123	120	117
75	117	121	121	121	121	124	125	122	120
80	120	123	123	123	123	126	127	124	122
85	123	126	125	125	125	128	129	126	124
90	126	128	127	127	127	130	130	128	125
95	129	130	129	129	129	131	132	130	127
100	132	131	131	130	131	133	133	132	128
105	—	133	132	131	132	134	135	133	—
110	—	134	134	133	133	135	136	135	—

Source: Reprinted from Seewald, R., Zelisko, D., Ramji, K., & Jamieson, D. 1991. *DSL 3.0 user's manual*. London, Ontario, Canada: The University of Western Ontario, with permission.

well to the use of probe-microphone measurements. This approach specifies **DSLs across frequency for the long-term speech spectrum**. For instance, if the hearing loss at 1000 Hz is 60 dB HL, the speech spectrum in the 1000-Hz region should be amplified to a sensation level (SL) of 23 dB. The gain of the hearing aid would need to be such that the input speech spectrum is amplified to a point 23 dB above the child's auditory threshold.

Hawkins, Morrison, Halligan, and Cooper (1989) described a procedure in which probe-microphone measurements are utilized in conjunction with the DSL approach. The attractiveness of the approach is that all measurements are specified as SPL in the ear canal. Auditory thresholds, amplified levels of the long-term speech spectrum, and RESR are all measured with a probe-microphone system. As a result, there are no conversions or corrections such as those described in Chapter 12. The limits of the dynamic range (the auditory threshold and the RESR), as well as how the amplified signal is packaged into this area, are all measured by the probe microphone and expressed in dB SPL in the ear canal.

The procedure is carried out in the following steps:

1. Determine the SPL in the ear canal at auditory threshold. To make this measurement, the probe tube is placed in the ear canal, the earphone is placed over the ear, and a pure tone is introduced at threshold. The SPL in the ear canal at threshold is measured by the probe microphone. This measurement defines the lower end of the dynamic range. Alternative methods of delivering the signal to the ear are an Etymotic ER-3A insert earphone attached to the child's own earmold (Stuart, Durieux-Smith, & Stenstrom, 1990) or a button-type hearing aid receiver coupled to the earmold (Gangne, Seewald, Zelisko, & Hudson, 1991; Zelisko, Seewald, & Gagne, 1990). These two methods avoid the potential problem of closing off the probe tube with pressure from the earphone cushion.

2. The prescribed DSLs (see Table 5–13) are added to the auditory threshold (in dB SPL) to determine the target level for the amplified speech spectrum. (Alternatively, these target levels can be found in Table 5–14 for standard earphone thresholds; use of these values, however, assumes the "average" child. Actual measurement with the probe would provide a more customized and accurate value.) For example, suppose the auditory threshold in dB HL was 60 dB HL, and the value measured in the ear canal by the probe was 64 dB SPL. The DSL for a 60 dB HL threshold at 1000 Hz is 23 dB. Therefore, 87 dB SPL (64 + 23) is the target level for the amplified speech spectrum in the ear canal at 1000 Hz. This procedure is repeated across

frequency, and target levels for the speech spectrum are determined.[1] Once the target levels for the amplified-speech spectrum are determined, the probe measurements can be made to adjust the hearing aid, leading to the third step.

3. A speech-spectrum noise with an overall level of 70 dB SPL is delivered to the child with the hearing aid on and the probe tube in the ear. The hearing aid is adjusted to best match to targets for output levels of the amplified-speech spectrum. Adjustments are made with the VCW and tone controls. If an acceptable match is not obtained, a different hearing aid is attached to the earmold, adjusted, and evaluated.

When the procedure is complete, the audiologist has data to confirm the following: (a) the maximum output the hearing aid is capable of delivering to the child's ear (RESR), (b) the width of the dynamic range across frequency (distance from the threshold to the RESR), (c) the sensation level of speech in each frequency region, and (d) the recommended VCW position and tone- and output-control settings to achieve the desired results.

For those who prefer an REIG approach to hearing aid fitting but are attracted to the DSL method, Seewald et al. (1991) have provided REIG values (Table 8–2) that should produce similar results to those described above.

CASE STUDIES

Hawkins, Morrison, Halligan, and Cooper (1989) presented four case studies with children that illustrate the usefulness of probe-microphone measurements and how they can be applied within the DSL approach. The four cases from this publication are presented and discussed here as each demonstrates some useful aspect of the procedure.

---

[1]A computerized program, compatible with IBM-based computers, is available from Richard Seewald, Hearing Health Care Research Unit, The University of Western Ontario, Department of Communicative Disorders, Elborne College, London, Ontario, Canada, N6G 1H1.

TABLE 8–2. REAL EAR INSERTION GAIN VALUES FOR THE DSL PROCEDURE

Threshold (dB HL)	Frequency (Hz)								
	250	500	750	1000	1500	2000	3000	4000	6000
0	0	0	0	0	0	0	0	0	0
5	0	0	0	0	0	0	1	1	1
10	0	1	1	2	2	3	3	3	3
15	1	2	2	4	4	5	6	6	6
20	2	3	4	6	7	8	9	9	9
25	4	5	6	9	10	11	12	12	12
30	6	7	8	12	13	14	15	15	16
35	9	10	11	15	16	17	19	19	19
40	12	13	14	19	20	20	22	22	23
45	16	16	17	22	23	24	26	26	27
50	19	19	21	26	27	28	30	30	32
55	23	23	25	29	31	31	34	34	36
60	27	26	28	33	35	35	37	37	40
65	31	30	32	37	38	38	41	44	44
70	35	34	36	41	42	42	45	45	48
75	40	38	39	44	46	45	48	48	52
80	43	41	43	48	49	49	52	52	55
85	47	45	47	51	53	52	55	55	58
90	51	49	50	54	56	55	58	59	61
95	54	52	53	57	59	58	61	62	64
100	57	55	56	60	62	60	64	65	66
105	—	58	59	62	64	63	66	68	—
110	—	61	61	64	67	65	68	71	—

Source: Reprinted from Seewald, R., Zelisko, D., Ramji, K., & Jamieson, D. 1991. *DSL 3.0 user's manual*. London, Ontario, Canada: The University of Western Ontario, with permission.

CASE 1: EXCESSIVE RESR AND LARGE 2-CM³ COUPLER/REAL-EAR DIFFERENCE

Figure 8–14 shows results from a 12-year-old child who was wearing a high-gain behind-the-ear hearing aid. In dB HL the audiogram was relatively flat with thresholds in the 80–85 dB HL region. The S —— S line represents the RESR of the child's hearing aid as she was wearing it. CS —— CS shows the 2-cm³ cou-

pler SSPL90 curve. Note that the RESR is much higher than the coupler values and exceeds 140 dB SPL in the 1000–3000 Hz region.

In spite of the severe hearing loss, the child was wearing the hearing aid at the minimum VCW position (#1 of 4 on this hearing aid), providing herself with only 20–25 dB of gain. When questioned, she said that if she turned it up any higher, the hearing aid hurt her ear. This was verified when the initial RESR curve was obtained at her use setting, as she winced

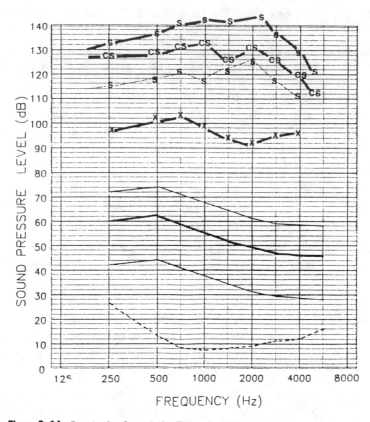

Figure 8–14. Results for Case 1. (In Figure 8–14 through 8–19, symbols are as follows: dashed line, normal auditory thresholds; solid line, long-term speech spectrum from Cox and Moore, 1988; X —— X or 0 —— 0, hearing thresholds in SPL in the ear canal; S —— S, RESR before hearing aid adjustment; S — — — S, RESR after adjustment; CS —— CS, 2-cm³ coupler SSPL90 for the hearing aid as set for the initial RESR measurements; ● —— ●, amplified speech spectrum target levels in the ear canal; A —— A, amplified speech levels.) See text for further explanation. (From Hawkins, D., Morrison, T., Halligan, P., & Cooper, W. 1989. Use of probe tube measurements in hearing aid selection for children: Some clinical experiences. *Ear and Hearing, 10,* 281–287, with permission.)

during the 90-dB SPL swept tone and complained that the signal hurt her ear. (A better approach, based on her complaint, would have been to lower the SSPL90 control before this initial measurement.) This case is an excellent example of a large real-ear/coupler difference occurring in a child. The overfitting resulted in the child adopting a maladaptive strategy (lowering the VCW and denying herself speech information) to deal with a loudness discomfort problem.

The target RESR values from Seewald et al. (1991) for this case are in the 120–127 dB SPL range. The post-adjustment curve shows the final RESR after changing the SSPL90 control. These levels are within 5 dB of the target values through 2000 Hz and leave a 20–30 dB dynamic range. These reduced levels are less likely to pose any threat to the child's residual hearing. With these output levels, the child did not object to the 90-dB SPL input and indicated that it no longer was uncomfortable. The

VCW then had to be rotated to #3 of 4 to achieve the desired target output levels; the child reported that this VCW setting was acceptable.

The final 2-cm³ coupler SSPL90 setting necessary to yield this RESR was approximately 110 dB SPL. This coupler value would certainly look restrictive if one was not aware of the real-ear/coupler difference for this child's ear.

CASE 2:
INADEQUATE SPEECH-SPECTRUM SENSATION LEVELS AND EXCESSIVE RESR

Figure 8–15 shows results from a 12-year-old boy with a sloping mild-to-profound sensorineural hearing loss. The child came to the clinic at the request of his school system for an evaluation of his high-gain behind-the-ear hearing aid. The RESR was excessively high in the 750–2000 Hz region, reaching 138 dB SPL at 2000 Hz. The solid circles represent the desired levels for the amplified-speech spectrum based on the DSLs. The A — — — A curve shows the levels to which the hearing aid was amplifying the speech spectrum as it was currently set. The goals for this case were to reduce the RESR, reduce the gain at 250 Hz, and increase the gain at 1500 and 2000 Hz. Given the 4000-Hz threshold of 125 dB SPL, it was deemed unrealistic to provide audible amplified-speech energy in that region.

The changes that resulted from modifications to the child's hearing aid are shown in Figure 8–16. The SSPL90 control was reduced

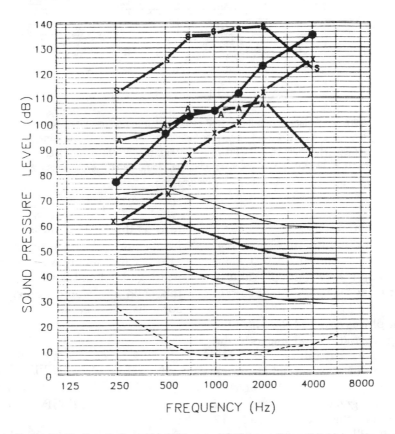

Figure 8–15. Initial results obtained in Case 2. See text for further explanation; see Figure 8–14 for explanation of symbols. (From Hawkins, D., Morrison, T., Halligan, P., & Cooper, W. 1989. Use of probe tube measurements in hearing aid selection for children: Some clinical experiences. *Ear and Hearing, 10,* 281–287, with permission.)

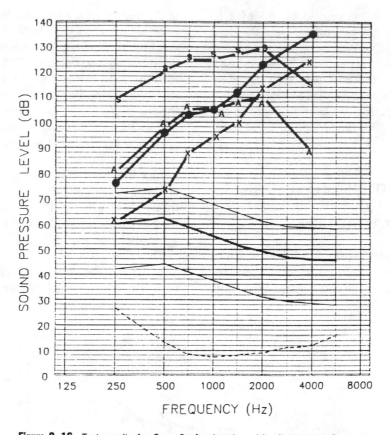

Figure 8–16. Test results for Case 2 after hearing aid adjustments. Symbols same as in Figure 8–14. See text for further explanation. (From Hawkins, D., Morrison, T., Halligan, P., & Cooper, W. 1989. Use of probe tube measurements in hearing aid selection for children: Some clinical experiences. *Ear and Hearing, 10,* 281–287, with permission.)

until the RESR shown by the S ——— S curve was obtained. The values are safer, more realistic, and yet still provide an adequate dynamic range. These output levels are all within 4 dB of the target values suggested by Seewald et al. (1991).

The tone control was adjusted to reduce the low-frequency gain, and a good match to the target levels was obtained through 1500 Hz. The average level of the amplified-speech spectrum was still 3 dB below threshold at 2000 Hz. However, given that the peaks of speech should exceed this average level by 12 dB, the child will still receive some information in the important 2000-Hz region. The 4000-Hz region is still clearly out of the pic-

ture, as the hearing aid is now limiting 10 dB below the child's threshold.

This information well illustrates what this hearing aid is and is not capable of providing this child and would be helpful for planning aural habilitation.

CASE 3:
INADEQUATE SPEECH SPECTRUM SENSATION LEVELS AND EXCESSIVE RESR

Figure 8–17 shows the initial test results for a 5-year-old boy wearing a high-gain behind-the-ear hearing aid. The pure-tone thresholds

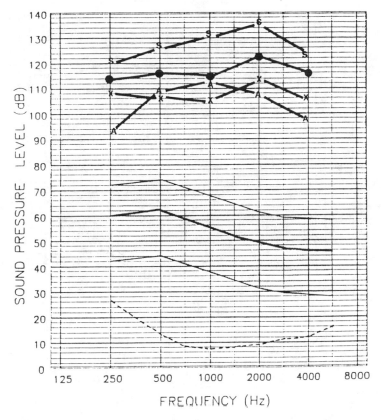

Figure 8-17. Initial test results obtained for Case 3. Symbols same as in Figure 8-14. See text for further explanation. (From Hawkins, D., Morrison, T., Halligan, P., & Cooper, W. 1989. Use of probe tube measurements in hearing aid selection for children: Some clinical experiences. *Ear and Hearing, 10,* 281–287, with permission.)

revealed a gently sloping severe sensorineural hearing loss. According to the target maximum output levels, the RESR was too restrictive in the 250-Hz region and slightly too high in the 2000-Hz region. The amplified level of the speech spectrum did not reach the targets at any of the tested frequencies. At 250, 2000, and 4000 Hz, the average level of speech was below auditory threshold. The goals in modifying the hearing aid's response were to (a) increase the RESR at 250 Hz and decrease it at 2000 Hz, and (b) increase the gain across frequency, especially at 250, 2000, and 4000 Hz, to achieve the DSLs.

The achieved results are shown in Figure 8–18. By adding a filtered earhook and adjusting the output control upward, the maximum output at 250 Hz increased, while the peak at 2000 Hz was reduced, providing an acceptable RESR (below 130 dB SPL) and keeping the dynamic range at a reasonable width. The resulting RESR is within 2 dB of target values through 2000 Hz.

By changing the VCW and tone control, the amplified-speech spectrum reached the targets at 500 and 1000 Hz but was still inadequate at 250, 2000, and 4000 Hz. While this modified fitting could be deemed more appropriate than the initial settings, one could argue that another hearing aid with more low-frequency gain should be evaluated on this child. More gain at 2000 Hz would also be a reasonable goal with a different hearing aid.

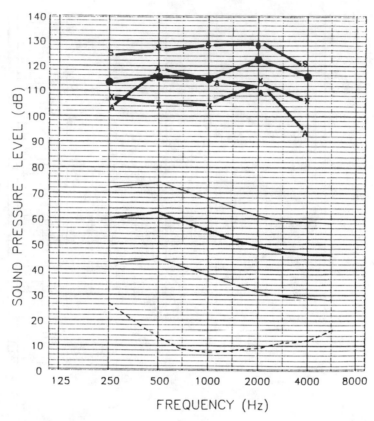

Figure 8–18. Test results obtained for Case 3 after hearing aid adjustments. Symbols same as in Figure 8–14. See text for further explanation. (From Hawkins, D., Morrison, T., Halligan, P., & Cooper, W. 1989. Use of probe tube measurements in hearing aid selection for children: Some clinical experiences. *Ear and Hearing, 10,* 281–287, with permission.)

CASE 4:
MINOR PROBLEMS WITH A RELATIVELY SUCCESSFUL FITTING

A quite different case is shown in Figure 8–19. This child had a very mild (20–30 dB HL) high-frequency sensorineural hearing loss and was wearing an in-the-ear hearing aid with a large vent that was completely closed. The output control was set to the maximum setting (highest SSPL90). Before obtaining the results shown in Figure 8–19, the vent plug was removed and the output control was set to yield the minimum SSPL90.

Notice that for this mild hearing loss, the DSL procedure required no gain through 1000

Hz (i.e., the amplified target levels are equal to the unaided speech spectrum). The amplified speech spectrum shows that no gain is present in the hearing aid through 1000 Hz. If the vent had remained plugged, there would have been an attenuation of the low-frequency input, as the unamplified low-frequency speech information would not have been able to enter unattenuated via the vent. Above 1000 Hz, the amplified speech-spectrum levels agree very well with the target levels.

The 2-cm³ coupler SSPL90 at the reduced setting looked appropriate for this hearing loss, with the maximum output reaching 104 dB SPL. However, the RESR reached 115 dB SPL at 2000 Hz, an excessive level for such a

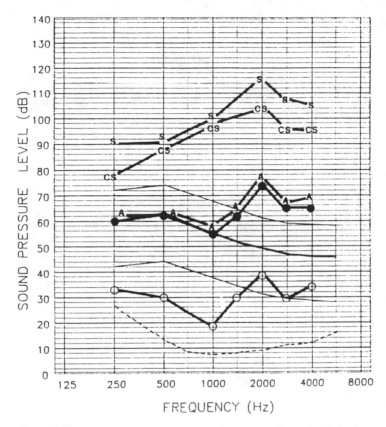

Figure 8–19. Test results for Case 4. Symbols same as in Figure 8–14. See text for further explanation. (From Hawkins, D., Morrison, T., Halligan, P., & Cooper, W. 1989. Use of probe tube measurements in hearing aid selection for children: Some clinical experiences. *Ear and Hearing, 10*, 281–287, with permission.)

mild hearing loss. The target RESR value at this frequency was 108 dB SPL. With the output control in its original highest SSPL90 position, SPLs greater than 120 in the real ear were possible. In summary, with the exception of the RESR being excessive in the 2000-Hz region, this fitting was considered appropriate (after the vent was unplugged and the output control reduced) and was easily verified with real-ear techniques.

CONCLUSIONS

Probe-microphone measurements offer the audiologist a powerful tool in selecting and fitting hearing aids for the pediatric population. Less time and less patient cooperation are required than for traditional soundfield hearing aid evaluation and testing. A desired RESR can be determined and the hearing aid quickly adjusted to produce acceptable values. A desired REIR can be determined and the hearing aid adjusted to match prescription values. The amplified long-term speech spectrum can be adjusted to desired sensation levels. These procedures can be accomplished very quickly for each child, taking into account the earmold, the residual volume of air, and the middle-ear impedance. Probe-microphone measurements can provide the audiologist with objective, reliable, and useful data for habilitation of the child with impaired hearing.

CHAPTER 9

Individualizing the Ordering of Custom Hearing Aids

■ H. GUSTAV MUELLER, Ph.D. ■

Much of the discussion throughout this text relates to the task of obtaining an "appropriate" real ear insertion response (REIR) or real ear aided response (REAR) when a hearing aid is fitted to a given individual. Chapter 5 described various prescriptive methods that can be used, and Chapter 6 reviewed the use of insertion gain to verify these prescriptive procedures. It is reasonable to assume that **the more user-specific information that is entered into the prescriptive method, the greater the likelihood that the resultant REIR or REAR will meet the desired target values**. For this reason, there is considerable interest in the use of probe-microphone measurement as a prefitting tool to provide individualized corrections to desired 2-cm³ coupler values for both hearing aid gain and output.

It is difficult to estimate how many audiologists use probe-microphone measurements to assist in selecting the appropriate 2-cm³ coupler response prior to the actual hearing aid fitting. One 1991 survey (Cranmer, 1991) of audiologist and nonaudiologist hearing aid dispensers revealed that approximately 50% of the respondents used probe-microphone equipment. Of this group, over half stated that they used this equipment for hearing aid prefitting measurements.

In apparent contrast to the findings of Cranmer (1991), other surveys have reported that nearly *90%* of orders for in-the-ear (ITE) and in-the-canal (ITC) hearing aids request that the manufacturer select the coupler values or hearing aid matrix, as only a pure tone audiogram is provided (Bratt & Sammeth, 1991; Valente, Valente, & Vass, 1991). These latter survey findings suggest that prefitting probe-microphone measurements are not frequently conducted, as it seems unlikely that an audiologist would make the effort to conduct these measures and then not use this information to select specific 2-cm³ coupler values or a hearing aid matrix. One explanation of the divergent survey results could be that those audiologists who actually conduct prefitting probe-microphone measurements simply do not order very many hearing aids.

There does seem to be a growing trend to use probe-microphone measurements in the prefitting process, however, and many manufacturers of probe-microphone systems have added software to their equipment to simplify these calculations. While individualized 2-cm^3 coupler corrections can be applied to both behind-the-ear (BTE) and ITE fittings, this chapter focuses primarily on the selection and ordering of custom ITE products, as individualized corrections have the widest application for this hearing aid style. With custom ITE hearing aids, especially the mini-canal models, there is limited flexibility in the adjustment of the frequency response and the output at the time that the hearing aid is fitted. Additionally, there usually **is only one model available to test** on a single patient. For these reasons, it is **critical that the 2-cm^3 coupler gain is a close approximation of what is required to obtain the desired real-ear results.**

The use of digitally programmable circuitry in ITE and ITC models potentially will reduce the need for some of the prefitting measurements. If the frequency response or output of an instrument needs to be altered to account for an unusual real ear unaided response (REUR) or real ear coupler difference (RECD), these changes can be made without returning the instrument to the manufacturer. It will be several years, however, before programmable custom hearing aids with this technology become standard.

ADVANTAGES OF INDIVIDUALIZED CORRECTIONS

The theory underlying the use of individualized corrections is that the prescriptive matrix or desired 2-cm^3 coupler values of a hearing aid must be altered if real ear results from an individual are other than average. If corrections are applied, a more acceptable REIR or REAR

should result. Besides the increased use of prescriptive methods and probe-microphone measurements in general, there are also two practical reasons why audiologists are beginning to use individualized corrections more frequently:

■ The continuing popularity of ITE hearing aids
■ Variances of ITE products within and among manufacturers when more haphazard ordering procedures are used.

POPULARITY OF ITE HEARING AIDS

Although there have been some reports of a "BTE comeback" (Kirkwood, 1990), it is apparent that ITE hearing aids will continue to occupy the largest share of the hearing aid market. Recent statistics suggest that there has been a leveling off, as the market share for ITE hearing aids has stayed around 80% since 1987. Table 9–1 from Kirkwood (1991) shows the ITE and BTE annual percentage of market share since 1982. Notice that the ITE market share has nearly doubled in less than 10 years. For

TABLE 9–1. PERCENTAGE OF TOTAL HEARING AID SALES REPRESENTED BY IN-THE-EAR AND BEHIND-THE-EAR INSTRUMENTS

Year	ITEs	BTEs
1982	42.0%	52.5%
1983	49.4%	46.7%
1984	58.2%	39.4%
1985	64.2%	33.7%
1986	70.5%	27.9%
1987	77.7%	21.1%
1988	79.7%	19.5%
1989	79.5%	19.7%
1990	78.4%	21.1%
1991	79.1%	20.5%

Source: Hearing Industries Association statistics. Percentages add up to less than 100% because a small percentage of hearing aids sold each year are eyeglass and bodyworn instruments. (From Kirkwood, D. 1991. 1991 U.S. hearing aid sales summary. *Hearing Journal, 44* (12), 9–15, with permission.)

1991, 28% of the ITE hearing aid sales were ITC instruments. In a few years, when most manufacturers will be offering programmable hearing aids in ITE (ITC) models, another spurt in the sales growth of this style would be expected.

The popularity of ITE hearing aids seems to be driven by demands from the consumer for a smaller, less visible device. In a 1988 article, Surr and Hawkins reported that, even when the advantages and disadvantages of both BTEs and ITEs were carefully explained to potential new hearing aid users, 73% selected the ITE style. In a similar study, Mueller and Budinger (1990) reported that 90% of their subjects selected the ITE (full-concha) style over a BTE instrument when they had compared the appearances of the two types of hearing aids.

When subjects are allowed to use their hearing aids for an extended period of time, it appears that the strong preference for the ITE style remains. Mueller, Bryant, Brown, & Budinger (1991), studied two matched-sample groups of new hearing aid users. One group of 52 subjects was fitted with BTE hearing aids, and the other group of 43 subjects was fitted with ITE instruments. All subjects in both groups were fitted binaurally. No subject in either group had experience with the other style of hearing aid. Mueller et al. (1991) reported that the **ITE user group was more satisfied with their hearing aids; ITE style users also were more frequent users of binaural hearing aids**. The strong preference for the ITE style was most apparent when the subjects from the two groups responded to 12 questions about the style they were *not* fitted with. As shown in Table 9–2, general dissatisfaction was expressed by the BTE users. Nearly 100% of them felt that the ITE hearing aids were less obvious, 88% believed that the ITE hearing aids were more modern, and 80% stated that they would use their hearing aids more often if they were the ITE style. In contrast, over 90% of the ITE users *disagreed* with these three statements.

The consumer's demand for a smaller hearing aid often works in opposition to the audiologist's desire to have a hearing aid that allows control of the frequency response and output parameters. In general, therefore, **the smaller the hearing aid, the greater the need for the audiologist to communicate clearly to the manufacturer about the desired circuitry of the instrument**.

CONSISTENCY AMONG AND WITHIN MANUFACTURERS

As discussed earlier, it is estimated that as many as **90% of custom hearing aids are ordered simply by providing the manufacturer the patient's pure-tone audiogram**. There are some distinct advantages to this approach for the audiologist:

■ Requires little time;
■ Little testing is necessary;
■ Practically no thinking is required;
■ Ordering easily can be handled by a clerical staff member.

This approach assumes, however, that the manufacturer knows better than the audiologist what is best for the patient, or at least that the manufacturer and the audiologist use the same prescriptive fitting rationale. It also assumes that, somehow, the manufacturer can predict a patient's loudness discomfort level (LDL) and resultant hearing aid output values from the pure-tone audiogram.

Angeli, Seestedt-Stanford, and Nerbonne (1990) studied the consistency among and within manufacturers regarding the electroacoustic properties of ITE instruments. These authors ordered two separate ITE hearing aids within a 6-month period from each of five different manufacturers. All 10 orders were made by supplying only an audiogram, and the same audiogram was used for all orders.

Angeli et al. (1990) reported that variations in high-frequency average (HFA) full-on gain (per the 2-cm^3 coupler) varied from 24 to 43 dB among manufacturers. The HFA SSPL90 values ranged from a low of 103 dB to a high of 113 dB. Variations in gain and SSPL90 between the two custom hearing aids supplied by each of the five manufacturers is shown in Figure 9–1. Notice that manufacturers A, C, and D had rel-

TABLE 9-2. HEARING AID USERS' RATINGS OF THE "OTHER STYLE"*

	Agree		Disagree	
	BTE Users	ITE Users	BTE Users	ITE Users
1. The other style of hearing aid would be less obvious to others.	94	2	2	91
2. The other style of hearing aid would cause less interference with my glasses.	94	0	2	93
3. The other style of hearing aid is more modern.	88	0	0	93
4. I would use my hearing aid(s) more if I had the other style of hearing aid.	80	0	10	91
5. The other style of hearing aid would be more comfortable to wear.	70	5	0	54
6. I would be more apt to use two hearing aids if I had the other style of hearing aids.	68	0	4	88
7. The other style of hearing aid would be easier to insert and remove.	58	14	4	68
8. The other style of hearing aid would be more stable.	46	0	0	41
9. The other style of hearing aid is more durable.	41	2	4	23
10. I could understand speech better with the other style of hearing aid.	26	2	0	51
11. The other style of hearing aid has better electronics.	24	7	0	32
12. The other style of hearing aid would have fewer repair problems.	24	0	2	22

*Percent BTE ($n = 52$) and ITE ($n = 43$) users responding in each category for the twelve statements. The "other style" refers to the instrument the patient was *not* fitted with.

Source: From Mueller, H., Bryant, M., Brown, W., & Budinger, A. 1991. Hearing aid selection for high-frequency hearing loss. In G. Studebaker, F. Bess, & L. Beck (Eds.), *The Vanderbilt hearing aid report II*, (pp. 269–287). Parkton, MD: York Press, with permission.

atively little variance. Manufacturer B, however, had a 11 dB difference in HFA gain between instruments, and manufacturer E had a 5 dB variance in SSPL90. As more manufacturers use computerized entry for circuit selection, differences in gain as large as that demonstrated by manufacturer B probably will occur less frequently.

The differences among manufacturers reported by Angeli et al. (1990) is interesting, but would be expected, as there is **no reason to believe that five different manufacturers would use the same fitting formula any more than** **one would expect five different audiologists to use the same fitting formula**. This verifies that either the audiologist must be very familiar with the prescriptive fitting method of each manufacturer, or that he or she must take some control of the hearing aid selection process.

It would seem that custom ITE manufacturers would welcome 2-cm³ coupler specifications provided by audiologists, as this would relieve them of making these decisions. At least one manufacturer appears to share this viewpoint, as at the conclusion of the Angeli et al. (1990) article, the following insightful com-

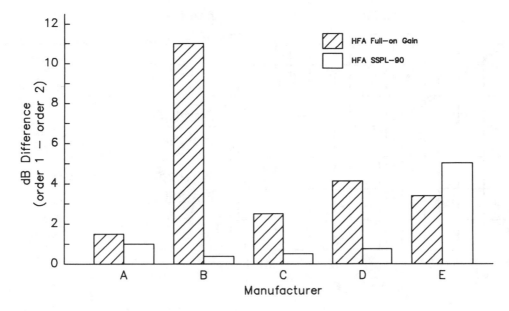

Figure 9–1. The difference in high-frequency average gain and SSPL90 for two custom ITE hearing aids ordered with identical audiograms from each of five manufacturers. (From Bratt, G., & Sammeth, C., 1991 [adapted from Angeli, Seestadt-Stanford, & Nerbonne, 1990]. Clinical implications of prescriptive formulas for hearing aid selection. In G. Studebaker, F. Bess, & L. Beck [Eds.], *The Vanderbilt hearing aid report II* [pp. 23–25]. Parkton, MD: York Press, with permission.)

ments were published from an anonymous reviewer involved in the manufacturing of custom ITE products:

The dispenser must clearly define the patient's needs and communicate these to the manufacturer. The manufacturer's role is to produce a product that meets these specifications. Without clearly defined specifications, or with incomplete data, too many assumptions must be made throughout the manufacturing process .... Only when clearly defined goals are established is it possible to determine whether they are achieved .... Completely defined specifications and improved lines of communication between the dispenser and the manufacturer should enable the hearing-impaired consumer to obtain the best possible amplification system. (p. 26)

ALTERNATIVE ORDERING METHODS

As audiologists begin to assume more responsibility in the selection of the desired frequency response and output for a custom hearing aid,

alternatives to the mail-in-the-audiogram approach need to be considered. Without employing probe-microphone measurements, there are methods of providing the manufacturer relatively complete information regarding the design specifications of the hearing aid.

MATRIX APPROXIMATION

Nearly all manufacturers provide a book that includes the 2-cm^3 coupler specifications that are available for all their custom ITE hearing aid models. A matrix is provided for each model defining such features as gain, SSPL90, slope, and frequency bandwidth. Usually, **manufacturers also provide a suggested fitting guide** based on the patient's pure-tone thresholds; **presumably the fitting guide is tied directly to the manufacturer's prescriptive fitting procedure**. Figure 9–2, for example, shows the full-on gain and SSPL90 curves for an ITC hearing aid with a matrix identification of 45/12/108/W.

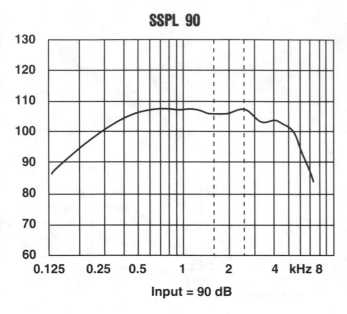

Input = 90 dB

Matrices

45 | 12 | 108 | W

Specifications

Peak Gain –	45dB $^{+5}_{-3}$
HFA Gain –	35dB
Peak SSPL 90 –	108dB ±5
HFA SSPL 90 –	105dB ±4

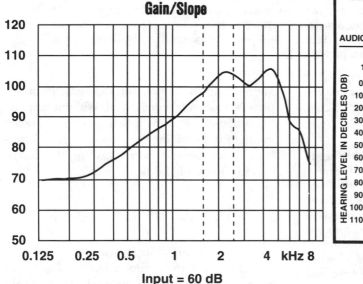

Input = 60 dB

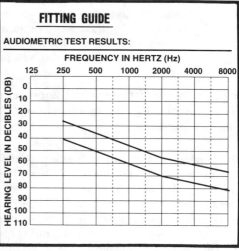

Figure 9–2. Sample matrix page from a hearing aid manufacturer for use in ordering custom in-the-ear (ITE) or in-the-canal (ITC) hearing aids. (Courtesy of Siemens Hearing Instruments, Inc., Piscataway, NJ)

In this case, 45 (dB) is the peak gain, 12 (dB) is the slope/octave of the frequency response, 108 (dB) is the peak SSPL90, and the W identifies that it is a wideband receiver. The fitting guide illustrates, according to this manufacturer's prescriptive fitting method, what hearing loss range would be best suited for this matrix.

Equipped with a matrix book, it is possible to look at a patient's pure-tone results, and then make a selection of the circuitry to be placed in the custom hearing aid. After some experimentation, audiologists usually find two or three favorite matrices and use these for the majority of their patients. In this approach, the matrix is not usually selected based on a formalized prescriptive method of the audiologist; rather, **the audiologist usually uses an approximation of some general fitting rule, the fitting guide furnished by the manufacturer, or simply an approach that has worked well in the past**.

Inexperienced audiologists often rely heavily on the fitting guidelines provided by the manufacturer. It is important to recognize, however, that the prescriptive method that manufacturers use to develop their fitting guide is not usually published, and in some cases it is proprietary. If the manufacturer's fitting guide is to be used, therefore, it is first necessary to determine if it agrees with your own prescriptive fitting philosophy.

PRESCRIBING 2-CM³ COUPLER GAIN

A step beyond the above method of semi-casual matrix selection, is to choose a formalized prescriptive method and then convert the resulting desired insertion gain to full-on gain 2-cm³ coupler values. Once this has been accomplished, these calculated 2-cm³ values can then be used to select the desired hearing aid matrix (or, if a matrix selection is not available, these 2-cm³ values, rather than an audiogram, can be mailed to the manufacturer). **This procedure involves making three decisions:**

■ The prescriptive fitting method to be used.
■ The amount of reserve gain.
■ The selection of the average correction factors used for the conversion to 2-cm³ values.

The **selection of correction factors**, discussed in Chapter 12, **probably requires the most thought**. Average coupler-to real-ear corrections have been referred to as CORFIGs (e.g., Killion & Monser, 1980). **These values**, which differ for different hearing aid styles and microphone locations, **can be conceptualized in two ways:**

■ The 2-cm³ response that will yield a flat REIR.
■ The values which must be added to the real

ear insertion gain (REIG) to determine desired 2-cm³ coupler gain.

In this chapter, CORFIGs are used as correction factors. The following is a protocol illustrating this use for calculating desired 2-cm³ values when ordering a custom ITE instrument:

1. Obtain desired REIG using a prescriptive fitting procedure.
2. Add reserve gain (e.g., 10 dB).
3. Apply CORFIGs to totals obtained in Step 2 to obtain desired 2-cm³ coupler full-on gain values.
4. Use calculated 2-cm³ values to select desired matrix, or provide actual 2-cm³ values to manufacturer for circuit selection.

An example of this process is shown in Table 9–3. In this case, the Australian National Acoustic Laboratories (NAL) prescriptive method (Byrne & Dillon, 1986) is used to obtain the desired REIG, 10 dB of reserve gain is included, and, in the final step, CORFIGs for a full-concha ITE are added. These CORFIGs are derived by Hawkins and published in Chapter 12.

The 2-cm³ values that are calculated in Table 9–3 can be used to select a desired matrix. One way to facilitate this selection is to develop a template of the manufacturer's matrix on clear acetate. Using a grease pencil, the desired 2-cm³ full-on gain curve can be plotted on the template; then, by overlaying the template on the published curves in the matrix book, a close approximation to the desired values can be found. For example, the matrix response shown in Figure 9–3 was selected for the patient whose results are displayed in Table 9–3. Unless matrix books from several manufacturers are used, the selection procedure becomes relatively simple after the first few cases. There also are computer programs that can be used in this process (e.g., Revit, 1990; Valente et al., 1991).

Byrne and Dillon (1986) included their own CORFIGs as part of the NAL prescriptive method. Although the specific CORFIG values are not shown, they are incorporated into Table 9–4. The values in this table *include 15 dB reserve gain*. Byrne and Dillon also have made com-

TABLE 9–3. CALCULATION OF DESIRED FULL-ON 2-CM^3 COUPLER GAIN USING THE NAL PRE-SCRIPTIVE METHOD

	Frequency (Hz)					
	.5k	1k	1.5k	2k	3k	4k
Pure-tone thresholds	35	40	45	45	50	50
Prescribed REIG (re: NAL)	9	19	21	19	20	20
Average CORFIG (ITE)	0	0	0	2	6	0
Desired 2-cm^3 at use VCW	9	19	21	21	26	20
Reserve gain	10	10	10	10	10	10
Desired full-on 2-cm^3 coupler gain	19	29	31	31	36	30

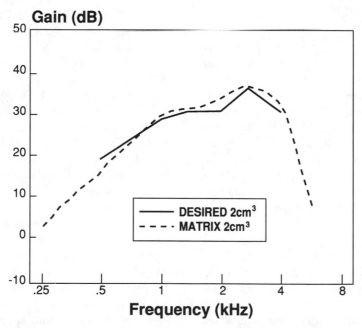

Figure 9–3. Illustration of a matrix 2-cm^3 response that was selected to match the calculated NAL prescriptive full-on coupler gain values (from Table 9–3).

TABLE 9-4. METHOD RECOMMENDED BY BYRNE AND DILLON (1986) FOR CALCULATING DESIRED 2-CM^3 COUPLER GAIN USING THE NAL PRESCRIPTIVE METHOD[a]

	2-cc Coupler[b]			Ear Simulator		
	BTE	ITE	Body	BTE	ITE	Body
1. Calculate $X = 0.05 (H_{500} + H_{1k} + H_{2k})$[c]						
2. $G_{250} = X + 0.31 H_{250} +$	1	−1	0	5	2	0
$G_{500} = X + 0.31 H_{500} +$	9	9	2	13	12	6
$G_{750} = X + 0.31 H_{750} +$	12	13	8	17	16	12
$G_{1k} = X + 0.31 H_{1k} +$	16	16	13	22	21	19
$G_{1.5k} = X + 0.31 H_{1.5k} +$	13	14	22	19	21	28
$G_{2k} = X + 0.31 H_{2k} +$	15	14	25	24	23	35
$G_{3k} = X + 0.31 H_{3k} +$	22	15	26	29	25	33
$G_{4k} = X + 0.31 H_{4k} +$	18	13	17	24	25	23
$G_{6k} = X + 0.31 H_{6k} +$	12	4		21	19	

1. Formulae predict approximate coupler gain expected to give required real ear gain.

[a]All formula refer to gain at maximum volume control and include a 15 dB reserve.

[b]2-cc Coupler data assume a HA2 style earmold simulator for the BTE and body aids, but a 2-mm I.D. tubing in the actual (fully occluded) earmold.

[c]H, HTL (ISO standard); G, coupler or ear simulator gain.

Source: From Byrne, D., & Dillon, H. 1986. The National Acoustic Laboratories' (NAL) new procedure for selecting the gain and frequency response of a hearing aid. *Ear and Hearing*, 7, 257–265, with permission.

mercially available a computer program and slide rules that can be used to simplify the calculations from hearing threshold to desired full-on 2-cm^3 coupler gain.

Applying average correction factors to prescriptive REIG targets to obtain desired 2-cm^3 coupler values for a custom ITE hearing aid design has several advantages over simply mailing in an audiogram. **This approach, however, is not without some limitations**. Differences in ear canal volume, resonance, and middle ear impedance potentially can have significant effects on an individual's real ear unaided response (REUR) and CORFIG. Using average values, therefore, could result in ordering an inappropriate hearing aid frequency response for someone whose REUR and/or CORFIG deviated significantly from normal. Probe-microphone measurements provide a convenient and reliable method to identify

such individuals and make appropriate adjustments in the real-ear-to-coupler corrections.

INDIVIDUALIZED 2-CM^3 COUPLER CORRECTIONS

When making individualized coupler corrections, there are two factors to consider: **the REUR and the CORFIG**. If a gain-based prescriptive method is used, which is usually the case (Martin & Morris, 1989), then the size and location of the peaks in the patient's REUR directly affect whether target gain is achieved. Hearing aids designed with a "canal resonance response," that is, a 2-cm^3 coupler peak around 3000 Hz, would not have a canal resonance response for someone whose REUR peaks below 2000 Hz. The REUR, however, is an open-ear measure; therefore, it might not relate directly to the individual's real-ear-to-coupler difference (RECD) or CORFIG, both of which incorporate a closed-ear measurement. **It is possible that someone with an average REUR could have an abnormal RECD, or vice versa.** For this reason, individual correction procedures have been designed using only the REUR, the REUR and the RECD, or only the RECD.

CORRECTIONS USING THE REUR

Much of the work in recent years concerning the design of earmolds and hearing aid circuitry has centered on methods to provide an amplified signal that corresponds to the configuration of the average REUR, that is, a peak in the 2-cm^3 coupler response in the 2700–3000 Hz region. It is generally believed, although not substantiated empirically, that if the configuration of the REAR resembles that of the REUR, not only will a more desirable REIR be present, but the patient will judge the sound quality as more favorable.

Upfold and Byrne (1988) established that the height and bandwidth of the REUR varies significantly among adult subjects. They reported mean values of: 2968 Hz for the peak frequency, and 18 dB for the primary peak height, with a bandwidth of 1.22 octaves. The range of responses, however, was as follows: 2000–3500 Hz for the primary peak frequency and 12–24 dB for the peak height, with the bandwidth varying from 0.33 to 2.33 octaves. Byrne and Upfold (1991) reported that average values were used for the NAL prescriptive method, as it was believed that adjustments could be made at the time of the hearing aid fitting to account for differences between coupler and real-ear values. The authors acknowledge, however, that for ITE and ITC fittings, it might be difficult to make the necessary adjustments for some patients, so it is more desirable *to get it right the first time*. The question then is, **What should the audiologist do when a given patient has an unusual REUR?**

One REUR correction method that has been proposed is to alter the desired 2-cm^3 coupler values by the amount that the REUR differs from average (Bratt, & Sammeth, 1991; Mueller, 1989; Valente, Valente, & Vass, 1990; Valente et al., 1991). This method attempts to formalize the general fitting practice of matching the configuration of the REAR to the REUR, which, in effect, is an REUR correction procedure. **Using individual REUR deviations from average REUR values to alter the desired 2-cm^3 coupler gain is based on the following assumptions**:

■ The audiologist's primary concern is the configuration of the *REIR*, not the *REAR*.
■ The average REUR is included in prescriptive gain calculations and CORFIGS.
■ There is a 1:1 relationship between the REUR and the REIG
■ There is a 1:1 relationship between 2-cm^3 coupler gain and the REIG.

If these assumptions are true, it is reasonable to assume that prescriptive target REIG will be attained more frequently if the desired 2-cm^3 coupler values are altered to the degree that the patient's REUR deviates from average. A sample protocol for using the REUR correction procedure is as follows:

1. Obtain desired REIG using a prescriptive fitting procedure.
2. Measure the patient's REUR; add or subtract deviations from the average REUR to the prescriptive REIG.
3. Add reserve gain (e.g., 10 dB).
4. Use CORFIGs to obtain desired 2-cm^3 couple full-on gain values.
5. Use calculated 2-cm^3 values to select desired matrix or provide actual 2-cm^3 coupler values to manufacturer for circuit selection.

Calculations using this protocol are shown in Table 9–5. This prescription is for the same patient as in Table 9–3, except with REUR corrections applied. This patient's REUR peaked in the 2000 Hz range and was approximately 10 dB greater than average at this frequency. At other key frequencies, the REUR was at or near average; therefore, no corrections were made. Ob-

TABLE 9–5. CALCULATION OF DESIRED FULL-ON 2-CM³ COUPLER GAIN USING THE NAL PRE-SCRIPTIVE METHOD WITH INDIVIDUAL REUR CORRECTIONS

	Frequency (Hz)					
	.5k	1k	1.5k	2k	3k	4k
Pure-tone thresholds	35	40	45	45	50	50
Prescribed REIG (re: NAL)	9	19	21	19	20	20
Individual REUR Deviation from average	0	0	+2	+10	−2	0
Average CORFIG (ITE)	0	0	0	+ 2	+6	0
Desired 2-cm³ at use VCW	9	19	23	31	24	20
Reserve gain	10	10	10	10	10	10
Desired full-on 2-cm³ coupler gain	19	29	33	41	34	30

serve that applying this REUR correction alters the matrix that would be selected for this patient. Figure 9–4 shows the matrix that would have been selected based on the calculations shown in Table 9–3 (Figure 9–4A), and the matrix that would appear to be most appropriate after REUR corrections (Figure 9–4B).

Some audiologists have adopted the practice of sending the patient's REUR to the manufacturer along with the audiogram when the hearing aid is ordered. This would seem to serve little purpose, as it tells the manufacturer very little concerning what alterations (if any) are necessary. When the audiologist uses these corrections (or some other correction method) directly to select a desired matrix, the guesswork for the manufacturer is eliminated, theoretically resulting in a more appropriate product for the patient. **A correction procedure using the REUR easily can be implemented into the hearing aid prefitting testing**. There are some exceptions to using this method and some potential measurement errors; these factors are discussed in the next sections.

Exceptions to REUR Corrections

Mueller (1989) pointed out that there are instances when it is **best to ignore the unusual REUR and *not* make a correction**, and he provided some examples when this would be the case. For instance, when there are known limitations in hearing aid circuitry, measurement corrections may not help. For example, it might be counterproductive to ask for less 2-cm³ gain at 4000 Hz if clinical experience has revealed that REIG at 4000 Hz consistently falls below prescriptive target for patients with average REURs.

Mueller and Bryant (1991) reported that the REUR correction method also has limitations for high-frequency hearing loss configurations, when ITE-IROS fittings are employed. The premise of the REUR correction procedure is that the patient's REUR will not be present when the hearing aid is fitted. That is, the real ear occluded response (REOR) will be at or below the input to the hearing aid. In an IROS fitting, however, a portion of the REUR usually remains; and therefore, the relationship between the REUR and REIG is not as straightforward as in a closed-mold fitting.

Mueller and Bryant (1991) examined the relationship between the REUR and REIG for ITE-IROS hearing aids by fitting 38 individuals with the same ITE hearing aid using a fixed volume control wheel (VCW) setting. Figure 9–5 illustrates the mean change in the REIG as a function of the REUR. Notice that, for 2000 Hz, a clear trend is present. As REUR values increase from less than 5 dB to over 20 dB, mean REIG *decreases* in a systematic manner. A

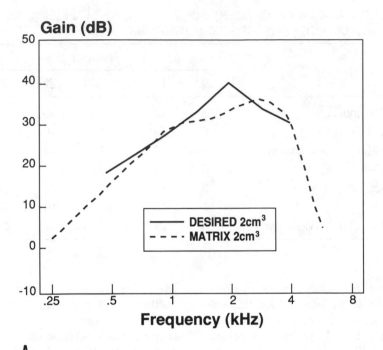

A

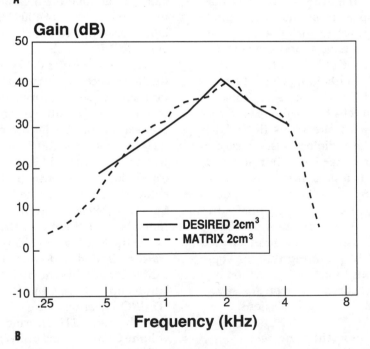

B

Figure 9–4. Panel A: Comparison of the previously selected matrix 2-cm³ response to the revised NAL desired coupler gain (see Table 9–5). Panel B: Comparison of the revised NAL desired coupler gain to a different matrix 2-cm³ response, which appears to be more appropriate.

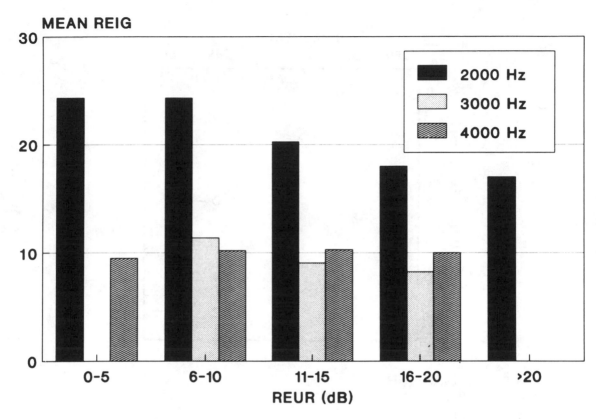

Figure 9–5. The relationship between real ear insertion gain (REIG) and the real ear unaided response (REUR) for 2000, 3000, and 4000 Hz for patients fitted with ITE-IROS hearing aids. (Reprinted from Mueller, H., & Bryant, M. 1991. Some commonly overlooked uses of probe microphone measurements. *Seminars in Hearing, 12,* 73–91, with permission.)

similar, although not as prominent, trend appears to be present for 3000 Hz. **For 4000 Hz, however, there is no significant relationship between the patient's REUR and REIG.** Mueller and Bryant wrote that even though a significant relationship was present between the REUR and REIG for 2000 and 3000 Hz, there was not a 1:1 change in the REIG. Roughly, a 2:1 inverse relationship was present. That is, a 10 dB *increase* in the REUR resulted in a 5 dB *decrease* in REIG. These findings suggest that it **might be difficult in some cases to apply REUR corrections when fitting ITE-IROS hearing aids**.

As mentioned earlier, there are cases when it simply is best to ignore an unusual REUR when calculating desired 2-cm³ prescriptive gain. For example, consider the patient whose audiogram and REUR are illustrated in Figure 9–6.

Regardless of what prescriptive fitting is utilized, the goal of this fitting would be to minimize REIG at 1500 and 2000 Hz and maximize REIR at 3000 and 4000 Hz. Note, however, that the REUR for this patient is at least 10 dB greater than average in the 2000 Hz region. Would it be wise to request an additional 10 dB of 2-cm³ coupler gain for this patient when ordering the hearing aid? Probably not, as it is likely that even without the correction, the REIG at 2000 Hz will exceed the prescriptive target.

The patient whose audiogram and REUR are shown in Figure 9–7 represents another situation when it might not be best to use the unusual REUR for 2-cm³ coupler corrections. Note that this hearing loss would result in prescriptive target gain that is greatest in the 3000–4000

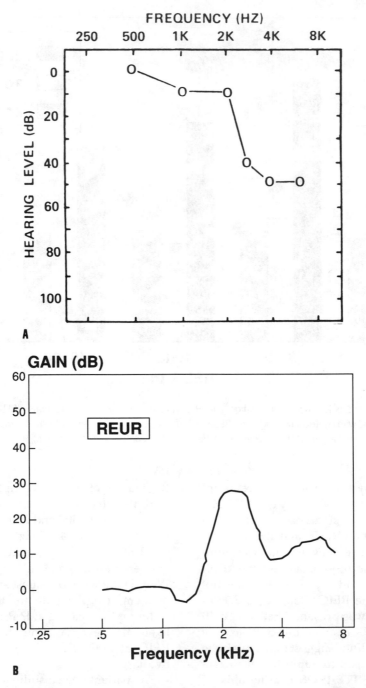

Figure 9–6. Audiogram (Panel A) and real ear unaided response (REUR) (Panel B) for a sample patient needing calculation of appropriate 2-cm³ coupler gain.

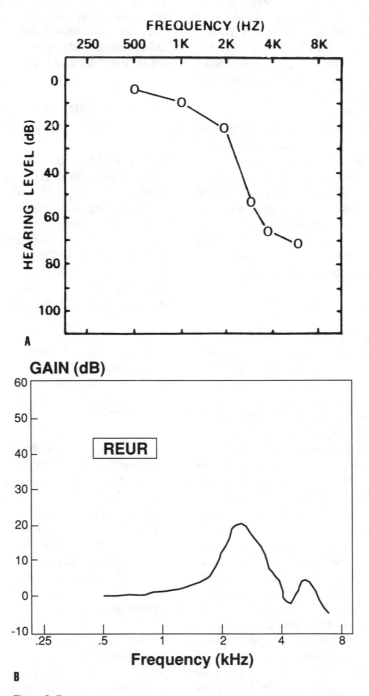

Figure 9–7. Audiogram (Panel A) and real ear unaided response (REUR) (Panel B) for a sample patient needing calculation of appropriate 2-cm³ coupler gain.

Hz region and, given that the hearing loss is only 65 dB for 4000 Hz, it is possible to make speech audible for this frequency. Consider, however, that this person's REUR for 4000 Hz is 0 dB, or about 12 dB less than average. Would it be wise to request 12 dB *less* 2-cm^3 coupler gain for this patient? Probably not, as exceeding prescriptive target gain at 4000 Hz rarely is a problem. In fact, **this person could be one of the few patient's for whom prescriptive target gain at 4000 Hz actually is achieved!**

These examples illustrate that **REUR corrections need to be considered on a case-by-case basis**, with consideration of the audiogram, prescriptive target gain, and limitations of ITE and ITC hearing aid circuitry. These variables often are not accounted for in the automated programs that facilitate these corrections.

Potential Measurement Error

If the REUR correction method is used, and difference values from the average REUR are applied, it is important to be **aware of potential errors that might be introduced due to procedural variables**. Some probe-microphone equipment has average (KEMAR) REUR values stored in memory, and the equipment will calculate REUR difference values for a given patient. It is important to know, however, what average REUR values are stored in the equipment that you are using. Most published REUR average data are referenced to the center of the head using the substitution method with a loudspeaker positioned at 0° azimuth (see Shaw, 1974 and Burkhard & Sachs, 1975). Using a modified-pressure method will result in slightly different REURs, and these values will vary as a result of the location of the reference microphone and loudspeaker azimuth (see Chapter 4). The measurement procedure used to establish a patient's REUR, therefore, easily could influence whether a REUR was judged as average. Fikret-Pasa and Revit (1992) suggested that a possible solution would be to have average-ear data available for the particular measurement method used (e.g., REURs measured with a KEMAR using your own equip-

ment) or to sample one's own group of patients and develop an "average" REUR. Another solution would be to use the individual's REUR in combination with another measure, as discussed in the following section.

CORRECTIONS USING THE REUR AND RECD

Rather than just using the REUR, as described above, it is possible to individualize the hearing aid order further by calculating the RECD (see Chapters 3 and 12). The REUR and RECD values then can be used with a prescriptive fitting approach. When ordering custom ITE hearing aids, the **REUR-RECD procedure**, as described by Punch, Chi, & Patterson (1990), **has two advantages over the average-REUR difference procedure described previously:**

■ Using the REUR directly eliminates the errors associated with comparison to an average REUR.
■ The RECD measurement eliminates the errors associated with using an average CORFIG.

The only apparent limitations of this procedure are that it requires more time than simply conducting an REUR, a supply of stock hearing aids with known 2-cm^3 values must be maintained, and the type of hearing aid (style, venting and microphone location) that is used for the RECD measurement should be the same as the hearing aid that will be fitted to the patient.

A protocol for using the REUR-RECD correction procedure, modified from Punch et al. (1990) is as follows:

1. Determine desired REIG values using a prescriptive fitting approach.
2. Measure the patient's REUR and REAR, then calculate the *REIR* using a hearing aid that is similar to the one that will be ordered (set the VCW to a mid position).
3. Remove the hearing aid and, without changing the VCW position, measure the 2-cm^3

coupler gain using the same input intensity that was used to measure the REAR.

4. Subtract the *REIR* from the 2-cm³ coupler gain, which will provide the customized CORFIG.
5. Add the CORFIG to the prescribed target REIG, which will yield the desired 2-cm³ coupler values for a use-gain setting.
6. Add reserve gain (e.g., 10 dB).
7. Use calculated 2-cm³ coupler values to select the desired matrix, or provide the manufacturer with actual 2-cm³ coupler values for circuit selection.

The above protocol (see Chapter 13 for more details) differs procedurally from that of **Punch et al. (1990), who recommended subtracting the RECD from the target REIG and adding the REUR. The same values will be obtained using either method**, although to understand both methods it is helpful to conduct the calculations using both for several cases.

An example of the REUR-RECD correction procedure is shown in Table 9–6, which again is based on the same patient as illustrated in Tables 9–3 and 9–5. Observe that in this instance, the values obtained using this type of correction are similar to the those for the REUR method; this is because this patient's RECD was close to average. Fikret-Pasa and Revit (1992) reported that RECDs were significantly different from average for 9 of the 18 ears tested in their study, including all ears with a his-

tory of conductive pathology. This finding emphasizes the importance of including RECD measurements in the test protocol when individualizing the hearing aid order.

CORRECTIONS USING THE RECD

The corrections that have been described using the REUR alone or the REUR and the RECD are designed to assist in achieving the prescriptive target REIG. Revit (1991d), suggests that **the individual's REUR might not be a relevant measure for the fitting of hearing aids**. He contended that, if prescription target REIG is based on earphone measures, which have an implied average-REUR reference, then the appropriate REUR to use when REIG measurements are made is the average REUR rather than the individual REUR. If this is so, then it is not necessary to correct for individual REUR variations. **Revit (1991d) recommended that the desired 2-cm³ coupler gain be determined by combining the prescriptive target REIG, the *average* REUR, the *measured* RECD, and the reserve gain** (plus any anticipated alteration due to earmold effects or microphone location).

Revit (1991d) summarizes his individualized selection procedure as follows:

The real ear **aided** response, not the real-ear insertion-gain response, is what is crucial to determining a proper fit. The suggested protocol accounts for

TABLE 9–6. CALCULATION OF DESIRED FULL-ON 2-CM³ COUPLER GAIN USING THE NAL PRESCRIPTIVE METHOD WITH REUR/RECD INDIVIDUAL CORRECTIONS

	Frequency (Hz)					
	.5k	*1k*	*1.5k*	*2k*	*3k*	*4k*
Pure-tone thresholds	35	40	45	45	50	50
Prescribed REIG (re: NAL)	9	19	21	19	20	20
Individual CORFIG (2-cm³ gain-REIG)	3	−4	2	11	3	2
Desired 2-cm³ at use VCW	12	15	23	30	23	22
Reserve gain	10	10	10	10	10	10
Desired full-on 2-cm³ coupler gain	22	25	33	40	33	32

the fact that earphone audiometry is based on an implied average REUR, and so the most defensible way to apply a fitting formula based on earphone audiometry would be to maintain the same implied reference throughout. If a correction for the individual REUR is desired, care should be taken to include the individual REUR in the entire process, either by evaluating the hearing loss in the soundfield, or by applying a "corrected" correction. (p. 11)

SELECTION OF SSPL90

This chapter has focused on various methods used to individualize the desired 2-cm^3 coupler response for ITE hearing aid fittings for the purpose of attaining target prescriptive gain. This is not to suggest, however, that it is not equally important to use probe-microphone measurement for individual selection of SSPL90. **Chapter 7 described a step-by-step method in which 2-cm^3 coupler values for desired SSPL90 can be reliably obtained for frequency specific LDLs** (Valente et al., 1991, described a similar procedure). These calculated SSPL90 values should be used jointly with the desired 2-cm^3 prescriptive gain when a matrix response is selected for a given individual.

CONCLUSIONS

At one time, it was not uncommon for audiologists to conduct testing with two, three, or more hearing aids at the time of the hearing aid evaluation. Today, hearing aid evaluations usually are conducted with only one instrument — the one that was custom ordered for the patient. In order to minimize failures during this verification process, **the efforts previously expended during the selection procedure now must be shifted to communicating the desired electroacoustic characteristics to the manufacturer via the hearing aid order.** Prefitting probe-microphone measurements offer a method for the audiologist to individualize the ordering procedure.

To date, research has not been conducted on a large number of subjects to determine if one custom hearing aid ordering procedure is superior to another. Work by Palmer (1992), with a limited number of subjects, suggests that the same correction procedure might not be best for all patients. It is reasonable to conclude, however, that the audiologist, rather than the manufacturer, is best able to determine the appropriate 2-cm^3 coupler response, and probe-microphone measurements are helpful in making this determination.

CHAPTER 10

Assessment of Fitting Arrangements, Special Circuitry, and Features

■ H. GUSTAV MUELLER, Ph.D. ■
■ DAVID B. HAWKINS, Ph.D. ■

In Chapters 6 and 7 we focused on the use of probe-microphone measurements for the selection and verification of real ear insertion gain (REIR) and the real ear saturation response (RESR). While these applications are the most common uses of probe-microphone technology, real ear observations of special performance features or fittings also are an important, and sometimes overlooked, use of probe-microphone instrumentation. It is somewhat **paradoxical that many hearing aids are fitted specifically because they have a given electroacoustic feature, yet the effectiveness of this feature is never tested formally while the patient is wearing the hearing aid**. This chapter

reviews how probe-microphone measurements can be used to assess the performance of different hearing aid fitting arrangements and to verify features such as directional microphones, compression circuitry, and automatic signal processing. Also discussed are the clinical applications when using probe-microphone measurements for fitting digitally programmable hearing aids, and when conducting other measures related to the hearing aid fitting.

HEARING AID ARRANGEMENTS

There are two different fitting arrangements which can be differentiated from the fitting of a single hearing aid: binaural and a CROS–BI-CROS system. Fortunately, for most audiologists, binaural amplification is now considered *the standard* hearing aid fitting; however, it is sometimes necessary to objectively evaluate the advantage provided. CROS and BICROS fittings also present a situation that requires a modification of the routine verification procedure. There are useful applications of probe-microphone measurements for both of these types of fitting arrangements.

BINAURAL HEARING AID FITTINGS

For the most part, as far as probe-microphone measurements are concerned, a binaural fitting simply is the process of conducting two separate monaural fittings (some fitting methods do prescribe slightly less gain for binaural: see Chapter 5). There are some unique uses of probe-microphone measurements, however, that have the greatest application for binaural fittings.

Aided Symmetry

It is generally believed that binaural fittings will be **most successful if the *aided* thresholds between ears for the speech frequencies are within 15 dB**. Success is moderate when the differences between ears in aided thresholds are 15–30 dB, and when interaural differences exceed 30 dB success reportedly is limited (Davis & Haggard, 1982; Mueller & Hawkins, 1990). At the conclusion of a binaural fitting, therefore, it is useful to consider the resulting aided thresholds to determine if the desired symmetry has been obtained. This can be accomplished by conducting aided thresholds in the soundfield; however, if REIRs already have been obtained, then one can simply subtract the real ear insertion gain (REIG) values from the unaided earphone thresholds to obtain an estimate of aided thresholds (see Mueller, Cuttie, & Shaw, 1990, for an example of this procedure). These estimates will be reasonably close to true aided thresholds.

Head Shadow Effect

Another use of probe-microphone measurements in binaural fittings relates more to patient education than the selection of specific hearing aid parameters. **One of the primary benefits of binaural amplification is the elimination of the head shadow effect** (Mueller & Hawkins, 1990). When only a single ear is fitted, the important high-frequency components of speech presented from the side of the unaided ear can be attenuated by 10–15 dB or more before reaching the hearing aid microphone of the aided ear. This attenuation effect is especially significant in monaural fittings whenever the hearing loss in the unaided ear is 35–45 dB HL or greater; since level will cause the average high-frequency speech sounds to be inaudible. If a hearing aid is fitted to both ears, the head shadow effect is no longer a problem unless there is a sizeable asymmetry in aided thresholds.

Probe-microphone measurements provide an excellent method to illustrate graphically the head shadow effect (and its elimination) to the patient considering the use of binaural hearing aids. To conduct these measures, it is necessary to use the substitution method, since with the modified-pressure method the regulating microphone will cause the equipment to try to correct the very effect that is being measured. The patient is positioned so that the loudspeaker is presenting the signal at either a 90° or 270° azimuth, and the probe-tube microphone is located at the opposite side of the head. Using this method it is possible to graphically demonstrate to the patient the attenuation effect of the head, and the advantage that is obtained by using a second hearing aid (see Chapter 12, Figure 12–6, for an example of this measurement). This method, in fact, is one of the only ways in a clinical setting to demonstrate objectively to the patient the advantage of a binaural fitting.

CROS AND BICROS

The traditional CROS or BICROS fitting is designed for someone with one unaidable ear and normal or aidable hearing in the other ear. A microphone is placed on the side of the head with the unaidable ear, and the input is then transferred to the good or better ear. The degree of gain provided to the better ear may be minimal (CROS with open-ear fitting) or more substantial (e.g., power BICROS). One of the primary objectives of these types of fittings, especially the minimal-gain CROS, is to provide the patient with better hearing for sounds originating from their bad side by eliminating the head shadow effect.

There are two ways in which probe-microphone measurements can be used in conjunction with a CROS or BICROS fitting. First, these measures can be used simply **to determine if the hearing aid is working appropriately, that is, if sounds from the bad side are being transferred to the aided ear**. It is sometimes difficult for patients to reliably report that a CROS hear-

ing aid is functioning, especially if their hearing in the aided ear is at or near normal. By positioning the patient so that the input to the hearing aid is directly toward their bad ear (azimuth of 90° or 270°), and placing the probe microphone in the aided ear, it is possible to quickly determine if the CROS or BICROS system is functioning as desired. Figure 10–1 illustrates typical probe-microphone measurements obtained for a CROS fitting. In this figure, the patient's real ear unaided response (REUR) for the right ear (obtained with the loudspeaker at a 270° azimuth off to the left side) is compared to the real ear aided response (REAR) obtained when the CROS hearing aid was fitted and adjusted to a use gain setting. Notice that the 270° azimuth REUR falls around 0 dB for this patient. This is because there is a cancellation between the external ear resonance and the head shadow effect. The REAR for the CROS instru-

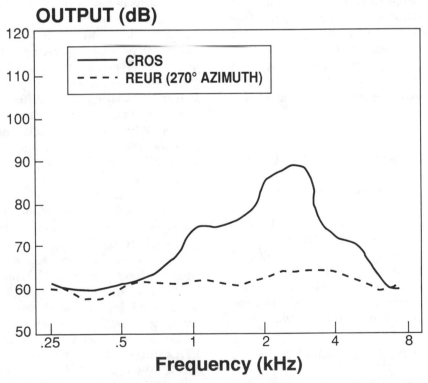

Figure 10–1. Output from a CROS-type hearing aid (stimulus presented to microphone side) compared to the patient's real ear unaided response (REUR) conducted at the same azimuth.

ment illustrates that the hearing aid is working as expected and that for this listening arrangement, an enhancement of the signal of 20–25 dB in the 2000 Hz range was obtained. This same technique also can be used to evaluate the off-side microphone for a BICROS fitting (see Mueller & Bryant, 1991).

Rather than simply using probe-micrphone measurements to determine if a CROS or BI-CROS system is working, it is possible to use these measurements to help determine if the desired REIR or REAR has been obtained. In general, prescriptive gain targets apply to CROS or BICROS fittings in much the same way as they apply to more conventional fitting arrangements.

An interesting application to consider is the fitting of a CROS hearing aid to someone who has excellent hearing in the aided ear — a situation in which the prescriptive target REIG is at or near 0 dB. **For this type of CROS fitting, one approach would be to use the patient's REUR obtained at 0° or 45° azimuth as the target for the real-ear aided signal delivered to that ear** *(the REAR)*, **but presented from a 270° azimuth** (Hawkins, Foley, Stelmachowicz, & New, 1992). It is necessary to use the substitution method of equalization when these measurements are conducted (see Chapter 3).

SPECIAL HEARING AID CIRCUITRY

Many hearing aids are selected and fitted because of their special circuitry. Until recently, it often was necessary for the audiologist to rely on the manufacturer's specifications or 2-cm^3 coupler measurements to assess the value of these features. A significant advantage of probe-microphone measurements is that this circuitry can now be systematically evaluated while the patient is wearing the hearing instrument.

DIRECTIONAL MICROPHONES

One type of special hearing aid feature that might be selected by the audiologist is a direc-

tional microphone. In the late 1970s, approximately 20% of all hearing aids dispensed in the United States contained a directional microphone. Today, partially due to the popularity of the smaller custom ITE instruments, the market share is much smaller. Surprisingly, even when a BTE is fitted, few audiologists presently select an instrument with a directional microphone. This fact is difficult to understand because nearly all research with directional microphones has shown that these hearing aids are superior to their omnidirectional counterparts (see Mueller, 1981, and Mueller & Hawkins, 1990, for review). In two recent studies, Jerger, Johnson, and Smith-Farach (1989) showed an advantage to using directional microphones in conjunction with compression, and Schum (1990) reported that directional microphones provided the same magnitude of benefit for understanding speech in noise as the newer automatic signal-processing systems.

The directional microphone hearing aid is designed to amplify acoustic signals originating from the front of the user to a greater degree than stimuli arriving from the rear quadrants. **When a directional hearing aid is fitted, therefore, it is necessary to determine if indeed the hearing aid is differentially sensitive to incoming signals from different azimuths.** While 2-cm^3 coupler measurements provide little or no information regarding the microphone's directionality, directional effects can be easily evaluated using a probe-microphone system.

A reasonable estimate of the directivity of a given hearing aid on a user's ear can be determined by conducting comparative REAR measurements. The first REAR is conducted with the loudspeaker at 0° azimuth. The patient is then rotated 180° and a second REAR is obtained for the same signal, now originating from behind the patient. For the standard nondirectional BTE instrument, the two REAR curves should be essentially identical. (Beck, 1983, reported that some nondirectional BTEs actually were most sensitive to sounds originating from *behind the user* — a condition we would not wish on our patients who are hearing impaired, or even people with normal hearing.)

When front-to-back REARs are compared for a directional microphone instrument, the 180 degree curve should fall 10–20 dB below that for the 0° signal, at least for the lower frequencies. **The amount of attenuation, however, varies among hearing aid manufacturers, hearing aid models, and earmold coupling systems; therefore, assessment of each individual fitting is important.**

An example of a BTE hearing aid with a good directional microphone design is illustrated in Figure 10–2. In Figure 10–2A, observe that the REAR for the 180° azimuth falls as much as 25 dB below the REAR obtained when the signal was presented from in front of the patient. These measurements were obtained with the loudspeaker positioned 0.5 m from the hearing aid user. The directional effect does diminish as a function of distance, as illustrated in Figure 10–2B. These REARs were obtained for the same hearing aid and gain setting with the patient seated 2 m from the sound source. The directional effect also will decrease to some extent in reverberation (Hawkins & Yacullo, 1984). While Figure 10–2 represents testing conducted in a sound suite, to enhance face validity the same measurements can be conducted in rooms with different reverberation characteristics.

Directional microphones have never enjoyed much popularity with custom ITE instruments. Presently, very few ITE manufacturers even offer the directional microphone as an option. One or two companies report success with this microphone arrangement, however, and an example of this construction is shown in Figure 10–3. Note the two inlet ports to the microphone, which is how the directional effect is accomplished.

Some manufacturers who do not offer a directional-microphone ITE hearing aid state simply that there is not a demand for this type of instrument from audiologists, which probably is true. This might be due in part to the notion that the microphone location of the ITE style hearing aid provides a directional effect and therefore, a directional microphone is not needed. A deep-seated ITE or in-the-canal (ITC) instrument does indeed provide a directional effect, as can be evaluated with comparative 0° and 180° REARs. As shown in Figure 10–4, a 0° versus 180° degree REAR difference or this low-profile ITE; however, there is no directional effect for the lower frequencies where the spectrum of background noise is the greatest. There is a minimal REAR difference present for the higher frequencies, presumably the result of pinna diffraction. For comparison purposes, the same patient was fitted with a directional microphone ITE hearing aid with similar gain characteristics. Figure 10–5 illustrates the REAR differences present for this instrument. The low frequency directional effects are not as great as shown earlier for the BTE hearing aid, but the potential for an improved signal-to-noise ratio for the patient clearly is present.

The examples shown effectively illustrate how a feature such as directional microphones can be evaluated rather precisely using probe-microphone measurements. **It is unlikely that the directional microphone effect would easily be detected using functional gain or soundfield speech audiometry, and 2-cm³ coupler measures do not represent real-ear or everyday listening situations.**

ACTIVE TONE CONTROL

For the past few years, hearing aids have been available with active tone control circuitry. Using a screwdriver controlled potentiometer, it is possible for the audiologist to make substantial changes in the slope of the hearing aid's frequency response at the time of the fitting. Probe-microphone measurements allow the audiologist to carefully monitor the real-ear effects of these adjustments, as a relatively minor rotation of the potentiometer dial can cause a 5–10 dB alteration of the low-frequency gain.

Active tone controls have not enjoyed the popularity that they deserve, as until recently,

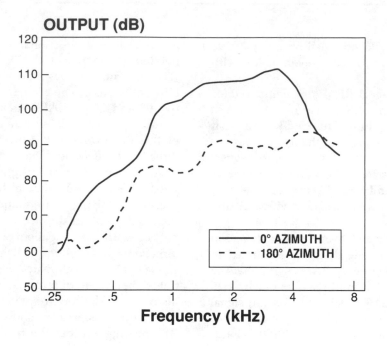

A

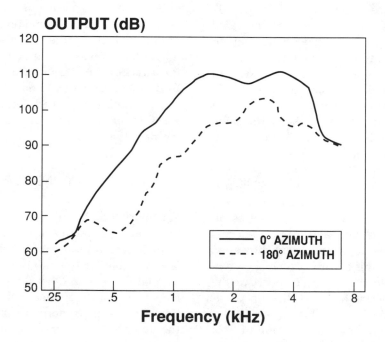

B

Figure 10–2. The real ear aided response (REAR) for a directional microphone hearing aid obtained at a 0° azimuth and at a 180° azimuth. REAR measurements obtained at a distance of 0.5 meters from the signal source (Panel A) and at 2 meters from the signal source (Panel B).

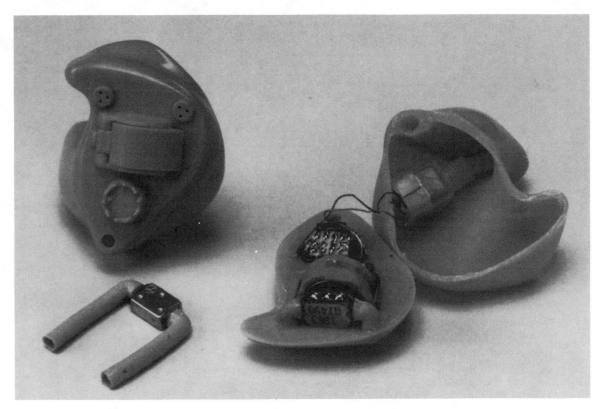

Figure 10–3. Illustration of a directional microphone ITE instrument. (Photo courtesy of Oto-Sonic, Inc.)

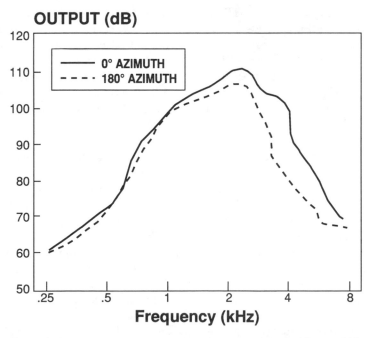

Figure 10–4. Real ear aided response (REAR) measurements at 0° and 180° azimuth for a nondirectional ITE hearing aid.

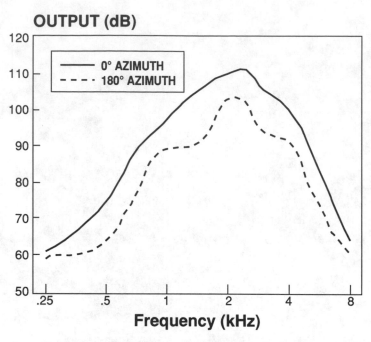

Figure 10-5. Real ear aided response (REAR) measurements at 0° and 180° azimuth for a directional ITE hearing aid.

this circuitry only was available in BTE instruments. **Today's technology, however, allows for combining active tone control circuitry with a Class D amplifier, housed in a small ITE instrument**. The higher frequency resonant peak of the Class D amplifier, coupled with the active tone control, provides an ability to match REIG with prescriptive target gain that previously was not possible with an ITE hearing aid (see review in Chapter 6). Figure 10-6 is an example of the range of REIG that is attainable with this type of circuitry in a ITE hearing aid. The dashed REIR illustrates maximum activation of the tone control circuitry. Clearly, this single ITE instrument could be adjusted to satisfy a wide range of prescriptive gain targets.

AUTOMATIC SIGNAL PROCESSING

In recent years there has been an increased interest in and use of automatic signal-processing (ASP) hearing aids. Traditionally, ASP

hearing aids have been used to reduce gain at high levels. The use of automatic gain control (AGC) rather than peak clipping results in less distortion for high-intensity speech signals. **Newer ASP circuitry has been designed not only for output limiting purposes, but also to alter automatically the gain and frequency response of the instrument**. The general approach has been to automatically vary the hearing aid's electroacoustic characteristics for different types of inputs in a manner that would theoretically improve speech understanding, especially in background noise, for the hearing aid user.

Because of the variety of ASP circuitry available, and the confusion that can occur when these circuits are discussed, Killion, Staab, and Preves (1990) proposed a classification system for these instruments. As shown in Figure 10-7, these authors have recommended that ASP circuitry be classified according to whether the hearing aid has a fixed frequency response or a level-dependent frequency response (LDFR).

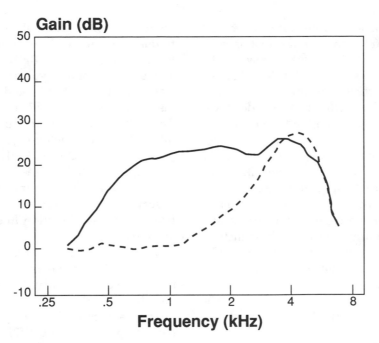

Figure 10–6. Illustration of the variation of real ear insertion gain (REIG) that is available from an ITE hearing aid with an active tone control and a Class D amplifier.

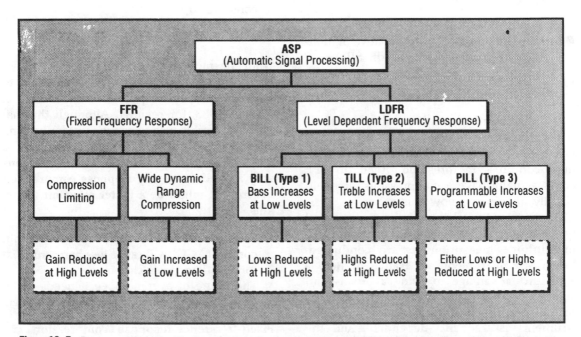

Figure 10–7. Recommended classification of automatic signal processing (ASP) hearing aids. (From Killion, M, Staab, W., & Preves, D. 1990. Classifying automatic signal processors. *Hearing Instruments, 41,* (8), 24–26, with permission.)

The LDFR circuits are further categorized according to the frequency range that is primarily affected: bass increases at low levels (BILL), treble increases at low levels (TILL), or programmable increases at low levels (PILL). A PILL can be either a BILL or a TILL depending on how it is programmed (See Figure 10–7). If this is starting to sound confusing, perhaps this quote from Dave Fabry (1991a, p. 71) will help: "PILL and BILL are just like TILL when they reduce their gain to nil."

Regardless of the acronyms that are used (or abused), probe-microphone measurements provide useful information when these instruments are assessed, especially for the verification of changes in the hearing aid's frequency response.

Procedural Considerations for ASP Instruments

The selection of input level becomes extremely critical whenever compression hearing aids are evaluated. Usually, it is best to measure REIRs or REARs at three different input levels:

- A relatively low level (50 dB SPL).
- A more intense level representative of moderately loud speech (60–70 dB SPL).
- A level intense enough to determine the RESR (90 dB SPL).

It is also important to remember that hearing aid circuitry tolerances are such that a hearing aid with specifications showing an input-compression threshold of 60 dB SPL could actually have a compression threshold slightly above or below this value.

As discussed in Chapter 4, there are several types of inputs that can be used when probe-microphone measurements are conducted. **When ASP instruments are evaluated, there is a distinct advantage to using a broad-band signal**. The sensor that controls the activation of the compression circuit of some AGC instruments is frequency-dependent, and the greatest AGC activation is present where gain is the greatest. Because many AGC instru-

ments have little gain below 1000 Hz, a low-frequency signal will cause little compression to occur. Hence, if an REIR was obtained for an instrument of this type using a pure-tone or warble-tone signal, it would appear that the instrument was a LDFR, more specifically a TILL. This response is an artifact of the probe-microphone test method, commonly referred to as *blooming* (Dolan, 1991; Ely, Curran, & Becker, 1979). If a broad-band signal is used, an appropriate input-output function will be observed, which is representative of how the hearing aid will function in everyday listening environments.

If the blooming artifact is not considered at the time that probe-microphone measurements are conducted, and a warble-tone stimulus is used, the frequency response of the hearing aid could be erroneously judged to have an inappropriate REIR configuration if inputs are used above the compression threshold. Blooming is most commonly observed in output-AGC instruments, but it also might be present with input-AGC, depending on the circuitry that is used and how the hearing aid is constructed.

Fixed Frequency Response ASP

Until the more recent development of LDFR circuits, compression circuitry was limited to fixed frequency responses (see Dillon & Walker, 1983, for review). Although the majority of audiologists continue to order hearing aids that use peak clipping as the method to limit the output, **there are at least two reasons why a fixed frequency response compression instrument might be a better selection** (Hawkins, 1986):

- Output limitation through automatic gain control (AGC) will cause less harmonic distortion than peak clipping.
- The range of average speech needs to be compressed into a narrowed dynamic range.

Fixed-frequency-response compression circuitry, either input or output controlled, can be selected and adjusted so that desired gain can be achieved for a variety of inputs without exceeding the patient's loudness discomfort level (LDL). When compression circuitry is selected, electroacoustic verification of this option becomes part of the hearing aid fitting procedure. To a large extent, this verification can be accomplished through 2-cm^3 measurements. **It usually is desirable, however, to observe these effects on the real ear, which also allows the patient to judge loudness at the same time that the probe-microphone measurements are taken.**

When input compression is present in a hearing aid, REIG is reduced systematically as input to the hearing aid increases, assuming that the threshold for compression has been exceeded. Figure 10–8 shows REIRs for an input compression hearing aid for five different input levels (50–90 dB). As shown, when an input of 90 dB was delivered to this hearing aid, only 10 dB of REIR was present in the 2000–4000 Hz region. As the input to the hearing aid was decreased in 10 dB steps, REIG increased

systematically (the compression knee of this instrument was set at 60–65 dB SPL).

As mentioned earlier, it is considered desirable to use limiting compression, such as output-AGC (AGC-O) rather than peak clipping to control the output of the hearing aid. In these cases, adjustment of the AGC is part of the LDL-RESR verification procedure. Figure 10–9 shows RESRs for a hearing aid that had an on/off control for the AGC-O. Observe that the RESR was lowered by approximately 8 dB when the AGC-O was activated. In many programmable units, the AGC-O can be adjusted in small steps, so that close agreement between the RESR and the patient's LDL can be obtained. Many probe-microphone units offer the option of conducting frequency-specific input-output functions. Figure 10–10 shows the real-ear input-output function at 2000 Hz for the same hearing aid shown in Figure 10–9.

Note in Figure 10–9 that the configuration of the frequency response remains essentially unchanged when the AGC–O is activated, as

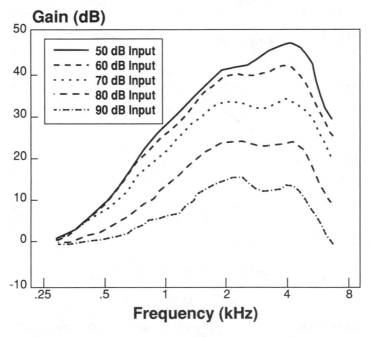

Figure 10–8. Real ear insertion responses (REIRs) for an input-controlled compression instrument for five different input levels.

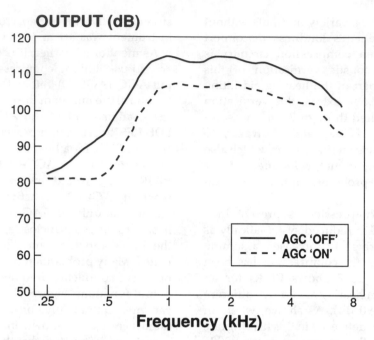

Figure 10–9. The effects of activation of automatic gain control (AGC) output-controlled compression. on the real ear saturation response (RESR).

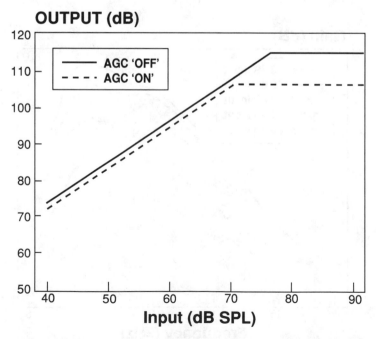

Figure 10–10. The effects of activation of automatic gain control (AGC) output-controlled compression on the real ear saturation response (RESR) at 2000 Hz.

expected for a compression circuit classified as fixed frequency response. If this patient's LDL was below the RESR at only a specific frequency region, such as 1500–2000 Hz, then it might not be desirable to reduce the output for the entire frequency range. As is discussed later, in the newer two- and three-channel programmable hearing aids (LDFR-ASP), it is possible to alter the output and the compression rate at specific frequency regions (this is why a PILL can be either a TILL or a BILL).

Level-Dependent Frequency Response ASP

As reviewed by Fabry (1991a), the use of LDFR circuits is based on the assumptions that:

■ There is no single frequency response that is optimal for every listening situation.
■ Nonlinear amplification should be used to prevent the hearing aid from reaching saturation.

The belief is that speech intelligibility will be maximized when these two assumptions are met using the appropriate circuitry. As mentioned, BILL and TILL (or PILL) are methods that attempt to achieve this goal.

BASS INCREASES FOR LOW LEVELS (BILL). As described by Fabry (1991a), BILL processing is used in the majority of so-called noise-reduction hearing aids, which also have been called adaptive-frequency-response, automatic signal processing, and automatic noise-reduction instruments. For BILL hearing aids, nonlinear amplification is activated by the overall level of background noise or by the intensity level of the noise (or other signals) at a specific frequency region. As the name indicates, the low frequencies are increased at low levels, or, otherwise stated, the low frequencies are decreased at high levels. This reduction in low-frequency amplification to some extent works as an automatic tone control and hence, has the potential to improve speech understanding in low - frequency background noise (Sigelman & Preves, 1987; Stach, Speerschneider, & Jerger, 1987).

One type of BILL hearing aid, the Siemens ASP, grew tremendously in popularity in 1987 and 1988 when it was announced to audiologists and the public (in *Parade Magazine*) that the President of the United States used this type of "noise-reduction" circuitry. This type of ASP circuitry is still commonly used today, with a greater success rate than in earlier years, as patients who can benefit from this type of hearing aid are now more carefully selected. The Argosy Manhattan circuit is another commonly used BILL type processing. Although this circuitry is somewhat different than that of the Siemens ASP, the Manhattan circuit effectively reduces gain in the low frequencies for inputs above 80 dB SPL.

Probe-microphone measurements provide a convenient method to assess the BILL processing in the real ear. Shown in Figure 10–11A are two REIRs for an ASP hearing aid with a 65 dB activation level. Notice that REIG in the low frequencies was reduced by 10–12 dB when the input to the hearing aid was increased to 80 dB. While it is usually best to assess ASP instruments with a composite noise signal, these comparative REIRs were conducted using a swept-warble tone, which at least demonstrate to the audiologist *and* the patient that the ASP circuitry is working appropriately. As shown in Figure 10–11B, **to add face validity to the measurements, it is possible to conduct REIRs with background noises of different levels in the listening environment**; a portable cassette player works well to deliver the noise signal. Another method is to disable the loudspeaker of the probe-microphone system and conduct a spectrum analysis for different inputs — a method described later in this chapter.

TREBLE INCREASES FOR LOW LEVELS (TILL) The only commercially available TILL circuitry is referred to as the K-AMP, and was designed by Killion (1988). **The circuitry is a four-stage amplifier, and was designed to provide the following features** (Killion, 1988a):

■ Substantial gain for low-intensity sounds
■ Decreasing gain for moderate-level sounds

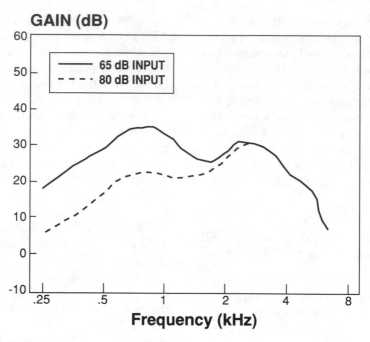

A

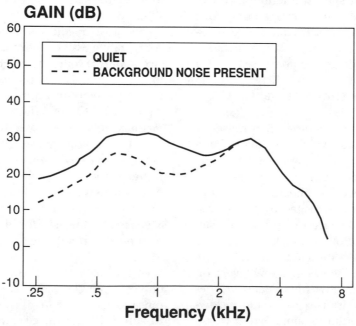

B

Figure 10–11. Real ear insertion response (REIR) measurements for a BILL-type automatic signal processing hearing aid. Results shown for two different input levels (Panel A) and comparative testing in quiet and when background noise was present (Panel B).

■ No gain (but no loss) for intense sounds
■ Compression limiting for the highest level sounds (to prevent peak clipping).

Figure 10–12, from Fabry (1991a), shows hypothetical REIR results that would be obtained from a TILL hearing aid (K-AMP, Figure 10–12A), compared with results from a hearing aid with BILL circuitry (Manhattan circuit, Figure 10–12B). As mentioned earlier, it is important that probe-microphone testing is conducted using several different input levels. For the K-AMP it is recommended that three or four different input levels are used when probe-microphone verification is conducted. This approach will help determine if the four design objectives have been met for the specific instrument that is being fitted.

While all manufacturers essentially use the same K-AMP circuitry, K-AMP hearing aids differ somewhat among manufacturers. Shown in Figure 10–13A are the REIRs (50 dB SPL input) for two different K-AMP hearing aids fitted to the same ear. Gain was adjusted for both instruments to equal 20 dB at 1000 Hz. Observe that the K-AMP hearing aid from manufacturer A provides a somewhat superior high-frequency REIG. Figure 10–13B shows the REIRs for the same two hearing aids (and gain settings) measured with a 90 dB SPL input. Recall that at a 90 dB SPL input the K-AMP hearing aid is designed to provide unity REIG — no gain but no loss. **Probe-microphone measurements offer an excellent method to determine if unity gain has been obtained for a given patient.** Consider, that this feature of the K-AMP hearing aid is directly related to the user's REUR. Figure 10–14 shows the REIRs (90 dB SPL input) for two different patients fitted with the same ITC K-AMP instrument; notice differences of 5 dB or more for some frequencies. These patients had average REURs; however, if someone had an extremely large REUR in the 1500–2000 region, it is probable that negative REIG would be present for that frequency range for a 90 dB input. This could be a reason for rejection of the K-AMP circuitry. It is important, therefore, to evaluate this feature at the time of the hearing aid fitting.

The differences in REIRs between manufacturers (Figure 10–13) could be due in part to the method used to create the acoustic horn effect, a component of the TILL response. Achieving an appropriate horn becomes increasingly difficult as K-AMPs are produced in the smaller ITC style. K-AMP hearing aids soon will be available with active tone-control circuitry, which will allow user-specific adjustment of gain in the lower frequencies. This might lead to more successful fittings of K-AMPs to individuals with high-frequency hearing loss.

PROGRAMMABLE HEARING AIDS

In recent years there has been a substantial increase in the production and use of digitally programmable hearing aids. Presently, this instrumentation is available from 10 or more different manufacturers, and some manufacturers are beginning to offer a complete product line of programmable units (see review by Bentler, 1991). Combining the fitting of programmable hearing aids with probe-microphone measurements has a special appeal to many audiologists. For the first time, especially with ITE and ITC hearing aid fittings, it is possible to make substantial changes in the electroacoustic characteristics of the hearing aid while it is being worn by the patient and simultaneously to measure, with a fair amount of precision, the magnitude of these changes in the ear canal. This puts the audiologist in control of the hearing aid fitting.

Many digitally programmable instruments do not represent new or different circuitry for processing the speech signal, but rather, they provide a digitally controlled method to easily manipulate circuitry that is available in similar nonprogrammable models. Digital control of such features as gain, frequency response slope, SSPL90, and compression threshold is common. For these hearing aids, the same probe-microphone measurement techniques and procedures that already have been discussed for nonprogrammable systems would apply. Sweetow and Mueller (1991a, 1991b) present examples of how probe-microphone measure-

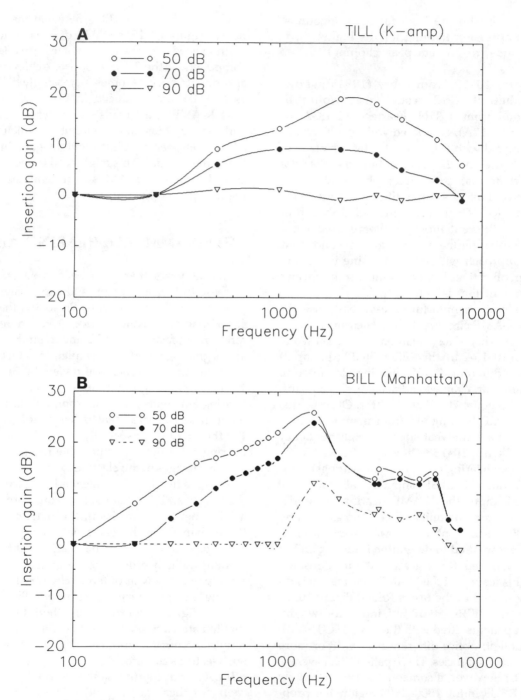

Figure 10–12. Panel A: Hypothetical insertion gain for K-AMP TILL hearing aid for three input levels. Panel B: Hypothetical insertion gain values for BILL-type hearing aid for three input levels. (From Fabry, D. 1991a. Programmable and automatic noise reduction in existing hearing aids. In G. Studebaker, F. Bess, & L. Beck [Eds.], *The Vanderbilt hearing aid report II* (pp. 65–75). Parkton, MD: York Press, with permission.)

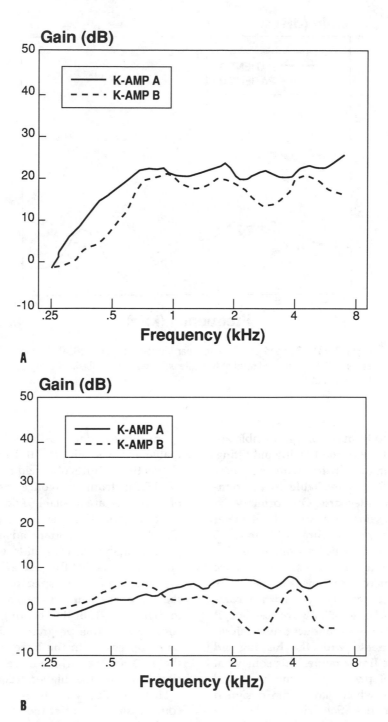

Figure 10–13. Comparison of the real ear insertion response (REIR) of two different K-AMPs fitted to the same person. Results shown for a 50 dB input (Panel A) and for a 90 dB input (Panel B).

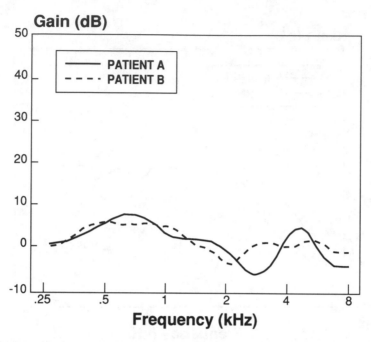

Figure 10–14. Comparison of the real ear insertion response (REIR) for the same K-AMP hearing aid fitted to two different ears. Results obtained using a 90 dB input.

ments can be used to make programmable adjustments at the time of the hearing aid fitting.

Some programmable instruments offer new technology that is not available in the nonprogrammable counterparts. One primary example is compression circuitry, where lower than normal compression thresholds (e.g., 45 dB SPL) and two- or three-channel adjustable compression options can have some influence on how probe-microphone measurements are conducted. **When hearing aids with a compression threshold of 45–55 dB are assessed, it might not be possible to conduct probe-microphone measurements with the hearing aid functioning in its linear mode.** This somewhat limits the use of prescriptive methods and REIR verification, which have been designed for linear instruments. (See Fabry, 1991b, for a review of the compression features of different programmable hearing aids.)

Many programmable instruments offer an adjustment of the hearing aid's frequency response that is not possible with nonprogrammable models. Figure 10–15A, for example, shows three REIRs obtained using a two-channel ITE instrument. Notice that a wide range of responses are available, and also that exceptionally good REIG is present through 4000 Hz. A second important advantage of using programmable hearing aids with more than one channel is that the **ASP effects can be programmed to be user-specific as a function of the frequency band.** As revealed in the REIRs in Figure 10–15B, this hearing aid with input compression was programmed to provide little compression in the lower frequency band (below 1500 Hz), with a more active compression ratio for the higher frequency band.

Hearing aids with two- or three-channel compression also **offer the opportunity for the audiologist to shape the SSPL90 curve or RESR to the patient's LDLs much the same way that the REIR is typically altered to match the prescriptive gain target.** As discussed in

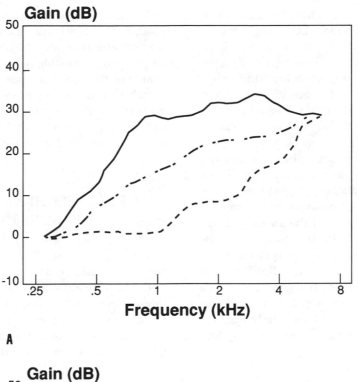

A

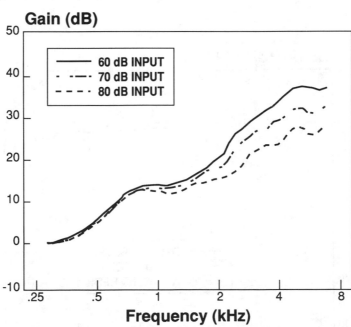

B

Figure 10–15. Panel A: Illustration of the range of real ear insertion gain (REIG) that can be obtained from a two-channel programmable hearing aid. Panel B: Illustration of the frequency-band compression effect that can be obtained from the same programmable hearing aid.

Chapter 3 and Chapter 7, the combined use of the RESR and behavioral LDL judgments allows the audiologist to properly adjust the maximum output of the hearing aid. In some instances, however, a peak in the RESR might exceed the patient's LDL at a specific frequency, although all other frequencies are judged as "Loud, but OK." In a single-channel instrument, it usually is necessary to lower the output for all frequencies, rather than only for a specific frequency range. As shown in Figure 10–16, with a three-channel programmable hearing aid it is possible to adjust one of the frequency bands to surround the area where the RESR exceeds the LDL and then lower the AGC-I threshold for this band. This will result in a lower and more acceptable RESR for this frequency region. Note in Figure 10–16 that the RESR values above and below the 1000–2500 Hz region are unchanged; hence, the overall dynamic range of the amplified speech signal is improved.

As the sophistication of the circuitry of programmable units increases, so will the reliance on probe-microphone measurements. For example, programmable hearing aids are already available that offer the user the capability to switch among four or more stored responses, each with different gain, power, and compression settings, require a well-thought-out fitting strategy and careful verification procedure.

RELATED HEARING AID MEASUREMENTS

In addition to the REIR, REAR, and RESR measurements used to assess the appropriateness of the hearing aid's electroacoustic characteristics or the functioning of special circuitry, there are several other measurements that can be conducted using probe-microphones at the time of the hearing aid fitting.

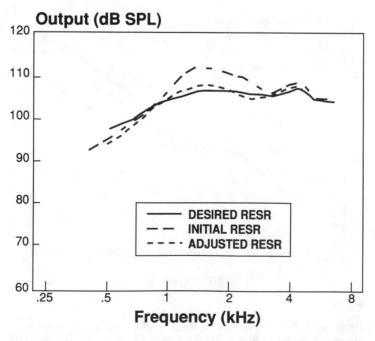

Figure 10–16. Comparative real ear saturation responses (RESRs) showing the ability to adjust the center band of a three-channel programmable instrument so that a match can be obtained between the RESR and the patient's loudness discomfort level (LDL).

HARMONIC DISTORTION

Harmonic distortion measured in a 2-cm³ coupler has long been an element of American National Standards Institute (ANSI) standards of hearing aid performance. Hearing aids that have excessive harmonic distortion are considered unacceptable, although it is not clearly known how much harmonic distortion is necessary to degrade speech intelligibility or even speech quality.

On occasion, however, patients report that distortion is present in a hearing aid when 2-cm³ coupler distortion values are low. This brings up the question of whether there is a hearing aid–real-ear interaction that could cause harmonic distortion in the ear canal from an otherwise nondistorting hearing aid. Although this would seem unlikely, it points out the practical appeal of conducting probe-microphone harmonic distortion measurements, and at least one or two probe-micro-phone systems offer this feature. The measurements are conducted in a similar manner as the REAR, and distortion values (1st and 2nd harmonic and total distortion) across frequencies are graphically displayed.

Few data are available regarding the reliability and validity of using probe-microphone equipment to make real-ear harmonic distortion measurements. Grimes and Mueller (1988) compared 2-cm³ coupler harmonic distortion to real ear distortion for nine BTE hearing aids using a Rastronics 10/3 probe-microphone system. Using the same VCW settings and input level, they reported that for all instruments, total harmonic distortion was 9–15% higher than coupler values when measured in the real ear. When a single hearing aid was measured in eight different ears, significantly different total harmonic distortion values were obtained, but only the low frequencies. The authors attributed this finding to variances in the amount of low-frequency gain, which caused a steep REIR slope in some cases. Of interest, Grimes and Mueller (1988) reported that when distortion values were calculated for the REUR of 12 ears, mean total harmonic distortion was 8%. This finding complicates the interpretation of the real-ear distortion values obtained with the

hearing aids. While real-ear harmonic distortion values are intriguing, and potentially could yield useful information, **we do not recommend that these measurements be used as a qualitative judgment of hearing aid performance until further reliability and validity data are available**.

REAL-EAR SPECTRUM ANALYSIS

In this context, *spectrum analysis* refers to the use of the probe-microphone system to analyze signals other than those produced by the equipment itself. Several probe-microphone systems have this option. By disabling the loudspeaker of the system (either through the software or by manually unhooking the speaker wires), recorded or live speech and environmental sounds, processed by the hearing aid, can be analyzed in the ear canal. A graphic representation of various amplified sounds can then be displayed.

There are two primary applications of using this type of probe-microphone measurement. First, if the audiologist is interested in how the hearing aid will respond in everyday listening conditions, this environment can be simulated in the clinic. The gain that is produced for speech or specific environmental sounds can be measured, or, speech and noise can be analyzed simultaneously.

A second application of this procedure is patient education. As described by Revit (1991b), speech sounds such as the [f] and [s] can be analyzed and compared, which is helpful in describing to the hearing aid user why he or she has problems discriminating between words containing these sounds. Environmental sounds or specific speech signals which might be annoying to the patient also can be measured, graphically displayed, and discussed. In general, **this approach fits nicely with the hearing aid orientation, as the spectrum analysis display is helpful in explaining the overall fitting rationale and potential problems**.

OCCLUSION EFFECT

Historically, the occlusion effect was associated with bone conduction audiometry. Studies have shown that when the ear is occluded with headphones, bone conducted signals in the 250 to 500 Hz range are enhanced by 15–20 dB (Hodgson & Tillman, 1966). Hearing aids and earmolds also cause occlusion, and in some cases the occlusion effect will prevent otherwise satisfied patients from using their hearing aids. Using a bone-conduction oscillator to present signals to the contralateral ear, Wimmer (1986) reported that the occlusion effect caused by earmolds was similar to that caused by headphones. Using probe-microphone equipment, Mueller and Bright (1992) studied the occlusion effect caused by hearing aids when the subjects vocalized the vowel /ee/ at 80 dB SPL. They reported a 13–15 dB occlusion effect for this speech sound at 250, 500 *and* 1000 Hz. These authors also reported that the occlusion effect does not vary significantly among subjects with different-sized ear canals. This suggests that nearly everyone fitted with hearing aids potentially could experience the occlusion effect.

The occlusion effect is the most annoying to hearing aid wearers when they talk or chew hard food (nacho-flavored Doritos have been reported to be especially bothersome). It also is particularly noticeable if the hearing aid user has relatively normal hearing for the frequencies of 500 Hz and below. Killion (1988b) discussed different methods to help eliminate, or at least reduce the occlusion effect:

■ Create a vent that is large enough to reduce the low frequency buildup of energy.
■ Use a Macrae vent (a two-stage acoustic filter that helps to reduce the feedback caused by venting).
■ Use a deep ear canal fitting.

Killion (1988b) also comments, however, that a common treatment of the problem is to tell the hearing aid user "Just wear it for a while and you'll get used to it." **One reason that occlusion-related complaints from hearing aid users were not always treated effectively in the past was that it was not possible easily to quantify the effect.**

Probe-microphone equipment has made measurement of the occlusion effect relatively simple. The following procedures can be used with most probe-microphone equipment to conduct these measures:

1. Disable the loudspeaker of system, either through the system's software or by unhooking the speaker wires.
2. Place the probe-tube in the open ear canal 25–30 mm from the tragal notch.
3. Have the patient vocalize; vowels such as /ee/ produce the greatest effect.
4. It is best to have the patient monitor the intensity of the vocalization; an inexpensive sound level meter works well for this purpose.
5. When the patient is producing the sound at the desired intensity (e.g., 80 dB SPL), conduct the open-ear (baseline) measure.
6. Place the hearing aid or earmold in the ear and repeat the above steps; usually the measurement is made with the hearing aid turned off.
7. The difference between the two measures is the occlusion effect.

Using the above procedure, it is possible to determine if a significant occlusion effect is present, and whether modifications are effective in eliminating or reducing the effect. Figure 10–17, from Revit (1991c), shows the decrease in the occlusion effect that can be obtained by enlarging the vent of an earmold. Shown is the spectrum of Larry's own voice, an /ee/sound, measured in the ear canal while he is wearing either a pin-hole or a medium vented earmold. Notice that the vent enlargement decreased the intensity of the speech in the ear canal by 10 dB at 250 Hz. If an open-ear response is first obtained, then the amount of occlusion that still remains also can be measured. Usually, however, it is not possible totally to eliminate the occlusion effect through venting, as the vent must be so large (e.g., a tube fitting using 2 mm tubing) that acoustic feedback is encountered which prevents the patient from obtaining the desired gain from the hearing aid.

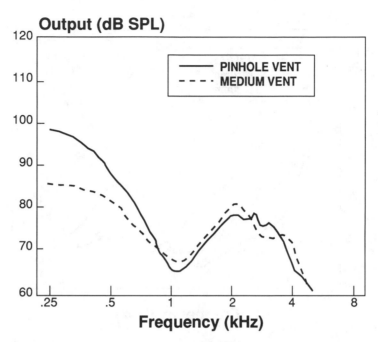

Figure 10–17. Measurement of the occlusion effect caused by a hearing aid earmold. The results shown illustrate the reduction in the occlusion effect that can be obtained by enlarging the vent size. (From Revit, L. 1991c. My voice sounds like it's in a barrel. *Larry's Corner*, Autumn, with permission.)

An alternative method of reducing the occlusion effect is to use long, deep-fitting canals on the earmold or ITE hearing aid. There are several reports concerning the effectiveness of this approach (e.g., Bryant, Mueller, & Northern, 1991; Killion, 1988; Orchick, 1990; Staab & Finlay, 1991). Figure 10–18A shows the open-ear response for the /ee/ sound (80 dB SPL) compared with the occlusion effect caused by standard earmolds with canal lengths of 10 mm and 20 mm. Observe that the earmold with the 10 mm canal length caused an occlusion effect of 20 dB for some frequencies. A substantial reduction in the occlusion effect occurred when the canal length was extended by 10 mm, although 5–10 dB of occlusion remained.

A special kind of earmold using minimal contact technology (MCT) is designed to reduce the occlusion effect by only making limited contact with the cartilaginous portion of the ear canal, and sealing around the perimeter at its medial tip. Figure 10–18B shows measurements similar to those displayed in Figure 10–18A, except that these comparisons were obtained using MCT earmolds. Note that, again, a significant difference was present between the 10 mm and 20 mm lengths; however, in Figure 10–18B **the occlusion effect was essentially eliminated when the 20 mm MCT earmold was used** (the reason that the occlusion measurements fall *below* the open ear response for the 3000 Hz region is that the ear canal resonance has been altered — these measurements were taken with the hearing aid turned off).

It is now possible easily to measure the occlusion effect caused by earmolds or hearing aids. These measurements are helpful in substantiating patient complaints and validating the effectiveness of venting or canal length alterations.

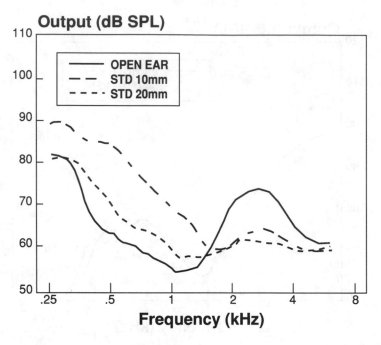

A

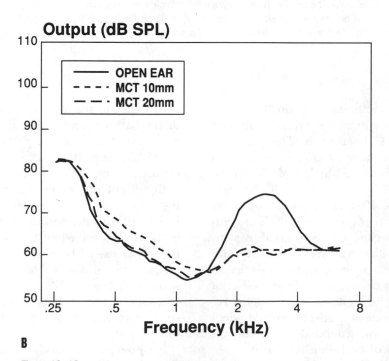

B

Figure 10–18. Measurement of the occlusion effect caused by earmolds as a function of the length of the earmold ear canal. Results are shown for standard (STD) earmolds (Panel A) and for earmolds constructed using minimal contact technology (MCT) (Panel B).

CONCLUSIONS

There are many uses of probe-microphone measurements which go beyond simply determining if the REIR or REAR agrees with a prescriptive fitting technique. In some instances, these measurements allow a level of assessment of hearing aid performance that is not possible in any other way. In other cases, the results confirm 2-cm^3 coupler data. **The scope of these probe-microphone measurements is limited only by the imagination of the audiologist**.

When these measures become a routine part of the hearing aid evaluation, a more complete picture of the overall hearing aid fitting can be realized. The graphic display provides a meaningful representation of whether the circuitry is performing the desired function and helps to predict the potential benefit a patient might expect to receive from a specific feature of the hearing aid. The patient's involvement in and observation of the measurement of these special features or fitting arrangements help to instill confidence in the instrument and the audiologist.

CHAPTER 11

Assessment of Telecoils and Assistive Listening Devices

■ H. GUSTAV MUELLER, Ph.D. ■

The increasing use of assistive listening devices (ALDs) for individuals with hearing impairment has sparked interest both in these systems, and in the role of the hearing aid telecoil as a means of interfacing ALDs with hearing aids. The selection and verification of the electroacoustic characteristics of hearing aid telecoils and ALDs rapidly is becoming an integral part of the overall hearing aid fitting procedure. This chapter discusses the clinical measurement of the hearing aid telecoil and ALDs, and, in particular, the important role that probe-microphone measures can play in determining the suitability of these instruments on an individual basis.

ASSESSMENT OF TELECOIL PERFORMANCE

With the passage of the Americans with Disabilities Act (ADA), which mandates commu-

nication accessibility, public and workplace accommodations for individuals with hearing impairment are becoming increasingly common. Many of these accommodations, including both telephone and wide-area ALD systems, function most successfully when the individual's hearing aids can be interfaced with the ALD via the hearing aid telecoil. Although induction coils have long been an optional feature of hearing aids, with the increasing use of ALDs, telecoils have assumed additional importance to the hearing aid user. Unfortunately, **many hearing aid users who require the assistance of telecoil circuitry either do not have telecoils in their hearing aids or the telecoils do not function with sufficient power and frequency bandwidth to be of significant benefit to the user**. Not infrequently, even when there is a telecoil present in the hearing aid, the user may not know how to use it. This situation commonly results in such problems as:

■ Poor speech understanding on the telephone.

■ Hearing aid feedback when using the telephone, which interferes with successful telephone use.
■ The need to remove the hearing aid to use the telephone.

These problems cause frustration for the patient, prompt the patient not to use his or her hearing aids when telephone use is anticipated, and often lead to a dissatisfaction with hearing aid use in general.

Inadequate telecoil function also results in the inability to access wide area assistive listening systems other than by removing the hearing aids and employing earphones. The selection and assessment of the hearing aid telecoil, therefore, can have an impact on the overall success of the hearing aid fitting. In addition to assuring appropriate gain and frequency response, **the attention given to the evaluation of the telecoil at the time of the hearing aid fitting also pays long-term dividends by improving patient understanding of the use and function of this feature.**

CLINICAL METHODS OF MEASURING TELECOIL PERFORMANCE

As outlined in the recent guidelines for hearing aid selection and fitting (Hawkins, Beck, Bratt, Fabry, Mueller, & Stelmachowicz, 1991) it is incumbent upon the audiologist to evaluate the function of the telecoil. Grimes and Mueller (1991a) cited several reasons why it is important to assess the function of the telecoil as a routine part of the hearing aid selection, evaluation, and verification procedure:

■ To ensure that the telecoil is capable of providing sufficient gain and adequate bandwidth for both telephone use and for interfacing with various types of ALDs.
■ To assist in determining which types of telephones and telephone amplifiers will interface most appropriately with the hearing aid.
■ To determine the best method of transmission from an ALD to the hearing aid (e.g.,

earphone, neckloop, silhouette, direct audio input).
■ To counsel and demonstrate to the patient the appropriate procedures for using the telephone and assistive devices with their hearing aids.

While concern for the patient's welfare would seem to be a substantial incentive to conduct routine telecoil measures, it is relevant to mention that there is potential legal liability if a medical device (i.e., hearing aid) is sold that is not fully functional.

The primary focus of this chapter is the probe-microphone measurement of telecoil function; however, it is important to review briefly two other measurement methods which also can be clinically useful. In general, these methods are used to complement the objective information obtained using probe-microphones.

2-cm³ Coupler Measures

Electroacoustic measurements of telecoil performance using a 2-cm^3 coupler, conducted according to the American National Standards Institute (ANSI, S3.22, 1987) provide comparisons with standard values supplied by manufacturers. **These measures allow for quality control within and among manufacturers and provide a relative estimate of telecoil strength.** The 2-cm^3 measurements conducted according to the ANSI standard, however, must be viewed with caution. In addition to the fact that these measurements are not reliable indicators of individual real-ear performance, there are several other factors that also limit the usefulness of this electroacoustic measurement (Beck & Nance, 1989). First, the ANSI standard requires that telecoil output be specified only at 1000 Hz, which might not be representative of gain at other frequency regions. Second, the measurement is made with the volume control wheel (VCW) in the full-on position. Finally, a tolerance value of ±6 dB from the manufacturer's specifications is allowed; hence, two identical models could vary in telecoil gain by up to 12 dB and still be considered "acceptable."

Another important factor, that limits the face validity of the 2-cm^3 telecoil measure, is that the standard requires that the hearing aid be oriented in the test box so that the maximum sound pressure level in the coupler is obtained; this procedure is not possible, or at least not practical, when the hearing aid is in the real ear (more on hearing aid orientation in a later section).

When conducted carefully, 2-cm^3 measures do provide useful *relative* information concerning the performance of the hearing aid's telecoil. Lewis, Feigin, Karasek, and Stelmachowicz (1991) have reviewed the evaluation and assessment of FM systems using 2-cm^3 measurements, and provided helpful guidelines. Many of their suggestions also apply to the evaluation of hearing aid telecoil performance.

Behavioral Assessment

A behavioral assessment using some type of speech material can be either formal or informal and involves a task which the patient completes while using the hearing aid in the telecoil mode. Formal behavioral assessment could include a standardized speech recognition test delivered via the telephone handset (e.g., the procedure described by Holmes and Frank, 1984) or a specifically designed test for the telephone such as the Telecoil Evaluation Procedure (Wallber, MacKenzie, & Clyme, 1987). **The use of standardized speech test materials provides the option of comparing hearing aid telecoil speech recognition or intelligibility scores with aided soundfield or unaided earphone measures.** If stock behind-the-ear (BTE) hearing aids are used for the evaluation, a standardized speech test also allows the audiologist to conduct paired-comparison testing of telecoil performance for different hearing aids. If only a single hearing aid is evaluated, however, as is usually the case in custom in-the-ear (ITE) fittings, then some pre-determined performance level must be used as a pass/fail criterion for the telecoil (e.g., the telecoil speech recognition score must be within X% of the aided soundfield speech recognition score).

While formal behavioral evaluation of telecoil performance would seem to offer some insightful findings, very few audiologists conduct this testing. This could be because the testing procedure is somewhat unconventional, or that the testing is viewed as too time-consuming. Another factor is that in ITE hearing aid fittings, an alternative choice is not readily available if the test results are unsatisfactory, as comparative testing with other models is not possible.

Informal behavioral assessment of telecoil performance is more popular and includes such approaches as asking the patient to judge the intelligibility of a recorded message delivered through the telephone or simply to listen to the loudness of the dial tone. **The advantages of the informal approach are its simplicity, speed, and the appearance of validity to the patient.** All that is required is a hearing aid-compatible telephone, and the patient has the experience of a real-life listening situation. One approach is to talk to the patient from a second office telephone. The patient then can determine if he or she is able to communicate using the hearing aid telecoil and compare the understanding of speech using the telecoil to that with an amplified headset.

The disadvantages of the informal telecoil assessment is the lack of a standard, controlled stimulus and the need to rely significantly on the hearing aid user's subjective report. The latter factor is particularly an issue with the new hearing aid user. It is helpful, therefore, to make an objective measure of telecoil function to assist in determining if the fitting is appropriate.

Probe-Microphone Measurements

Real-ear measures of telecoil performance provide specific information regarding how the telecoil response is influenced by the patient's own external ear characteristics. These measures also provide information related to the coupling of the hearing aid to the ear. For instance, an earmold or ITE hearing aid that is vented (intentional or unintentional by way of a slit leak) might result in a telecoil real ear aided response (REAR) that has significantly less gain (especially for the lower frequencies) than suggested by 2-cm^3 coupler measures.

Another advantage of probe-microphone measures of telecoil performance is the ability to assess the effects of orientation of the telecoil itself within the hearing aid case (for review, see Beck & Nance, 1989). While coupler measurements specify that the hearing aid should be oriented in the magnetic field so that the maximum gain is realized, in the real ear the position of the coil is determined not only by its placement in the hearing aid, but also by the hearing aid's placement on or in the ear. The directivity of the coil, therefore, must be aligned appropriately in relation to the device that is generating the magnetic field. **An undesirable orientation may cause a substantial reduction in sensitivity for a given device, such as the telephone, yet an acceptable coupler response may be present**. This factor is especially important for ITE instruments, as **manufacturers sometimes are not able to place the telecoil in the most desirable position; often, the telecoil simply is placed *wherever there is room***.

Beck and Nance (1989), in their review of the hearing aid telecoil, reported that the maximum pickup strength of the induction coil is located at the perpendicular ends of the coil's central axis. These authors presented the example that a telecoil with a front-to-back orientation would have maximum pickup for communication situation using an auditory room loop; whereas a lateral, or side-to-side, orientation would be more effective for transmissions from a telephone handset. Compton (1991) suggested that if a given person desires to use the telecoil next to the telephone receiver, but also will be using ALDs, then it is best to mount the telecoil vertically and teach the user how to angle the telephone receiver for the best reception.

For custom hearing aids, it is helpful if the audiologist considers how the telecoil will be used when the hearing aid is selected; and in some instances, this information must be passed along to the manufacturer. This approach requires close cooperation and frequent communication between the manufacturer and the audiologist. Verification that the hearing aid was built as specified is necessary at the time of the fitting. Probe-microphone measures offer a simple method of assessing many of the variables associated with telecoil orientation, and such measures are quickly and easily performed.

Because of the popularity of ITE hearing aids, and the fact that each year these hearing aids are fitted to individuals with increasingly greater hearing loss, it is important to comment further on telecoil circuitry for this hearing aid style. There seems to be a certain percentage of audiologists who simply believe that "telecoils in ITE hearing aids don't work." This belief is often given as a reason not to order telecoils in ITE instruments, not to evaluate telecoil performance when ITE hearing aids are fitted, or to choose a BTE instrument when a telecoil is necessary. While ITE hearing aid telecoils seldom have the degree of strength available in their BTE counterparts, the strength is adequate for many individuals. The patient who requires a telecoil and desires the ITE style, therefore, often may be fitted successfully without compromise by the audiologist. With ITE fittings, however, it is even more important to conduct probe-microphone measurements at the time of the fitting. **The shape and available space within the ITE hearing aid shell easily can influence important factors such as:**

- The size of the telecoil.
- The positioning of the telecoil in the instrument.
- Whether a pre-amplifier can be utilized.

All three of these factors will affect the performance of the hearing aid in the real ear. As shown in the following section, clinical test paradigms can be designed to evaluate the above variables on an individual basis.

APPLICATIONS OF PROBE-MICROPHONE MEASUREMENTS

Minor adaptations or adjustments normally are required to assess telecoil function using standard probe-microphone equipment, and several different approaches can be used. To some extent, the approach selected is dependent on the specific aspect of telecoil function that is in question. This section discusses three different methods in which probe-microphone measures can be used to evaluate and compare hearing aid telecoil performance on an individual basis.

Use of an FM or Hard-Wired System

A personal FM system, or a hard-wired ALD such as a Pocket Talker, coupled to the hearing aid with a neckloop or silhouette can be employed to measure telecoil performance (see Hawkins, 1987a). To conduct this measure, the ALD microphone is placed at the aided ear, near the monitoring microphone of the probe-microphone system if the modified-pressure method is used. This should assure that a constant input is used when different hearing aids

are evaluated. (See Lewis et al., 1991, for a suggested procedure for using the Fonix probe-microphone equipment.)

Hawkins (1987a) recommends using an 80 dB SPL input signal for a swept pure tone. Lewis et al. (1991) state that a 75 dB SPL signal more closely corresponds to the 85 dB SPL overall level of speech at the microphone of the FM system. **If the purpose of the testing is to evaluate the performance of the hearing aid telecoil, not the personal FM system in a typical use situation, lower intensity input signals are appropriate** (See Chapter 13 for a step-by-step test protocol.)

The acoustical signal from the probe-microphone equipment is converted by the personal FM system to an electromagnetic signal through the use of a neckloop or silhouette receiver (see Figure 11–1). The electromagnetic signal is received by the hearing aid tele-

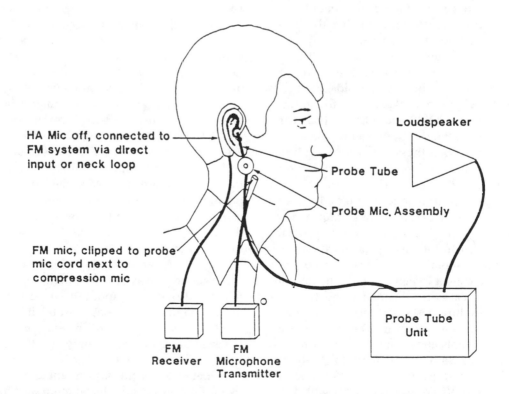

Figure 11–1. Schematic illustration of the procedure for conducting probe-microphone measurements of a personal FM system. (From Hawkins, D. 1987a. Assessment of FM systems with an ear canal probe tube microphone system. *Ear and Hearing, 8,* 301–303, with permission.)

coil, and the output of the hearing aid is then measured in the ear canal of the user. In this way, not only can the telecoil response itself be assessed, or several telecoil responses from different hearing aids be evaluated, but the effects of one ALD receiver versus another can be compared.

Using the above procedure, comparisons of telecoil response between hearing aids easily can be made. One reason for conducting these measures might be to assure that the telecoil REAR or real ear insertion response (REIR) is appropriate for the patient's hearing loss. **While it is common for audiologists to expend a great deal of time and effort matching the conventional REIR to a prescriptive gain target, the telecoil real-ear response often is ignored**. Perhaps audiologists believe that the telecoil REIR can be predicted from the 2-cm³ coupler results, that the telecoil response is the same as the microphone response, or that the telecoil response is the same for all instruments. As shown in in the following examples, these assumptions are not always true.

Mueller, Budinger, and Grimes (1990) compared the telecoil responses of different custom ITE hearing aids. The hearing aids were all ordered for a hypothetical patient with a gradually sloping 60 to 80 dB hearing loss. The hearing aids were obtained from leading manufacturers by supplying them with desired full-on gain 2-cm³ coupler values, based on the National Acoustic Laboratories (NAL) prescriptive method and recommended coupler correction factors. The manufacturers were informed of the purpose of the order and asked to provide their best telecoil for this hypothetical patient.

The first comparisons of these telecoil responses are shown in Figure 11–2. The telecoil REIR measures were obtained using the FM system procedure described earlier, with a silhouette induction receiver. The gain for all three instruments shown here was adjusted to approximately 30 dB at 1000 Hz for both the microphone and telecoil REIRs (for telecoil measures, the VCW was set to full-on). Observe that for these three custom ITE hearing aids, all ordered using the same desired 2-cm³

coupler gain, **telecoil real ear insertion gain (REIG) at an important frequency such as 3000 Hz varies from *0 dB* for ITE C to over 20 dB for ITE A and ITE B**. Clearly, the microphone REIR does not accurately predict the REIR of the telecoil (at least not for this type of induction field). While there is a general similarity between the microphone and telecoil REIRs, for all three instruments the frequency range of the telecoil response is narrower when compared with the microphone REIR. In particular, a difference in gain as great as 15 dB is present for ITE B in the low frequencies.

The REIRs shown in Figure 11–2 help explain why telecoils in ITE hearing aids receive mixed reviews. The differences between models are great enough to determine success or failure with the instrument. To further illustrate, observe the comparison of the two ITE hearing aid telecoil REIRs shown in Figure 11–3. Note that **when the REIG was adjusted to equivalent gain in the 1500 Hz region for both instruments, differences as large as 20 dB were present at other important frequencies**. If these differences also occurred for a telephone conducted signal, this factor easily could determine whether a hearing aid was accepted or rejected for telephone use. (As might be predicted from Figure 11–3, the 2-cm³ telecoil gain at 1000 Hz for these two instruments was essentially identical.) As is discussed in a later section, this type of probe-microphone assessment using a personal FM system can be supplemented with probe-microphone measures using an actual telephone receiver to assure that a specific induction field does not change the real-ear response significantly.

In addition to the configuration of the REIR, the absolute gain available from the hearing aid telecoil also is an important concern. When evaluating maximum telecoil REIG, it is important to consider the specific listening condition. For example, if the patient only uses the telecoil in conjunction with an ALD that has its own amplifier and volume adjustment, the sensitivity of the hearing aid telecoil might not be that important an issue. For this listening situation, the strength of the magnetic field can be in-

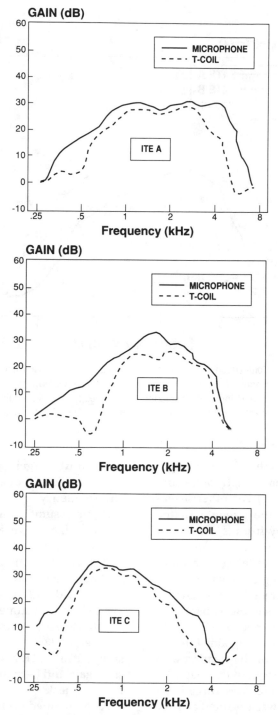

Figure 11–2. Comparison of the real ear insertion response (REIR) for the microphone and telecoil for three different in-the-ear (ITE) hearing aids measured on the same ear. (Adapted from Mueller, H., & Bryant, M. 1991. Some commonly overlooked uses of probe microphone measurements. *Seminars in Hearing, 12,* 73–91.)

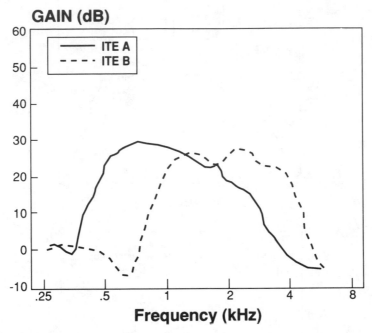

Figure 11-3. Comparison of the telecoil real ear insertion response (REIR) for two in-the-ear (ITE) hearing aids measured on the same ear. (Adapted from Grimes, A., & Mueller, H. 1991a. Using probe-microphone measures to assess telecoils and ALDs. Part I: Assessment of telecoil performance. *Hearing Journal, 44,* 16–21.)

creased to compensate for the reduced strength of the telecoil. (This approach might cause substantial distortion, however.) For other listening conditions in which the strength of the magnetic field is relatively fixed, such as in a looped room or listening on the telephone, the sensitivity of the hearing aid telecoil becomes more critical. Many hearing aid users need to turn their VCW to a higher setting or even full-on gain for this type of listening situation.

Figure 11–4 displays the telecoil REIRs obtained from five different hearing aids fitted to the same individual. One of the hearing aids was a BTE model; the strength of the magnetic field (neckloop induction receiver) was adjusted so that 50 dB of REIG was obtained at 1000 Hz when this instrument was set to full-on gain. In comparison, **observe that the maximum gain obtained from the *best* ITE hearing aid falls 20 dB below the BTE model REIR.** Three of the four ITE hearing aids have less

than 10 dB of gain below 1000 Hz, and the REIG of ITE B does not exceed 10 dB at any frequency.

If one assumes that a looped room or telephone might have a stronger field strength than the level used for the comparison shown in Figure 11–4, then it is possible that these findings exaggerate the BTE–ITE and ITE–ITE hearing aid differences. These results, however, clearly illustrate why patients might prefer the telecoil of one ITE hearing aid over another, and why in some instances it is necessary to use a BTE instrument to obtain the desired gain and frequency response for a specific listening task.

As mentioned earlier, the positioning of the telecoil in the hearing aid shell can have a significant effect on the sensitivity for specific magnetic field orientations. This important factor can be measured using the personal FM system with different coupling systems. Figure

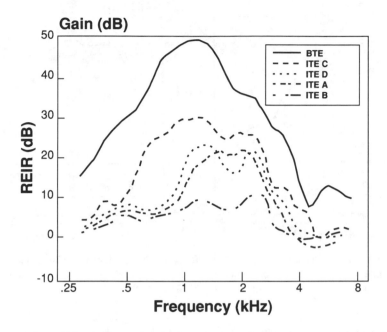

Figure 11–4. Comparison of the telecoil real ear insertion response (REIR) of a behind-the-ear (BTE) hearing aid and four in-the-ear (ITE) hearing aids from different manufacturers. All REIRs were conducted using an equal input produced from a personal FM system. (Adapted from Mueller, H., Budinger, A., & Grimes, A. 1990. Insertion gain comparisons of ITE telecoils. *Reports in Hearing Instrumentation and Technology, 2,* 11–15.)

11–5, from Mueller and Bryant (1991), illustrates the importance of conducting this measurement. Shown are the REIRs of two different custom ITE hearing aids fitted to the same individual and adjusted to produce maximum gain for two different coupling receivers, a postauricular silhouette and a neckloop. Observe that one of the ITE hearing aids revealed no significant difference in telecoil REIR as a function of the coupling method (left panel). For the other hearing aid, however, note that the maximum gain available via the neckloop falls 10–15 dB below the REIR obtained using the silhouette receiver (right panel). Mueller and Bryant (1991) reported that it was possible to increase the REIR substantially for this hearing aid simply by lifting the neckloop to a position horizontal to the ear. **These findings again point out the importance of tailoring the probe-**

microphone measurements to specific listening situations that might be experienced by the hearing aid user. This type of comparison also is useful for selecting the best coupling method for the hearing aid.

In ordering an ITE with a telecoil, another important consideration is whether to request a pre-amplifier for the telecoil circuit. Many manufacturers recommended that all ITE telecoils include a pre-amplifier, if space permits. Does the pre-amplifier provide a substantial increase in REIG? According to Grimes and Mueller (1991a), it does, at least based on the product from one manufacturer. To evaluate the benefit of this option, these authors ordered two custom ITE instruments, one with and one without a telecoil pre-amplifier circuit, from the same manufacturer. Again, using the personal FM system procedure previously de-

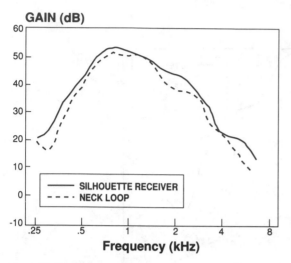
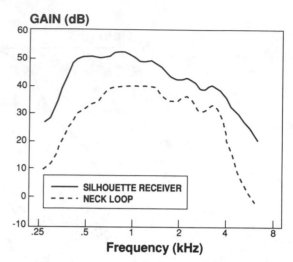

Figure 11–5. Comparison of the real ear insertion response (REIR) for two different in-the-ear (ITE) hearing aids measured using both a silhouette and a neckloop receiver. (Adapted from Mueller, H., & Bryant, M. 1991. Some commonly overlooked uses of probe microphone measurements. *Seminars in Hearing, 12*, 73–91.)

scribed, with a neckloop, probe-microphone insertion gain measures were conducted.

Figure 11–6 illustrates the difference in the REIRs for the two ITE hearing aids, both set at maximum gain. As shown, nearly 20 dB more gain was available from the hearing aid equipped with the pre-amplifier (ITE A). As can be seen from the examples in the preceding figures, careful assessment of the user's hearing aid telecoil as it will be utilized with the specific assistive device(s) is an important part of the hearing aid evaluation. Significant interactions between hearing aid and assistive device may affect how successful the hearing aid fitting ultimately is judged to be. **Also, appropriate counseling of the hearing aid user in how best to utilize the hearing aid with various assistive devices cannot be made without specific knowledge of how the telecoil functions in each situation.**

Use of an Induction-Field Loop

A second method which can be used to conduct probe-microphone measurements of hearing aid telecoil function is to set up a small induction field around the patient. Portable induction loop systems can be used for this purpose, although a more **ideal method is to use a wire loop that is specially designed to attach to your probe-microphone system** (not all probe-microphone systems offer this option, see Chapter 2 for review). The wire that is attached to the probe system is formed into a loop which encircles the area in which the patient is seated. The strength of the magnetic field that is created can be measured and monitored using a field strength meter. Gilmore and Lederman (1989) reported that a desirable field strength is approximately 100 mA/m, which is consistent with the strength of a typical induction-loop system (ILS).

Once the probe-microphone system has been configured in this manner, the electromagnetic signal is received by the hearing aid telecoil, and the output of the hearing aid can be measured in a manner similar to that used for conventional loudspeaker transduced signals. An advantage to this method of measurement is that it simulates an actual ILS; therefore, it is particularly suited for the person who frequently uses an ILS in meetings, as the orientation of the magnetic field is similar for both the probe-microphone arrangement and the ILS environment.

Although the induction loop option has been available for use with probe-microphone systems for the past several years, it does not seem to be used widely, and little has been published on the effectiveness of this approach. Grimes

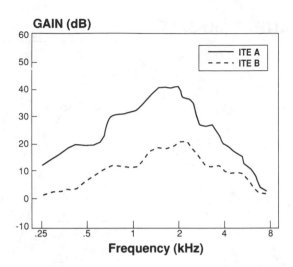

Figure 11-6. Telecoil real ear insertion responses (REIRs) for two in-the-ear (ITE) hearing aids; one with a pre-amplifier (ITE A) and the other without (ITE B). (Adapted from Grimes, A., & Mueller, H. 1991a. Using probe-microphone measures to assess telecoils and ALDs. Part I: Assessment of telecoil performance. *Hearing Journal, 44*, 16–21.)

and Mueller (1991a) used the induction-loop method to compare the telecoil performance of three different ITE hearing aids ordered for the same patient. Shown in Figure 11–7 are the REARs for these instruments. Observe that the output and bandwidth differ significantly for the three hearing aids. The peak output for ITE B is 10–20 dB less at 1500 Hz than that of ITE A or ITE C. Additionally, the REARs of ITEs A and C are notably different, with ITE A showing substantially more low-frequency output than ITE C.

The differences among telecoil REAR shown in Figure 11–7 would appear to be significant enough to affect a patient's communication ability, and easily could determine which instrument would be fitted. From a more practical standpoint, **these finding also could determine which custom hearing aid manufacturer would be used when a good telecoil is needed**. The decision is not always straightforward, however. The next section discusses how these same hearing aids might be rank-ordered differently if a different testing approach were used.

Use of a Telephone Receiver

A third method that can be used to measure real-ear hearing aid telecoil performance uti-

lizes a signal originating from an actual telephone receiver, much as occurs in everyday telephone use. While there is no standardized stimulus for performing this measure, Grimes and Mueller (1991a) reported one approach that can be used easily in a typical clinic or dispensing office. Speech spectrum noise (70 dB SPL) was led from a clinical audiometer, via an earphone held tightly on a telephone receiver (if necessary, the earphone and headset can be fixed together with masking tape). This telephone then "called" another telephone within the clinic, located in close proximity to the probe-microphone system. In this way, a uniform signal was continuously available from an actual telephone receiver, which was then used by the patient. Relative comparisons of telephone receivers, the positioning of the telephone, telephone amplifiers, and hearing aids (both microphone responses and telecoil responses) were then made. To conduct these measures, it was necessary to disable the loudspeaker of the probe-microphone equipment, allowing direct SPL output measures to be made with the probe microphone. For some equipment, disabling the loudspeaker is a software adjustment, while for other units the wires must be physically unhooked. (This modification of the probe-microphone equip-

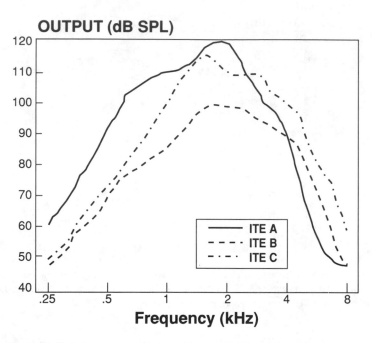

Figure 11–7. Telecoil real ear aided response (REAR) of three different in-the-ear (ITE) hearing aids. Measurements conducted using an induction-loop system. (Adapted from Grimes, A., & Mueller, H. 1991a. Using probe-microphone measures to assess telecoils and ALDs. Part I: Assessment of telecoil performance. *Hearing Journal, 44,* 21–29.)

ment also is discussed in Chapter 10 in the section regarding measurement of the occlusion effect).

This telephone procedure can be used to compare the telecoil gain available from different hearing instruments for a given patient for telephone use. If only one hearing aid is available, as in an ITE hearing aid fitting, then the output can be compared to a predetermined clinical standard or target. Grimes and Mueller (1991a) reported using this method to compare the telecoil responses of the same three ITE hearing aids that were discussed in the previous section (see Figure 11–7). Again, the hearing aids were set at maximum gain and tested in the same ear. The telephone handset was positioned to obtain the maximum output for each hearing aid. As shown in Figure 11–8, the output levels and frequency responses of the three instruments again varied substantially. The lowest powered instrument in the

ILS measurement (ITE B, see Figure 11–7), however, was not the lowest powered instrument when using the telephone-conducted speech noise (ITE C was). ITE A, which had the greatest low-frequency output in the ILS condition, also demonstrated the best low-frequency response using this method. The differences among ITE hearing aids demonstrated in Figure 11–8 indicate that for a telephone-conducted signal, **large differences in output potentially are present among ITE hearing aid manufacturers, and significant differences in the recognition of speech through the telephone certainly could be expected to occur.**

SUMMARY

The first half of this chapter has presented some background information and clinical protocols for the routine assessment of hearing aid

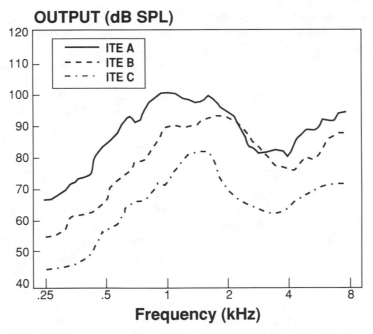

Figure 11–8. Telecoil real ear aided response (REAR) of three different in-the-ear (ITE) hearing aids. Measurements conducted using telephone transduced speech-spectrum noise. (Adapted from Grimes, A., & Mueller, H. 1991a. Using probe-microphone measures to assess telecoils and ALDs. Part I: Assessment of telecoil performance *Hearing Journal, 44,* 21–29.)

telecoil function. As the impact of the ADA continues to underline the importance of ALDs, greater importance will be placed on the function of the hearing aid telecoil. Probe-microphone measurements can play a prominent role in assuring that an appropriate telecoil selection has been made for each patient. This is particularly important when fitting custom ITE hearing aids, in which variations in the size and positioning of the telecoil may cause significant variations among instruments.

It is helpful to conduct probe-microphone measures using test conditions that most closely represent the real-life use of the telecoil: in a looped room space if the hearing aid user frequently is in an ILS listening environment, with a personal FM system if such a system commonly is used, or using a telephone-transduced signal, with the telephone held in a realistic position, if telephone accessibility is a major concern.

A final issue concerns the practical application of these measurements when ITE fittings are involved. How do you establish a clinic standard for "satisfactory" ITE hearing aid telecoil function? Do you send an ITE hearing aid back to the manufacturer because the telecoil does not meet your clinic standard? How do you know if there is anything the manufacturer can do to improve the hearing aid's telecoil performance? These are all important questions with no easy answers available. Based on our experience, the following recommendations are offered to help maximize the occurrence of successful ITE telecoil fittings:

■ Inform the manufacturer that you are concerned about the performance of the telecoil.
■ Discuss the positioning of the telecoil within the shell with the manufacturer.
■ Order a pre-amplifier circuit for the telecoil whenever space permits.

■ Through the use of probe-microphone measurements, critically evaluate and compare the telecoil performance from different manufacturers.

■ Select one or two manufacturers who consistently produce the best custom ITE telecoil response.

ASSESSMENT OF TELEPHONES, TELEPHONE AMPLIFIERS, AND ASSISTIVE LISTENING DEVICES

The preceding section discussed the importance of the hearing aid telecoil; without question, this feature is a key element in the successful coupling of a listening device to an impaired ear. The other equally important element is the function of the sound source itself, such as the telephone, the telephone amplifier, or other ALDs. The latter includes infrared or FM receivers and hard-wired personal communication devices.

In the 1980s, there was substantial growth in the availability and use of ALDs, and an understanding of these amplification systems is important for the audiologist (see Compton, 1989, 1991, for a review of these systems). ALDs are used in a variety of situations in the home, at work, and in wide area applications such as theaters and places of worship. **The primary advantage of assistive devices over hearing aids accrue in situations of noise, distance, or reverberation, as these devices can significantly improve the signal-to-noise ratio to the user's ear.**

Given the documented advantages of ALDs, it is somewhat surprising that these devices occupy a relatively small market share of this country's hearing health care industry income. Compton (1989) wrote that this small acceptance could be the result of several factors and suggested that, perhaps, audiologists know too little about the technology to be comfortable dispensing it or have too little time to become involved in the multitude of devices and systems. As is illustrated in the next few pages of this chapter, probe-microphone measures offer a method to gain confidence in the fitting of

ALDs, as the advantages (or disadvantages) of various systems readily are observable. An important peripheral benefit is that the measurement process itself promotes a greater understanding of these devices for both the audiologist and the ALD user.

ALDs may be used in place of, or in conjunction with, personal hearing aids. When used in conjunction with personal hearing aids, the coupling is provided either inductively via the hearing aid telecoil (utilizing a room loop, neckloop, or silhouette induction receiver) or by employing direct audio input. The various other hearing aid and receiver options that presently are available are shown in Figure 11–9, taken from a recent publication by Compton (1991).

For most people who are fitted with ALDs, decisions regarding SSPL90, gain, frequency response, and distortion are as important as if the person were fitted with conventional hearing aids. **In many states, ALDs are considered medical devices, and hence, the same evaluation procedures that apply to hearing aids (Hawkins et al., 1991) also apply to these amplification systems.** Probe-microphone measures might be even more important for the fitting of an ALD, since typically there is little or no electroacoustic information provided by the manufacturer. In addition, since many ALDs utilize lightweight headphones, traditional 2-cm^3 coupler measures are not practical since there is no easy or reliable way to place and seal the receiver to the coupler. In using telephones and telephone amplifiers (with or without a hearing aid telecoil), the output from the telephone receiver is also a critical factor in ensuring adequate telephone use. The remainder of this chapter, therefore, presents some clinical methods for using probe-microphone measurements in the assessment of telephone receivers, telephone amplifiers, and ALDs.

TELEPHONE AMPLIFIERS AND DEVICES

Both telephones and telephone amplifiers can be evaluated using some of the same ap-

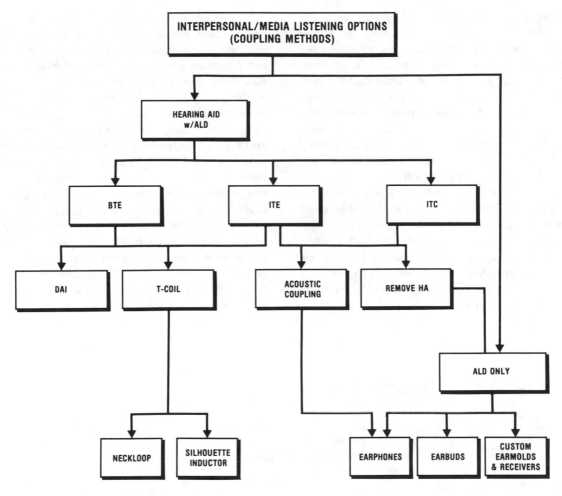

ALD = ASSISTIVE LISTENING DEVICE

Figure 11–9. Illustration of interpersonal/media listening options: Coupling methods. (From Compton, C. 1991. Clinical management of assistive technology users. In G. Studebaker, F. Bess, & L. Beck [Eds.], *The Vanderbilt hearing aid report II* (pp. 301–318). Parkton, MD: York Press, with permission.)

proaches by which hearing aid telecoil performance is assessed: behaviorally (formal or informal) and using probe-microphone measures. Electroacoustic assessment using 2-cm³ coupler measures usually is not feasible.

Grimes and Mueller (1991b) evaluated a variety of telephones, telephone amplifiers, and acoustic telephone devices, using probe-microphone measures of a telephone-transduced noise (as described earlier in this chapter). The following examples, adapted from Grimes and Mueller (1991b), illustrate how this procedure easily can be used for comparisons of telephone receivers, telephone amplifiers, and hearing aids coupled to telephones (in terms of both microphone and telecoil responses).

Comparison of Telephone Receivers

The effect of the telephone receiver on the signal delivered to the eardrum can be assessed using a probe-microphone system with the loudspeaker disabled. In this way, the probe system becomes a spectrum analyzer, and the intensity of any sound or noise can be measured in the ear canal (assuming that the output is sufficient). It is possible, therefore, to use this equipment to compare telephones independently of hearing aids. This measurement has direct application to the fitting of hearing aids, since in some instances, the inability of the patient to understand telephone-transduced speech with the hearing aid is due to a poorly functioning telephone. This has been increasingly a problem in recent years with the advent of poor-quality discount telephones, and the greater use of cordless telephones. These telephones often have little or no magnetic field, high internal noise levels and relatively high distortion.

To illustrate the potential effects of the telephone itself, Figure 11–10 compares two telephones, one judged to be of high quality and the other an inexpensive "throw-away" type (the kind that arrives free-of-charge for subscribing to your favorite magazine). The two responses shown in Figure 11–10 represent the output from the high quality office telephone and the disposable telephone. The sound pressure level of the telephone-transduced speech noise was measured in the ear canal without the hearing aid in place. It is not necessary to make this measure in the ear canal, and the same relative differences between the outputs of the telephones would be expected if the probe tube simply had been held near the receiver. The final shape of the speech signal, however, will be affected by the individual's real ear unaided response (REUR). Addition-

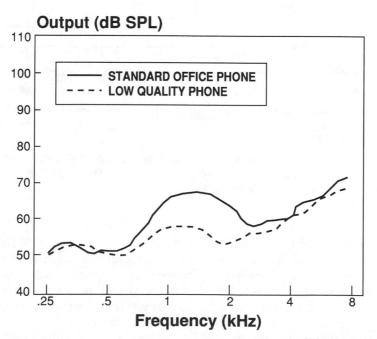

Figure 11–10. Comparison of the real-ear output (db SPL) of speech-spectrum noise produced by two different telephones. (Adapted from Grimes, A., & Mueller, H. 1991b. Using probe-microphone measures to assess telecoils and ALDs. Part II: Assessment of ALDs, telephones, and telephone amplifiers. *Hearing Journal, 44,* 21–29.)

ally, it is helpful for counseling if the patient is actively involved in the measurement, as it adds a bit more realism to the comparison process.

As shown in Figure 11–10, the inexpensive telephone clearly has reduced gain when compared with the standard office telephone. This difference in output, which is as great as 10–15 dB at some frequencies, easily could have a significant effect on an individual's speech understanding ability, especially for patients who do not have telecoils in their hearing aids and rely on a strong acoustic output. **When troubleshooting complaints concerning telephone use, it might be helpful to conduct these types of probe-microphone measures using the hearing aid user's own telephone**.

Comparison of Telephone Amplifiers

In recent years, various types of telephone amplifiers have become available to the general public. The effectiveness of these telephone amplifiers can be compared using probe microphone measurements in the same manner as discussed in the preceding section. In Figure 11–11, for example, the output from one type of purported high-frequency-emphasis telephone receiver is displayed; the SPL values shown represent the output of the speech-spectrum noise measured in the real ear. This type of telephone amplifier is advertised to increase high-frequency gain at a greater rate than low-frequency gain as the volume wheel is rotated higher.

The two output responses shown in Figure 11–11 reveal that, although this telephone amplifier does increase the signal by 5–10 dB when the volume control is rotated, this particular model provides relatively greater *low-frequency* amplification as the overall gain is increased. As a result, when compared to the maximum output of similar commercially avail-

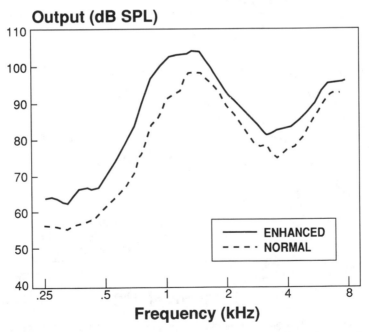

Figure 11–11. Real-ear output (dB SPL) of a telephone amplifier in the normal and in the enhanced listening settings (Adapted from Grimes, A., & Mueller, H. 1991b. Using probe-microphone measures to assess telecoils and ALDs. Part II: Assessment of ALDs, telephones, and telephone amplifiers. *Hearing Journal, 44,* 21–29.)

able units, this telephone amplifier has 10–15 dB *less* gain in the 1500–2000 Hz region — which may be sufficient cause for sugggesting that a patient purchase a different system.

Adjunct (in-line) or strap-on acoustical telephone amplifiers can be evaluated in a similar fashion. Maximum gain, frequency response, and linearity of the VCW all can be assessed in the real ear. Frequently, this assessment information is useful for patient instruction and counseling. For instance, one type of telephone amplifier that is widely distributed by telephone companies has a volume control slider that allows the patient to vary the output from the minimum to maximum setting. This amplifier, however, actually performs as an attenuator when the slider is positioned in the minimum setting.

Figure 11–12 compares the effects of the two extreme amplifier settings to the output ob-

tained from the telephone without the amplifier attached. **For the patient whose results are shown in Figure 11–12, it was necessary to adjust the "amplifier" to mid-volume just to equal the intensity obtained using the telephone alone.** Clearly, this type of information is important in educating patients about how to use such devices.

Assessment of Receiver Attachments

Increasingly popular are the paste-on "donut" or snap-on plastic extension devices, which are attached to the telephone receiver for using the telephone with an ITE hearing aid (without a telecoil). The reported value of using this type of device is to reduce feedback, enabling greater hearing aid gain for telephone use to increase the intensity of the speech signal. Probe-microphone measures provide a simple method to evaluate, on an individual basis, whether

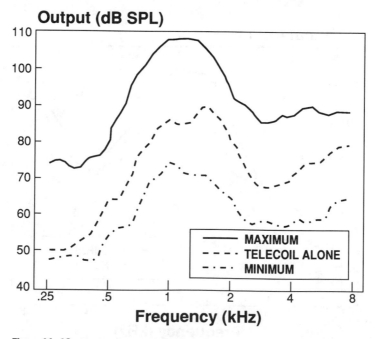

Figure 11–12. Real-ear output (dB SPL) of a hearing aid telecoil used with a telephone amplifier adjusted to the maximum and minimum settings. Also shown is the real-ear response obtained using the hearing aid telecoil without amplifier. (Adapted from Grimes, A., & Mueller, H. 1991b. Using probe-microphone measures to assess telecoils and ALDs. Part II: Assessment of ALDs, telephones, and telephone amplifiers. *Hearing Journal, 44,* 21–29.)

these devices provide the desired improvement of the telephone-transduced speech signal. Despite the popularity of these devices, little data are available regarding their effectiveness.

A comparison of the effects of two such devices is shown in Figure 11–13. The measurements were conducted for telephone-transduced speech noise for a patient fitted with an ITE model hearing aid. Displayed is the maximum gain possible prior to feedback using the two different telephone attachments. Also shown, for comparison, is the maximum gain possible when simply holding the telephone up to the hearing aid microphone without any receiver attachment. **For this patient, both attachments offered improved real-ear gain, and the greatest gain was obtained with the plastic snap-on device.** In general, we have observed that at least some benefit is present

from these devices for all users, although the degree is variable; therefore, routine measurement of this option is advised.

For hearing aid users who use the telephone, particularly in their work, the selection and real-ear assessment of the optimal telephone arrangement is very important in the hearing aid fitting process. Whether to use a telecoil, direct audio input, telephone amplifier, or feedback-reduction device, or simply to remove the hearing aid when using the telephone must be assessed in order for the individual to attain maximum speech understanding on the telephone.

ASSISTIVE LISTENING DEVICES

In recommending or dispensing ALDs, it is helpful to measure the performance of the de-

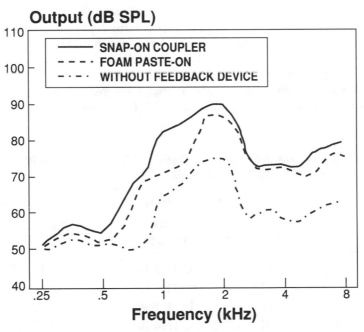

Figure 11–13. Maximum real-ear output (dB SPL) obtained just below feedback for two different telephone receiver attachments. Also shown is the maximum real-ear output (dB SPL) obtained just below feedback using the telephone receiver without either device. (Adapted from Grimes, A., & Mueller, H. 1991b. Using probe-microphone measures to assess telecoils and ALDs. Part II: Assessment of ALDs, telephones, and telephone amplifiers. *Hearing Journal*, *44*, 21–29.)

vice on the individual user. Specific devices, and the choice of receiver style used to couple the device to the ear or to the hearing aid, all have the potential to affect greatly the power and frequency response of the speech signal reaching the ear. ALD assessment using probe-microphone measures can be made directly (when using an acoustic receiver or earphone), or, as recommended by Hawkins (1987a), the ALD can be measured as it interfaces with the hearing aid (via silhouette, neckloop, induction receiver, or direct audio input). If the assistive device has a remote or extension microphone, placing this microphone at the monitor microphone of the probe-microphone system and using a relatively high input (such as 75 or 80 dB SPL) would be appropriate. If, however, the device has an internal or rigid microphone placement, then it is probably best simply to conduct the probe-microphone measurements with the ALD microphone in the position in which it normally would be located for communication.

Real-Ear Comparison of ALD Systems

As mentioned at the beginning of this chapter, ALDs often arrive from the manufacturer with little or no electroacoustic information avail-

able. This is especially unfortunate for the consumer, as in most states these devices can be purchased over the counter or through the mail and are not controlled by hearing aid dispensing regulations. Some of these devices retail for as little as $19.95, which attracts the attention of many individuals with impaired hearing. As expected, **many of these low-budget ALDs have sharply peaked frequency response curves, low gain, and high distortion.** Perhaps even worse, **some of these devices have extremely high output, to the extent that acoustic trauma could potentially result.** All of these factors further emphasize the importance of probe-microphone measures when ALDs are dispensed. Patients who have purchased ALDs through other sources should be encouraged to bring in their system so that it can be assessed properly.

The variability of these over the counter ALD devices was illustrated in a report by Brooks and Grimes (1989). These authors conducted probe-microphone measurements for six different commercially available hard-wired ALDs, assessing the REIR, peak REIG, and the real ear saturation response (RESR). Table 11–1 displays the results of these measurements; significant differences in the REIG and RESR

TABLE 11–1. SUMMARY OF THE MAXIMUM REAL EAR INSERTION GAIN (REIG) AND REAL EAR SATURATION RESPONSE (RESR) FOR SIX DIFFERENT ASSISTIVE LISTENING DEVICES*

ALD System	Maximum REIG (70 dB Input)		RESR (90 dB Input)	
	Average dB (1, 1.6, 2.5 kHz)	Peak (Frequency)	Average dB (1, 1.6, 2.5 kHz)	Peak (Frequency)
1	15	32 (667 Hz)	107	115 (4490 Hz)
2	34	46 (375 Hz)	131	134 (1624 Hz)
3	25	42 (397 Hz)	110	114 (502 Hz)
4	36	46 (794 Hz)	103	124 (3175 Hz)
5	32	42 (1000 Hz)	112	115 (375 Hz)
6	12	24 (375 Hz)	106	112 (375 Hz)

*REIG measures were conducted using maximum rotation of the volume control wheel or the point of maximum gain before feedback occurred.

Source: Adapted from Brooks, W., & Grimes, A. 1989. *Real ear assessment of personal communication devices.* Paper presented at the Annual Convention of the American Speech-Language-Hearing Association, St. Louis, MO.

findings among these devices are obvious. First, notice that almost all units have peak REIG below 800 Hz, a response not common or normally desired in today's hearing aids. Second, observe that the average gain varies by more than 20 dB among systems. **Finally and perhaps of greatest importance for the consumer, the RESR values differ by as much as 28 dB among units, and one device produced a real-ear peak output of *134 dB SPL*.** These RESR values, obtained in an adult ear, could be significantly higher if these systems had been fitted to a young child (see Chapters 7 and 8).

Comparison of ALD Receivers

As shown in Table 11–1, there is considerable variability in electroacoustic characteristics among ALDs. As a result, these devices must be selected carefully to match the patient's degree of hearing loss, loudness discomfort levels, and other amplification needs. When these decisions are made, it also is important to consider the type of receiver that the patient will be using. The variability in gain, output, and frequency response that can result from the ALD receiver is as great, if not greater, than among ALDs themselves.

Brooks and Grimes (1989) compared the differences in the REIRs obtained when using a single ALD with different receivers. The three receivers tested were lightweight headphones (Walkman type), hard earbud, and soft earbud. The measurements were obtained using a constant VCW setting for the ALD at a 70 dB SPL input (the microphone of ALD was placed at the regulating microphone of the probe-microphone system).

The REIRs obtained for the different receivers are shown in Figure 11–14. Notice that the

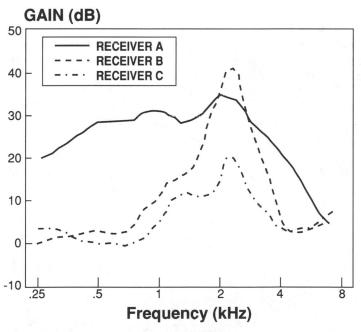

Figure 11–14. Real ear insertion response (REIR) obtained using three different receivers fitted to the same ALD. (Adapted from Brooks, W., & Grimes A. 1989. *Real ear assessment of personal communication devices.* Paper presented at the Annual Convention of the American Speech-Language-Hearing Association, St. Louis, MO.)

style of receiver alters significantly the amount and configuration of the gain delivered to the ear. While it is possible that the REIR obtained with receiver C (lightweight headphones) would be adequate for someone with a mild high-frequency impairment, most ALD users would require more low-frequency gain than available using either this receiver or receiver B (hard earbud). **This large variability among receivers illustrates the importance of evaluating individual receivers, as well as the ALD itself, whenever these systems are fitted**.

Frequency Response Selection

A final issue, related to the data presented in the preceding section, concerns the overall appropriateness of the frequency response of the ALD. **If the device is used in place of a hearing aid, then presumably the prescriptive formulae normally used for fitting hearing aids**

also would be applicable to fitting ALDs. As with hearing aid fittings, probe-microphone measurements can be used to determine if the REIR or REAR is within acceptable tolerances of target.

In Figure 11–15, adapted from Mueller and Bryant (1991), NAL prescriptive target gain for a typical high-frequency presbycusic-type hearing loss is compared with the REIRs achieved by two different, popular, commercially available hard-wired personal communication devices. The gain of each device was adjusted so that REIG equaled target gain at 1000 Hz, using a 70 dB input (swept pure tone). The resulting REIR-prescriptive target gain comparisons shown in Figure 11–15 illustrate that, while both systems provide limited gain above 2000 Hz, one of the ALDs is clearly more appropriate in terms of meeting target gain than the other. It is important to consider that, depending on the ALD microphone loca-

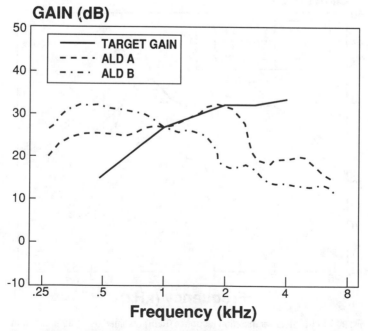

Figure 11–15. Real ear insertion response (REIR) of two different ALDs fitted to the same individual. Target prescriptive gain for this patient also is shown. (Adapted from Mueller, H., & Bryant, M. 1991. Some commonly overlooked uses of probe microphone measurements. *Seminars in Hearing, 12*, 73–91.)

tion, the input to the ALD might be much higher than to a hearing aid, and therefore, less gain will be needed. The desired configuration of the ALD REIR, however, would remain the same. **While NAL target gain might not be the appropriate "gold standard" for all users of ALDs, it seems reasonable to establish some criterion by which the performance of the ALD system can be judged.**

SUMMARY

In general, probe-microphone measurements have been underutilized in the evaluation of telecoil circuitry and ALDs. This is partly because there are no standard protocols for conducting these measures; consequently, **audiologists must often learn the best evaluation method through experimentation. While this trial-and-error procedure is sometimes frustrating, it also encourages innovation, which often leads to the discovery of new and meaningful ways to utilize the probe-microphone technology.**

There are several important factors to consider in achieving successful hearing aid–ALD–telephone usage. As the use and popularity of ALDs continues to grow, the clinical assessment of the hearing aid telecoil and the ALD device itself will become a routine part of the hearing aid evaluation. Once the factors that have been discussed in this chapter have been considered, it becomes clear that **probe-microphone measurements provide the most effective and reliable method to validate the selection of hearing aid telecoils, telephone amplifiers, and other assistive listening devices.**

CHAPTER 12

Corrections and Transformations Relevant to Hearing Aid Selection

■ DAVID B. HAWKINS, Ph.D. ■

The audiologist working with hearing aids must constantly blend together the art and science of selection and fitting, taking into account everything from acoustics to personality. This chapter is concerned with the vast array of acoustic transformations that occur with hearing aids and hearing aid-related decisions. Unfortunately, our field uses a variety of different references and couplers for hearing loss in soundfield, hearing loss under earphones, the calibration of earphones, the measurements of hearing aid characteristics, output in a real ear, and so forth. In selecting and fitting hearing aids, many of these acoustic transformations merge together.

This chapter describes a variety of corrections and transformations relevant to hearing aid decisions and serves as a reference source for the audiologist involved with hearing aids.

Publications by Skinner (1988) and Bentler and Pavlovic (1989) greatly facilitated collection of these values, and the interested reader is encouraged to study these papers. It should be noted that slightly different values have been published for many of these corrections. The choice of which data to present in this chapter is based on the procedures used and the relevance to clinical decisions.

THE ENVIRONMENT

AMBIENT NOISE LEVELS

If the audiologist chooses to obtain functional gain measurements in place of, or in addition to, probe-microphone measures, care must be taken to ensure that the acoustic environment is acceptable. ANSI standard S3.1-1977 (1977), entitled "Criteria for Permissible Ambient Noise During Audiometric Testing," provides information concerning the allowable noise levels for testing hearing in the soundfield. Table 12–1 shows the maximum permissible ambient noise levels in octave and third-octave bands to allow testing down to 0 dB HL. As an example, to test to 0 dB HL at 500 Hz, the ambient noise level in the test booth would have to be less than 14.5 dB sound pressure level (SPL) in an octave band centered at 500 Hz. If the actual measured ambient noise level was 24.5 dB SPL (10 dB above the maximum for 0 dB HL), then testing could be accomplished to a level of 10 dB HL. Unless testing is being done in a relatively poor sound booth, and/or there are rather high ambient noise levels outside the test booth, these issues become important mainly for persons with normal or near-normal hearing sensitivity in some portion of the frequency range.

When making probe-microphone measurements, the issue of acceptable ambient noise levels is rarely a problem unless the test environment is noisy. The signal levels involved are typically in the 50–90 dB SPL range, well above the ambient noise levels in the environments that most audiologists would use for hearing aid selection purposes.

MASKED AIDED THRESHOLDS

A second issue concerning environmental effects on functional gain involves the possibility of the aided threshold being masked by the amplified room noise and/or circuit noise in the hearing aid. Either or both of these sources of noise can produce a certain amount of effective masking and limit the aided threshold that can be obtained. For instance, if the amplified room noise through the hearing aid created 15 dB of effective masking at 500 Hz, then no matter how much gain the hearing aid had at 500 Hz, the best possible aided threshold is 15 dB HL. For example, if the unaided threshold is 25 dB HL and the hearing aid has 20 dB of gain, the correct aided threshold is 5 dB HL, indicating 20 dB of functional gain. However, given the effective masking level of 15 dB, functional gain would be in error with only 10 dB of gain; that is, 25 dB (unaided threshold) − 15 dB (effective masking level) = 10 dB.

Macrae and Frazer (1980) and Macrae (1982) have suggested that aided thresholds be viewed suspiciously if unaided thresholds are less than 30 dB HL. To determine if an aided threshold is in fact a masked threshold, repeat the aided threshold with a higher volume control wheel (VCW) setting. If the threshold improves, the first threshold was real; if the threshold stays the same or gets worse (due to the increased circuit noise in the hearing aid at the higher volume setting), the first threshold could have been contaminated by masking.

Masked aided thresholds are not a concern when making probe-microphone measurements since behavioral thresholds are not involved. This is a significant advantage of probe-tube measurements when assessing real-ear performance of persons with normal or near-normal hearing in certain frequency regions.

TABLE 12–1. MAXIMUM PERMISSIBLE AMBIENT NOISE LEVELS (dB SPL) IN OCTAVE AND THIRD-OCTAVE BANDS FOR TESTING TO 0 dB HL

	Frequency (Hz)				
	250	500	1000	2000	4000
Octave band levels	18.5	14.5	14.0	8.5	9.0
Third-octave band levels	13.5	9.5	9.0	3.5	15.5

Note: Values from ANSI S3.1-1977.

SOUNDFIELD CALIBRATION VALUES

If unaided and aided soundfield thresholds are expressed in dB HL and plotted on an audiogram, it is necessary that the sound field be calibrated appropriately. Since the ANSI audiometer calibration standard does not provide reference levels for soundfield testing, data from the available literature must be used. The most systematic approach to soundfield calibration is described by Walker, Dillon, and Byrne (1984). Their recommendations for soundfield calibration values are given in Table 12–2 for loudspeakers located at 0° and 90° azimuths. Data for a 45° azimuth loudspeaker location are from Morgan, Dirks, and Bower (1979). The values in this table must be added to the HL dial reading to determine the appropriate SPL in the soundfield for proper calibration; for example, if a 45° azimuth loudspeaker is used at 500 Hz with a 70 dB HL signal, then 79 dB SPL (70 + 9) should be measured in the soundfield with a sound-level meter at the calibrated location.

STANDARD EARPHONE MEASUREMENTS

CONVERSION OF dB HL TO COUPLER SPL

The basic measurements that precede any hearing aid selection and fitting are made during the audiological evaluation. These typically include air- and bone-conduction thresholds, speech reception thresholds, most comfortable loudness levels, loudness discomfort levels (LDLs), word-recognition scores, and immittance testing. The most common transducer used is the TDH series earphone mounted in a supra-aural earphone cushion (MX-41/AR). Since audiometer attenuators are calibrated in dB HL, the values obtained for most of these measurements are expressed in Hearing Level (HL), not sound pressure level (SPL). When dealing with hearing aids, however, it is neces-

TABLE 12–2. REFERENCE EQUIVALENT THRESHOLD SPLs FOR SOUNDFIELD TESTING WITH THREE LOUDSPEAKER AZIMUTHS

Frequency (Hz)	Loudspeaker Azimuth		
	0°[a]	45°[b]	90°[a]
250	16.0	20.5	16.0
500	9.5	9.0	7.5
1000	5.5	0.9	3.5
1500	4.5	2.0	2.0
2000	2.5	−0.5	4.0
3000	0.5	−4.1	0.5
4000	1.5	−3.1	1.0
6000	7.5	3.8	1.5
Speech	16.5	12.5	15.0

[a]Values from Walker et al. (1984).
[b]Values from Morgan et al. (1979).

sary to have values expressed in dB SPL. There are several conversions that can be applied. For instance, the most obvious and common transformations applied to dB HL values are to convert them to dB SPL as measured in the NBS-9A 6-cm^3 coupler that is used to calibrate the earphone. These are the values in the ANSI calibration standard (ANSI S3.6-1989), and they are shown in Table 12–3 for TDH-39, TDH-49, TDH-50, and Telex 1470A earphones. The values in this table are added to the dB HL dial reading to convert to dB SPL. For instance, if the LDL was obtained at 100 dB HL at 1000 Hz with a TDH-39 earphone, the LDL would be 107 dB SPL as measured in a 6-cm^3 coupler.

If speech is used as the stimulus, the conversion from dB HL to dB SPL involves adding 12.5 dB plus the reference value at 1000 Hz. For example, if a TDH-49 earphone were being used, the speech conversion would be 12.5 + 7.5 (the reference value at 1000 Hz for the TDH-49) or 20 dB. If the LDL was obtained with spondaic words at 90 dB HL, the LDL would be 110 dB SPL. Conversions such as these are common when selecting the SSPL90 of hearing aids.

There are problems when conversions from dB HL to dB SPL in a 6-cm^3 coupler are utilized

TABLE 12–3. STANDARD REFERENCE EQUIVALENT THRESHOLD SPLs FOR VARIOUS EARPHONES ON THE NBS-9A 6-CM^3 COUPLER

Frequency (Hz)	TDH-39	TDH-49 and TDH-50	Telex 1470A
125	45.0	47.5	47.0
250	25.5	26.5	27.5
500	11.5	13.5	13.0
750	8.0	8.5	8.5
1000	7.0	7.5	6.5
1500	6.5	7.5	5.0
2000	9.0	11.0	8.0
3000	10.0	9.5	7.5
4000	9.5	10.5	9.0
6000	15.5	13.5	17.5
8000	13.0	13.0	17.5

Note: Values from ANSI S3.6-1989.

for hearing aid purposes. The electroacoustic characteristics of hearing aids are specified as output in an HA-1 or HA-2 2-cm^3 coupler. As a result, it is not possible to utilize an LDL obtained through a standard earphone and specified as dB SPL in a 6-cm^3 coupler and precisely select the SSPL90 of a hearing aid when the maximum output has been measured in a 2-cm^3 coupler. In an attempt to deal with this problem, Hawkins, Cooper, and Thompson (1990) made measurements in 30 adults to determine the dB HL to 2-cm^3 coupler SPL conversions when standard earphones are used. Their results are shown in Table 12–4 for TDH-39, TDH-49, and TDH-50 earphones. These values are useful in that they allow the audiologist to measure LDLs under standard earphones and then convert to dB SPL in a 2-cm^3 coupler for purposes of selecting the SSPL90 for a behind-the-ear (BTE) hearing aid or specifying the SSPL90 in an in-the-ear (ITE) hearing aid order. For example, if LDLs were obtained with TDH-39 earphones at 95 dB HL at 500 and 1000 Hz and at 100 dB HL at 2000 and 4000 Hz, the desired SSPL90 would be 105 dB SPL at 500 Hz (95 + 9.9), 101 dB SPL at 1000 Hz (95 + 5.5), 105 dB SPL at 2000 Hz (100 + 5.2), and 100 dB SPL (100 + −0.5) at 4000 Hz. Given

that SSPL90 curves cannot typically be tailored this closely across frequency, an appropriate selection is to specify an SSPL90 curve of approximately 105 dB SPL and request an output control with a range of 10–15 dB down from 105. This enables the SSPL90 to be reduced if the person experiences loudness discomfort due to the SSPL90 slightly exceeding the LDLs in the 1000- and 4000-Hz regions.

REAL-EAR FREQUENCY RESPONSE OF A TDH-39 EARPHONE

Word-recognition scores obtained by audiologists are often viewed as representing "optimal performance." Given the emphasis on selective amplification in the hearing aid literature in recent years, the implication is that the hearing aid frequency response needs to be tailored to the individual hearing loss configuration to provide best speech understanding. The frequency response that is commonly shown for the TDH-39 earphone is the flat response measured in an NBS-9A 6-cm^3 coupler and shown in Figure 12-1. The 6-cm^3 coupler, however, does not accurately represent the real-ear response of the earphone. Figure 12-2 shows

TABLE 12–4. CONVERSION VALUES FROM dB HL
TO dB SPL IN A 2-CM^3 COUPLER FOR TDH-39, TDH-
49, AND TDH-50 EARPHONES

Frequency (Hz)	TDH-39	TDH-49 and 50
250	20.7	21.7
500	9.9	11.9
750	7.3	7.8
1000	5.5	6.0
1500	2.5	3.5
2000	5.2	7.2
3000	5.7	5.2
4000	−0.5	0.5
6000	−0.2	−2.2

Note: Based on data from Hawkins et al. (1990).

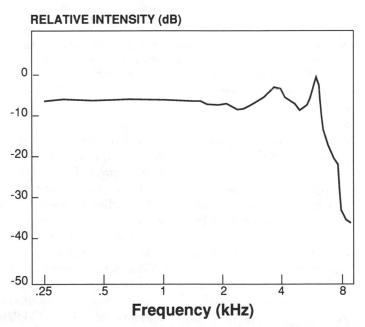

Figure 12–1. Frequency response of a TDH-39 earphone as measured on an
NBS-9A 6-cm^3 coupler. (Adapted from Sanders, J. 1964. Masking in audiometry. *Archives of Otolaryngology, 80,* 541–556.)

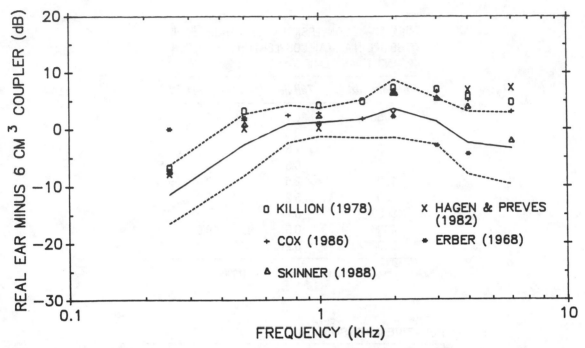

Figure 12–2. Real-ear frequency response of a TDH-39 earphone. The solid line represents the mean of 30 subjects from Hawkins et al. (1990) and the dotted line is ±1 standard deviation. Also plotted are results from five other studies. (From Hawkins, D., Cooper, W., & Thompson, D. 1990. Comparisons among SPLs in real ears, 2-cm³ and 6-cm³ couplers. *Journal of American Academy of Audiology, 1,* 154–161, with permission.)

the real-ear response of the TDH-39 earphone from the Hawkins, et al. (1990) study as well as from five other studies. Unlike the 6-cm³ coupler response, the real-ear frequency response rolls off in the lows due to leakage around the cushion (acting like a vent) and has a peak in the 2000-Hz region. Notice that the real-ear frequency response of the earphone is similar to a typical hearing aid response rather than the classic 6-cm³ coupler frequency response.

ALTERNATIVE EARPHONE MEASUREMENTS

CONVERSION OF dB HL TO 2-CM³ COUPLER SPL

In recent years, an alternative earphone, the **Etymotic ER-3A**, has become available for stan-

dard audiometric testing. This insert earphone is coupled to the ear canal via a soft plastic tip or a compressible foam plug. It has several distinct advantages over the traditional TDH series, such as **eliminating the possibility of collapsed ear canals** during testing, **increased interaural attenuation** (reducing masking difficulties), and **listener comfort**.

The advantage of the ER-3A earphone for hearing aid applications is that it is **calibrated in a 2-cm³ coupler**. The interim reference values for conversion from dB HL to dB SPL in a 2-cm³ coupler are shown in Table 12–5 (ANSI, 1989). If LDLs are obtained with the ER-3A earphone, the values in Table 12–5 can be simply added to the dB HL dial reading, and the LDL is then expressed in the appropriate terms for SSPL90 selection. For instance, if LDLs were obtained with the ER-3A earphone at 100 dB HL at 500, 1000, and 2000 Hz, the SSPL90 in a 2-cm³ cou-

TABLE 12–5. INTERIM REFERENCE EQUIVALENT THRESHOLD SPLs FOR THE ETYMOTIC ER-3A INSERT EARPHONE ON THE HA-1 2-CM^3 COUPLER

Frequency (Hz)	125	250	500	1000	2000	3000	4000	6000	8000
Equivalent Threshold (SPL)	27.5	15.5	8.5	3.5	6.5	5.5	1.5	−1.5	−4.0

Note: Values from ANSI S3.6-1989.

pler would be specified as 109 dB SPL (100 + 8.5), 104 dB SPL (100 + 3.5), and 107 dB SPL (100 + 6.5), respectively. The advantage of being calibrated in the 2-cm^3 coupler, along with the increased comfort of this earphone compared with the supra-aural cushion of the TDH series, makes the ER-3A earphone a very attractive alternative for the clinical audiologist working with hearing aids.

REAL-EAR FREQUENCY RESPONSE OF AN ER-3A INSERT EARPHONE

The ER-3A insert earphone was designed to simulate the response of the TDH earphone. As a result, the real-ear frequency response is quite similar. Figure 12–3 (taken from ER-3A specifications) shows the real-ear response of the ER-3A with the TDH-39 and TDH-49 responses included for comparison. The increased low-frequency response of the ER-3A is reduced when the foam plug does not create a tight seal.

TRANSFER FUNCTIONS FROM THE SOUNDFIELD TO VARIOUS LOCATIONS RELEVANT TO HEARING AIDS

There are a variety of points on the head at which sound can be measured that have relevance to hearing aid fitting. The SPL measured at these points can be affected by diffraction of sound off the head and body and by resonances created by the external ear. The changes that occur to sound as it progresses from the field to these locations

are discussed in this section. The locations that are relevant include (a) the microphone of the BTE hearing aid, (b) the microphone of the full-shell ITE hearing aid, (c) the microphone of the in-the-canal (ITC) hearing aid, (d) the tympanic membrane, (e) the hearing aid microphone location when a sound originates from the same side of the head (head baffle), and (f) the hearing aid microphone location when the sound originates from the opposite side of the head (head shadow).

FIELD-TO-BTE-MICROPHONE TRANSFER FUNCTION

The transformation of sound is relatively minor as it travels from the field to the BTE microphone location above the ear. Figure 12–4 shows the field-to-BTE-microphone transfer function obtained by Kuhn (1979). The SPL is increased only slightly at the BTE microphone due to head diffraction effects, with the largest increase being 3 dB at 2000 Hz. In other words, there is little increase in SPL at the BTE microphone due to its location over the ear.

FIELD-TO-ITE-MICROPHONE TRANSFER FUNCTION

In contrast to the BTE microphone location, there are sizeable increases in SPL at the ITE microphone location relative to the field. These are due to the in-the-concha location of the microphone. To derive this transfer function, the difference values between the BTE and ITE microphone locations reported by Cox and Risberg (1986) are added to the transfer function of Kuhn

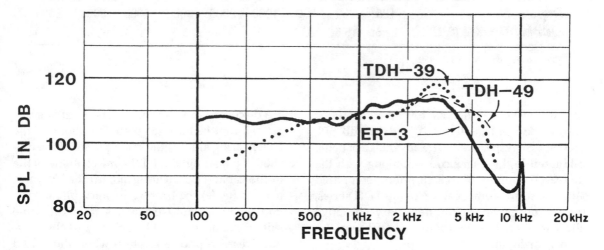

Figure 12–3. Estimated real-ear frequency response of the ER-3A insert earphone. (From Etymotic Research ER-3A specifications, with permission.)

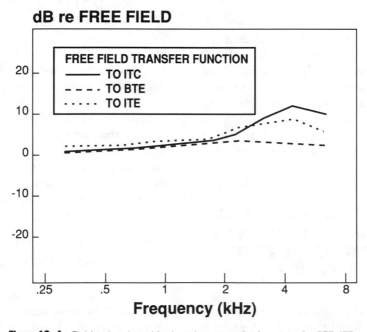

Figure 12–4. Field-to-hearing-aid-microphone transfer functions for BTE, ITE, and ITC hearing aids. BTE and ITC data are from Kuhn (1979), and ITE data are from Kuhn (1979) with modifications from Cox and Risberg (1986).

(1979). The resulting values are shown in Figure 12–4 and represent the field-to-ITE-microphone transfer function. Note the increase in the SPL arriving at the ITE hearing aid microphone compared with the BTE. This is especially true in the higher frequencies, where the concha location serves to increase the high-frequency input to the ITE hearing aid microphone by 6–8 dB in the 2000- to 4000-Hz region. This is an important phenomenon and **explains why different 2-cm³ coupler gain values are needed for the same real ear insertion gain (REIG) for BTE and ITE hearing aids.** If the input is greater in the higher frequencies at the ITE microphone, then less hearing aid gain is needed to achieve the same desired REIG.

FIELD-TO-ITC-MICROPHONE TRANSFER FUNCTION

With an ITC hearing aid, the concha is open and free to resonate. As a result, the SPL at the hearing aid microphone is increased even further in the higher frequencies. The field-to-ITC-microphone location was taken from a field-to-blocked-ear-canal-entrance transfer function measured by Kuhn (1979) and shown in Figure 12–4. Compared with the ITE transfer function, there is an increased input to the ITC hearing aid microphone in the 3000–6000 Hz region. This rather sizeable increase means that less coupler gain will be needed in the higher frequencies with an ITC than with an ITE or BTE to achieve the same amount of REIG. These findings led Sullivan (1989a, 1989b) to conclude that "smaller is better" in terms of acoustic efficiency. The term "better" is not related to speech understanding but to the fact that the smaller the ITE, the less the necessary coupler gain to achieve the same REIG.

FIELD-TO-TYMPANIC-MEMBRANE TRANSFER FUNCTION

As sound travels from the soundfield to the tympanic membrane, there is a large increase in SPL in the higher frequencies due to the combined resonances of the concha and ear canal. With the concha resonating as in Figure 12–4, and the ear canal acting as a quarter-wavelength resonator with a peak in the 2500–3000 Hz region, the combined transfer function shows a broad increase in the higher frequencies, peaking at 17 dB at 2700 Hz. The classic field-to-tympanic-membrane transfer function (called the real ear unaided response, or REUR, in probe-microphone terminology) from Shaw (1974) is shown in Figure 12–5 for sounds originating from azimuths of 0°, 45°, and 90°.

There can be **large individual differences in the REUR,** a finding that argues for individual assessment of this function in probe-microphone measurements. Both the location of the peak resonant frequency, as well as the amplitude of the peak, can vary widely across adults and children.

The REUR is important in hearing aid selection and fitting because this "natural amplification" is lost when the ear is occluded by an earmold or ITE hearing aid. Some selection and fitting procedures measure this function with probe-microphone systems to compensate individually for the lost resonance. (See Chapters 3, 4, 6, 8, and 9 for information on the REUR, how it varies as a function of age, loudspeaker azimuth, and regulating microphone location, and how the REUR can be incorporated into assessment and selection of hearing aids with probe-microphone measurements.)

FIELD-TO-HEARING-AID MICROPHONE ON THE SAME SIDE OF THE HEAD

When a person is wearing a hearing aid on the right ear and sound originates from the right side of the head (such as a 90° azimuth), an increase in SPL occurs at the hearing aid microphone due to a **head baffle effect.** The magnitude of this effect is shown in Figure 12–6 from a study by Hawkins, Foley, Stelmachowicz, and New (1992). An increase of approximately 5–7 dB occurs through the mid frequencies,

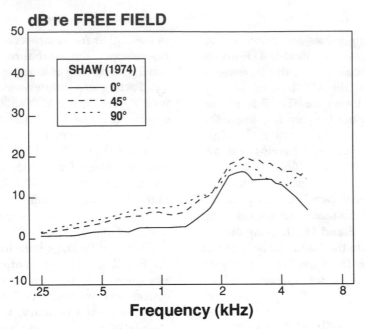

Figure 12-5. Field-to-tympanic-membrane transfer functions for loudspeaker azimuths of 0°, 45°, and 90°. Data are from Shaw (1974).

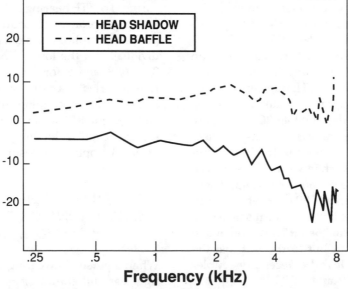

Figure 12-6. Head baffle and head shadow effects. The head baffle effect shows the increase in SPL present at the location of a BTE microphone (re: a vacant field) for a 90° azimuth source. The head shadow effect shows the decrease in SPL present at the location of a BTE microphone (re: a vacant field) for a 270° azimuth source. (Adapted from Hawkins, D., Foley, J., Stelmachowicz, P., & New, T. 1992. Desired frequency response characteristics of CROS hearing aids. Study in progress.)

then decreases in the higher frequencies. As a result, the input to the hearing aid microphone is increased for sounds originating from the same side of the head, and less gain may be appropriate. This may explain the habit of some persons who are hearing-impaired turning the side of their head toward the speaker in an attempt to hear better.

FIELD-TO-HEARING-AID MICROPHONE FROM THE OPPOSITE SIDE OF THE HEAD.

When a person is wearing a hearing aid on the right ear and sound originates from the left side of the head (270° azimuth), there is a decrease in SPL arriving at the right ear in the higher frequencies. This is due to the **head shadow** phenomenon, where the head casts a sound shadow for frequencies whose wavelength is less than the dimensions of the head. Given the average width of the adult head, the decrease in sound at the far ear begins to occur around 1500 Hz. Figure 12–6 also shows the amount of decrease that occurs as a result of the head shadow. It represents a significant reduction in higher frequencies, reaching 10 dB at 4000 Hz.

This decrease in SPL due to the head shadow is partially responsible for the difficulties experienced by monaural hearing aid users and is the phenomenon that contralateral routing of signals (CROS) hearing aids attempt to circumvent.

DIFFERENCES BETWEEN OUTPUT IN THE REAL EAR AND THE 2-CM³ COUPLER: THE REAL EAR COUPLER DIFFERENCE (RECD)

It would be convenient if the SPL output measured in a 2-cm³ coupler were identical to that measured in the real ear. Unfortunately, this is not the case. As discussed in Chapters 3, 7, and 9, this difference between hearing aid output (not gain) in a real ear and a 2-cm³ coupler is called the real ear coupler difference,

or RECD. There are several reasons why the absolute SPL output in a real ear (the real ear aided response, or REAR) is greater than that measured in a 2-cm³ coupler. First, the volume of the coupler (2-cm³) is not equal to the volume found in the typical ear canal. The **actual volume in adults is approximately 1.26 cm³; in children it is 0.66 cm³** (Bratt, 1980). The smaller volumes of real ear canals result in increased SPL compared with that of the 2-cm³ coupler. The second factor is that the impedance of the 2-cm³ coupler is not representative of the average human ear, again resulting in more SPL in the real ear than in the coupler. When these two factors are combined, a **significant increase in SPL is evident in the ear canal relative to the 2-cm³ coupler**, especially in the higher frequencies. Figure 12–7 from Hawkins et al. (1990) shows results of several studies that have measured the difference between output in adult ear canals and in a 2-cm³ coupler. (See Chapter 8 for RECD information in children.) Below 1000 Hz, there are only minor differences between output in the real ear and the 2-cm³ coupler. The data from Hawkins et al. (1990) and Feigin, Kopun, Stelmachowicz, and Gorga (1989) suggest that below 500 Hz there is slightly less output in the real ear canal than the 2-cm³ coupler. Above 1000 Hz, there is increasingly more output in the real ear canal, reaching 10–15 dB more at 6000 Hz.

Table 12–6 shows the RECDs in numerical form. These numbers represent the average of the data from Hawkins et al. (1990) and Feigin et al. (1989). The numbers in Table 12–6 are added to the 2-cm³ coupler output to yield predicted real-ear output.

These results have direct implications for predicting maximum output in the real ear from 2-cm³ coupler measurements. For instance, based on the data in Table 12–6, if a hearing aid had a 2-cm³ coupler SSPL90 of 110 dB SPL at 2000 Hz, then the predicted real ear saturation response (RESR) would be approximately 115 dB SPL. While these mean conversions are useful, the standard deviations are large enough to represent a compelling argument for the use of probe-microphone measurements to make the actual assessment of output in the real ear.

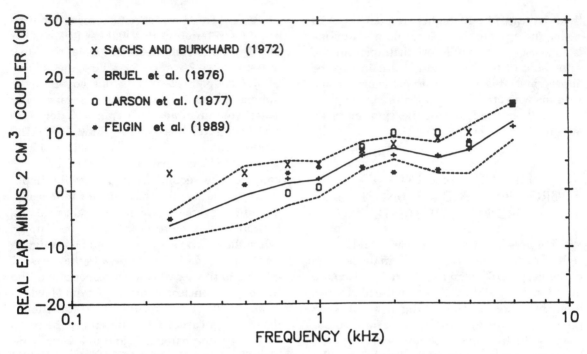

Figure 12-7. The difference between the output in a real ear (REAR) and a 2-cm³ coupler. Values above the 0 line indicate more output in a real ear than in a 2-cm³ coupler. The solid line represents the mean of 30 subjects from Hawkins et al. (1990) and the dotted line is ±1 standard deviation. Also plotted are results from four other studies. (From Hawkins, D., Cooper, W., & Thompson, D. 1990. Comparisons among SPLs in real ears, 2-cm³ and 6-cm³ couplers. *Journal of American Academy of Audiology, 1,* 154–161, with permission.)

TABLE 12-6. DIFFERENCES BETWEEN OUTPUT IN A REAL EAR AND A 2-CM³ COUPLER

			Frequency (Hz)				
250	500	1000	1500	2000	3000	4000	6000
−6	0	3	5	5	5	8	13

Numbers should be added to 2-cm³ coupler output to predict output in an average adult real ear. Values represent data averaged from Feigin et al. (1989) and Hawkins et al. (1990).

The differences between output in an ear canal and a 2-cm³ coupler (RECDs) are generally larger for children than those shown for adults in Figure 12–7 and Table 12–6. Data on these differences for children are presented in Chapter 8.

DIFFERENCES BETWEEN REIG AND 2-CM³ COUPLER GAIN

A comparison between **gain** in the real ear canal (REIG) and in the 2-cm³ coupler is quite a different issue than **output** in the real ear (REAR)

and a 2-cm^3 coupler. Since many gain and frequency response selection schemes specify desired REIG and then convert to 2-cm^3 coupler gain for BTE selection or ITE ordering, the actual conversion factors from REIG to 2-cm^3 coupler are important. The term often used to represent these conversion factors from 2-cm^3 gain to REIG is **CORFIG**, which can stand for either *COupler Response for Flat Insertion Gain* or *CORrection FIGure* (Killion & Monser, 1980)

There are three main factors that must be considered in the theoretical generation of a CORFIG to convert REIG to 2-cm^3 coupler gain. First, the field-to-tympanic-membrane transfer function (the REUR) will be lost when the ear is occluded with the hearing aid or earmold. Therefore, the transfer function shown in Figure 12–5 must be added to the desired REIG.

Second, there will be an increase in the SPL entering the hearing aid microphone when it is on a real ear, as compared with the testing in a 2-cm^3 coupler. This is due to the field-to-hearing aid microphone transfer functions described earlier and shown in Figure 12–4. Since these transfer functions represent an increase in SPL, these values, which will be different depending on whether a BTE, ITE, or ITC hearing aid is used, will be subtracted from the desired REIG. Because this factor differs with the style of hearing aid, it is necessary to calculate three different CORFIGs, one each for BTE, ITE, and ITC hearing aids.

A third factor involved in the generation of a CORFIG is that more output SPL is developed in a real ear than a 2-cm^3 coupler, as shown in Figure 12–7 and Table 12–6. This factor can be subtracted from the desired REIG, as more output is present in the real ear.

In summary, the CORFIG for converting REIG to 2-cm^3 coupler gain involves adding the REUR to the desired REIG, then subtracting the field-to-hearing-aid-microphone transfer function and the REAR/2-cm^3 coupler difference. The final **CORFIG represents the difference that is expected between REIG and 2-cm^3 coupler gain for the average person.** A CORFIG can be determined on an individual person by measuring REIG with a probe-microphone system and then measuring hearing aid gain at the same VCW setting on a 2-cm^3 coupler. This method is useful in customizing the hearing aid selection process and is discussed in detail in Chapter 9.

CORFIGs FOR BTE HEARING AIDS

CORFIGs have been determined behaviorally for BTE hearing aids by measuring functional gain and 2-cm^3 coupler gain on a number of adult subjects. Examples of this approach were described by Zemplenyi, Dirks, and Gilman (1985) employing 15 subjects and by Hawkins, Montgomery, Prosek, and Walden (1987) using 20 subjects. Their results, along with data obtained on a Knowles Electronics Manikin for Acoustic Research (KEMAR) by Burnett (1989), are shown in Figure 12–8. The differences in the lower frequencies are probably due to an excellent earmold seal on the manikin and the typical less-than-perfect earmold seal on real people.

The BTE CORFIGs suggest that REIG will be substantially less than 2-cm^3 coupler gain in the 2000–4000 Hz region. For example, at 4000 Hz, if the desired REIG were 25 dB, then approximately 35 dB of 2-cm^3 coupler gain would have to be present in the hearing aid. The corrections shown in Figure 12–8 agree well with clinical experience with BTE hearing aids. Other theoretical or KEMAR-measured CORFIGs for BTE hearing aids (e.g., Lybarger & Teder, 1986) show only minor differences between REIG and 2-cm^3 coupler gain, a finding hard to reconcile with clinical experience and the behavioral studies.

CORFIGs FOR ITE HEARING AIDS

Due to the more advantageous microphone location with the ITE hearing aid, the CORFIG is different, with smaller differences between REIG and 2-cm^3 coupler gain than with the BTE. The results of a behavioral study compar-

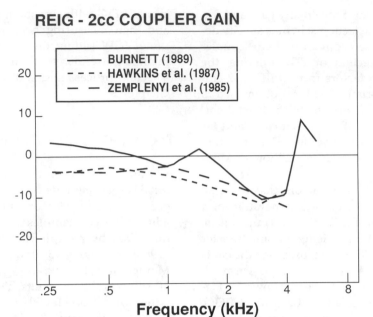

Figure 12–8. The CORFIGs for a BTE hearing aid from three studies. Values below the 0 line indicate less REIG than 2-cm³ coupler gain.

ing real-ear to 2-cm³ coupler gain (Mason & Popelka, 1986) are shown in Figure 12–9 along with the KEMAR-derived curve from Burnett and Beck (1987). The agreement is close, with the main discrepancy being in the low frequencies, where again there may have been venting effects in the behavioral data but not in the KEMAR data.

CORFIGs FOR ITC HEARING AIDS

To date there are no behavioral studies that have determined CORFIGs for ITC hearing aids. Two theoretical curves have been published (Bentler & Pavlovic, 1989; Lybarger & Teder, 1986) and are shown in Figure 12–10. From these data, it can be concluded that for an ITC hearing aid the REIG is very similar to 2-cm³ coupler gain through 3000 Hz, with more gain in the real ear at 4000 Hz and above. This high-frequency effect is in sharp contrast to the BTE CORFIG, where substantially less real-ear gain than 2-cm³ coupler gain is present. This differ-

ence is due to the **more favorable location of the ITC hearing aid microphone**. The same amount of REIG can be achieved with an ITC as a BTE in the higher frequencies with much less 2-cm³ coupler gain.

CORFIG SUMMARY

Table 12–7 provides a summary of the CORFIGs for the three types of hearing aids. These values represent this author's best guess as to clinical CORFIGs that could be used by the audiologist to convert from desired REIG values to necessary 2-cm³ coupler gains or to predict REIGs from 2-cm³ coupler gain values.

There is confusion as to whether these numbers are added or subtracted. This decision depends on which direction the conversion is being made. If one has a 2-cm³ coupler gain curve and wants to predict the amount of REIG, the numbers in Table 12–7 are added to the 2-cm³ coupler gain. For instance, if a BTE hearing aid had 30 dB of 2-cm³ gain at 3000 Hz, the pre-

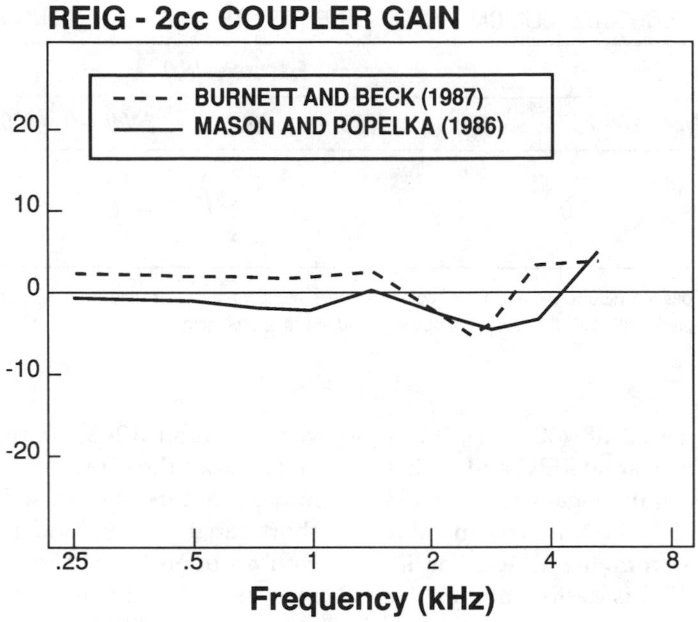

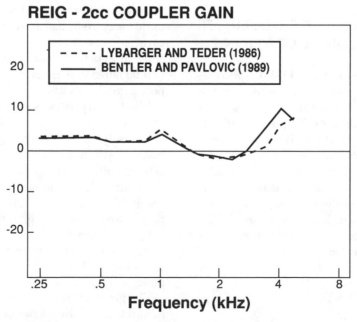

REIG - 2cc COUPLER GAIN

Figure 12–9. The CORFIGs for an ITE hearing aid from two studies. Values below the 0 line indicate less REIG than 2-cm³ coupler gain.

REIG - 2cc COUPLER GAIN

Figure 12–10. The CORFIGs for an ITC hearing aid from two studies. Values below the 0 line indicate less REIG than 2-cm³ coupler gain.

TABLE 12–7. SUGGESTED CLINICAL CORFIGs FOR BTE, ITE, AND ITC HEARING AIDS

Hearing Aid Type	Frequency (Hz)						
	250	500	1000	2000	3000	4000	6000
BTE	−3	−2	−2	−7	−10	−10	0
ITE	0	0	0	−2	− 6	0	3
ITC	0	0	0	−2	− 3	3	7

Note: To convert desired REIG to 2-cm³ coupler gain, the above numbers are subtracted from REIG. To convert 2-cm³ coupler gain to predicted REIG, the above numbers are added to 2-cm³ gain.

dicted REIG would be 20 dB (30 + (−10) = 20). If one has a desired target REIG and wishes to know the 2-cm³ coupler gain that should yield the desired REIG, the numbers in Table 12–7 are subtracted from the REIG. For instance, if 20 dB of REIG is desired at 3000 Hz with an ITE hearing aid, the predicted 2-cm³ coupler gain to yield this REIG would be 26 dB (20 − (−6) = 26). If predictions need to be made to or from 2-cm³ full-on gain values, an extra 10 or 15 dB needs to be included in the computation for reserve gain.

REAL-EAR EFFECTS OF DIFFERENT EARMOLD CONFIGURATIONS

It is important to realize that CORFIGs and prescription procedure formulas assume an **unvented earmold** with a canal bore of a specific dimension, typically 2 or 3 mm. These conditions are not always met in the actual hearing aid fitting. As a result, to select or order a hearing aid with the best probability of producing the desired real-ear response, it is necessary to include the effects of the earmold and venting configuration that are likely to be used. This requires knowledge of the real-ear effects of various earmold alterations.

VENTING

Lybarger (1985) provided the most comprehensive data on the real-ear effects of earmold venting. Table 12–8, adapted from Lybarger's data, shows the effect of vents of 1-, 2-, and 3-mm diameters when used with medium and short canal lengths and a short canal length with an open bore. The values in Table 12–8 represent the changes as compared with an unvented condition. Negative numbers indicate that the vent causes attenuation, and positive numbers indicate that more SPL is present relative to the unvented condition. While the latter may sound contradictory, a vent can increase SPL through vent-associated reactance resonance. Fortunately, these increases are generally not present in the real ear canal when minor leaks (slit leaks) are present around the earmold. For practical purposes, one can assume most of the positive numbers in Table 12–8 will be close to 0, meaning that little amplification actually occurs as a result of a vent.

What is surprising is the actual insignificance of the venting effect and that **this effect is confined only to the very low frequencies**. For instance, when a medium-canal-length earmold is used with an average vent diameter (2 mm), the vent only attenuates below 400 Hz. Electronic filtering is a far more effective way to reduce low-frequency gain than venting. Other subjective benefits, however, such as wearer comfort and reduction of the occlusion effect, often justify the presence of a vent in the earmold or ITE hearing aid.

The greatest amount of low-frequency attenuation occurs when a nonoccluding earmold is employed, which acts like a large vent. The amount of low-frequency attenuation present

TABLE 12–8. REAL-EAR EFFECTS OF PARALLEL VENTS (VENTED MINUS UNVENTED RESPONSE) FOR THREE EARMOLD CONFIGURATIONS

Earmold type	Vent (mm)	Frequency (Hz)						
		200	400	500	800	1000	1250	1600
Medium canal	1	0	4	2	1	1	0	0
length (17 mm)	2	−15	0	9	2	3	2	1
	3	−23	−10	− 4	3	3	4	2
Short canal	1	− 2	5	3	−1	1	0	0
length (12 mm)	2	−17	− 2	6	3	3	2	1
	3	−25	−12	− 6	4	3	4	3
Very short canal	1	− 8	8	6	1	1	1	0
(6 mm) and	2	−22	− 9	− 2	5	4	3	2
open bore	3	−29	−16	−11	1	1	4	3

Note: Based on data from Lybarger (1985).

TABLE 12–9. REAL-EAR EFFECT OF A NONOCCLUDING EARMOLD (OCCLUDING MINUS NONOCCLUDING RESPONSE) FOR TWO TUBING INSERTION DEPTHS

Insertion depth	Frequency (Hz)								
	200	400	500	800	1000	1600	2000	3000	4000
Short (1 mm)	−46	−34	−30	−22	−18	−11	−7	1	−2
Long (14 mm)	−37	−25	−21	−13	− 9	− 2	1	5	3

Note: Based on data from Lybarger (1985).

in a real ear with a nonoccluding earmold has been quantified by Lybarger (1985). These values are shown in Table 12–9. Note that the nonoccluding earmold begins attenuating below 2000 Hz. The attenuation increases as frequency decreases, reaching 46 dB at 200 Hz for the short insertion depth.

INTERNAL EARMOLD DIMENSIONS

Dillon (1985) provided the most complete set of data concerning the effects of changing the internal dimensions of the earmold. Table 12–10 shows some of these data. All of the values are changes from HA-2 earmold values (25 mm of #13 tubing cemented into the bore, followed by 18 mm of a 3-mm inner-diameter bore), the type used in the 2-cm^3 coupler for ANSI measurements and equivalent to a 3-mm Libby horn. (Specific dimensions of each of these types of earmolds are given in the Dillon, 1985, article.) It is clear that rather large changes can occur in the high-frequency response of the hearing aid through altering the internal dimensions of the earmold.

TABLE 12–10. EFFECTS OF EARMOLD CHANGES RELATIVE TO HA-2 EARMOLD RESPONSE

Earmold	Frequency (Hz)								
	250	500	1000	1500	2000	3000	4000	5000	6000
#13 tubing to tip	0	1	1	0	0	− 2	− 5	− 8	− 7
Llbby (3 mm)	0	0	0	1	1	3	2	0	− 4
Libby (4 mm)	−1	−1	−2	0	0	2	3	0	0
6R12	0	0	0	0	0	0	0	2	1
8CR	−1	−2	−3	−1	0	5	− 3	− 5	− 2
6B10	0	0	0	0	0	1	3	− 5	− 2
6B0	0	1	1	0	0	− 2	− 5	− 8	− 7
6C5	1	2	1	1	2	− 5	−10	−13	−16
6C10	1	3	0	−1	−3	−11	−17	−19	−22

Note: Based on data from Dillon (1985).

CONCLUSIONS

This chapter serves as a reference for a variety of corrections and transformations that are relevant to hearing aid selection and fitting. While it is not possible for the audiologist to remember all the specific numerical values, knowledge of the presence and interactions of the appropriate corrections and transformations is quite useful in understanding and increasing the scientific aspects of hearing aid selection and fitting.

CHAPTER 13

Test Protocols for Probe-Microphone Measurements

■ DAVID B. HAWKINS, Ph.D. ■

■ H. GUSTAV MUELLER, Ph.D. ■

The following test protocols are provided as quick references when conducting various probe-microphone measurements. Each type of measurement has a specific abbreviated test protocol, clinical applications, and chapter references.

The protocols have been written in a step-by-step manner. There may be some steps that will vary depending on what probe-microphone equipment is being employed. In particular, the initial soundfield equalization and probe-tube calibration procedures differ among equipment. We recommend that you consult the operation manual for aspects that are equipment-specific.

REAL EAR UNAIDED RESPONSE (REUR)

TEST PROTOCOL

- Equalize soundfield and calibrate probe tube.
- Place probe tube in ear canal 25–30 mm past the tragal notch.
- Select stimulus type and intensity. It is best to select stimulus and intensity that will later be used for real ear insertion response (REIR) measurement. If above the room noise floor, 60 dB SPL is acceptable.
- Conduct measurement.

CLINICAL APPLICATION

- Provides reference for the REIR measurement.
- Can be used in selecting the appropriate 2-cm^3 coupler gain based on target real ear insertion gain (REIG); that is, the REUR is used to "customize" the conversion from prescribed REIG to 2-cm^3 coupler gain.
- Unusual configuration could indicate tympanic membrane perforation, external or middle ear pathology, or excessive cerumen.

REFERENCE

- Chapters 3, 4, 6, and 9.

REAL EAR AIDED RESPONSE (REAR) AS PART OF REAL EAR INSERTION RESPONSE (REIR)

TEST PROTOCOL

- Keep probe tube at same location in ear canal as was used for REUR measurement.
- Place hearing aid on the patient and adjust volume control wheel (VCW) to desired position.
- Select same stimulus and intensity as used in REUR measurement.
- Conduct measurement and repeat until desired response is obtained.

CLINICAL APPLICATION

- Serves as aided response from which the REIR is derived.

- Serves as indication of amplified sound pressure level (SPL) in the ear canal for a given input level.
- Used in determining the real ear to coupler difference (RECD).

REFERENCE

- Chapters 3, 4, 6, 7, and 9.

REAR AS PART OF AMPLIFIED-SPEECH SPECTRUM APPROACH

TEST PROTOCOL

- Equalize soundfield and calibrate probe tube.
- Place probe tube in ear canal 25–30 mm past the tragal notch (15–20 mm with a child).
- Select stimulus type and intensity. Speech-weighted noise at 70 dB SPL best represents typical inputs.
- Place hearing aid on the patient and adjust VCW to desired position.
- Conduct measurement and repeat until desired response is obtained, that is, targets for the amplified speech spectrum are most closely approximated.

CLINICAL APPLICATION

- Used to adjust the hearing aid to make speech audible and at desired sensation levels` (DSLs).
- Particularly appealing for pediatric population.

REFERENCE

- Chapters 5 and 8.

TELECOIL REAR USING INPUT FROM TELEPHONE

TEST PROTOCOL

- Disable loudspeaker, either through the system's software or by manually unhooking wires leading to loudspeaker. Ready system to measure a signal.

- Place probe tube in ear canal 25–30 mm past the tragal notch.
- Place hearing aid on the patient and set to T to activate telecoil.
- Adjust VCW to full-on.
- Connect two telephone lines within the clinic (use one line to "call" another).
- Route speech noise from audiometer earphone at 60 dB HL to the transmitting telephone, which is received by the other telephone, located near the probe-microphone equipment.
- Place headset of receiving telephone at desired position near the hearing aid; rotation of headset may be required to obtain most output.
- Conduct measurement.

CLINICAL APPLICATION

- Determine if telecoil response is appropriate.
- Allows comparison of one telecoil response to another.
- Allows comparison of one telephone to another.
- Determines the effects of telephone-amplifying systems.
- Determines sensitivity of the telecoil as a function of positioning of the headset.

REFERENCE

- Chapter 11.

REAR OF AN ASSISTIVE LISTENING DEVICE (ALD) OR FM SYSTEM

TEST PROTOCOL

- Place ALD microphone in the calibrated or equalized soundfield location. If possible, use the substitution method and equalize the field, then locate ALD microphone in the vacant soundfield at the calibrated location. If using modi-fied-comparison method, place the ALD microphone near the regulating microphone.
- Place probe tube in ear canal 25–30 mm past the tragal notch.
- Fit receiver of ALD (e.g., earbud or headphones) to the ear.
- Adjust ALD VCW to desired position.
- Assuming the ALD will be used with the microphone 6–8 in. from the speak-er's mouth, select either a speech-weighted noise at 80 dB SPL or a swept frequency-specific signal at 75 dB SPL.
- Conduct measurement.

CLINICAL APPLICATION

- Determines if ALD response is appropriate.
- Allows comparison of one ALD to another.
- Allows comparison of the effects of different ALD receivers.

REFERENCE

- Chapter 11.

REAL EAR INSERTION RESPONSE (REIR)

TEST PROTOCOL

- Equalize soundfield and calibrate probe tube.
- Place probe tube in ear canal 25–30 mm past the tragal notch.
- Select stimulus type and intensity.
- Complete REUR and REAR as described earlier.
- REIR is typically automatically displayed by subtracting the REUR from the REAR.
- Make adjustments using digital programming potentiometer(s), VCW, venting, and so on. Repeat measurements until best match to target REIG values is obtained.

CLINICAL APPLICATION

- Provides verification of target REIG values.
- Determines acceptability of hearing aid gain and frequency response.

REFERENCE

- Chapters 3, 4, 5, 6, 9, 10, and 11.

REAL EAR SATURATION RESPONSE (RESR)

TEST PROTOCOL

- Equalize soundfield and calibrate probe tube.

- Adjust hearing aid output control to minimum SSPL90 setting.
- Place probe tube in ear canal 25–30 mm past the tragal notch.
- Place hearing aid on patient and adjust VCW to highest position before feedback or projected use setting if hearing aid has input compression.
- Select swept pure-tone or warble-tone signal at 90 dB SPL.
- Conduct measurement; curve will represent minimum RESR for the instrument.
- Increase SSPL90 control and repeat measurement until desired RESR is obtained.

CLINICAL APPLICATION

- Determines the maximum SPL the hearing aid is capable of delivering to the user's ear.
- Allows proper adjustment of SSPL90.
- Provides information relevant to concerns about overamplification.
- Provides documentation for any litigation concerning overamplification.

REFERENCE

- Chapters 4, 7, and 8.

REAL EAR AND 2-CM³ LOUDNESS DISCOMFORT LEVELS (LDLs)

TEST PROTOCOL

- Calibrate probe tube if necessary.
- Disable loudspeaker, either through the system's software or by manually unhooking wires leading to loudspeaker. Ready system to measure a signal.
- Place probe tube in ear canal 25–30 mm past the tragal notch.
- Place a portable audiometer with ER-3A earphones next to the probe-microphone system.
- Using a foam insert, put the ER-3A on the patient's ear (probe tube can be threaded through the foam to help maintain proper position in the ear canal).
- Obtain LDLs for pure tones at 500, 1000, and 2000 Hz.
- At the determined point of loudness discomfort at each frequency, turn the pure tone on continuously and measure the SPL in the ear canal at the LDL.
- Record the LDLs in dB HL and convert to dB SPL in a 2-cm³ coupler. These conversions are obtained by calibrating the ER-3A in an HA-1 2-cm³ coupler; for instance, if 70 dB HL on the audiometer dial produces 75 dB SPL in the

2-cm3 coupler, then 5 dB is added to the earphone dB HL LDL to give the LDL in 2-cm^3 dB SPL.

CLINICAL APPLICATION

■ Provides target 2-cm^3 coupler SSPL90 values based on LDLs for use in selecting behind-the-ear (BTE) hearing aids or ordering in-the-ear (ITE) hearing aids.
■ Provides target RESR values for use in adjusting the output control and setting the SSPL90 at the hearing aid fitting.

REFERENCE

■ Chapter 7.

PREDICTED REAL EAR SATURATION RESPONSE (RESR)

TEST PROTOCOL

■ Equalize soundfield and calibrate probe tube.
■ Place probe tube in ear canal 25–30 mm past the tragal notch.
■ Place hearing aid on the patient and adjust the VCW to a mid position.
■ Obtain REAR with a 60- or 70-dB SPL signal.
■ Without changing the VCW, remove the hearing aid and measure the 2-cm^3 coupler output using the same input intensity as was used for the REAR.
■ Obtain a real ear to coupler difference (RECD) by subtracting the 2-cm^3 response from the REAR.
■ Turn the VCW full-on and measure an SSPL90 curve in the 2-cm^3 coupler.
■ Add the RECD to the 2-cm^3 coupler SSPL90 curve; the result is the predicted RESR.

CLINICAL APPLICATION

■ Determines the maximum predicted SPL the hearing aid is capable of delivering to the user's ear.
■ Allows proper adjustment of SSPL90.
■ Provides information relevant to concerns about overamplification.
■ Provides documentation for any litigation concerning overamplification.

REFERENCE

- Chapter 7.

REAL EAR OCCLUDED RESPONSE (REOR)

TEST PROTOCOL

- Equalize soundfield and calibrate probe tube.
- Place probe tube in ear canal 25–30 mm past the tragal notch.
- Conduct REUR measurement.
- Place ITE hearing aid or BTE and earmold in the ear with the hearing aid turned off.
- Conduct measurement using the same input intensity as was used for the REUR.
- Compare REOR to the REUR and the input level used.

CLINICAL APPLICATION

- Determines the degree that the hearing aid or earmold is attenuating direct input sound, that is, is venting allowing sound to pass through at desired frequencies.
- Determines if increased gain is present in the lower frequencies due to vent resonance.

REFERENCE

- Chapters 3 and 6.

OCCLUSION EFFECT CAUSED BY HEARING AID OR EARMOLD

TEST PROTOCOL

- Disable loudspeaker, either through the system's software or by manually unhooking wires leading to loudspeaker. Ready system to measure a signal.
- Place probe tube in ear canal 25–30 mm past the tragal notch.
- Have patient vocalize a vowel such as /ee/.

- Have patient monitor vocal intensity by observing a sound-level meter.
- When patient sustains vocalization at a desired level, for example, 80 dB SPL at 12 in., measure SPL in the unaided ear canal.
- Place ITE hearing aid or BTE with earmold on the patient with the hearing aid turned off; repeat the measurement.
- Compare the difference between the two measurements, which is the occlusion effect.

CLINICAL APPLICATION

- Determines if a hearing aid or earmold is causing an occlusion effect for the patient's voice.
- Determines if alterations in venting or canal length reduce the occlusion effect.

REFERENCE

- Chapter 10.

REAL EAR COUPLER DIFFERENCE (RECD)

TEST PROTOCOL

- Equalize soundfield and calibrate probe tube.
- Place probe tube in ear canal 25–30 mm past the tragal notch.
- Place hearing aid on the patient and set the VCW to a mid position. Obtain an REAR with a 60- or 70-dB SPL signal (level is important only in that the hearing aid should not be in saturation).
- Remove the hearing aid without changing the VCW.
- Measure the output of the hearing aid in a 2-cm^3 coupler with the same input intensity as used in the REAR measurement.
- Subtract the 2-cm^3 coupler output from the REAR, producing the RECD.

CLINICAL APPLICATION

- Can be used in selecting the appropriate 2-cm^3 coupler gain based on target REIG, that is, the RECD can be used to "customize" the conversion from prescribed REIG to 2-cm^3 coupler gain.
- Can be used in obtaining the predicted RESR.

REFERENCE

■ Chapters 7, 9, and 12.

DETERMINING DESIRED 2-CM³ COUPLER GAIN THROUGH USE OF CUSTOMIZED CORRECTION VALUES (CORFIGs)

TEST PROTOCOL

■ Equalize soundfield and calibrate probe tube.
■ Place probe tube in ear canal 25–30 mm past the tragal notch.
■ Measure the REUR.
■ Place hearing aid on the patient, preferably the type that will be selected or ordered, and set the VCW to a mid position.
■ Measure the REAR and thus determine the REIR.
■ Remove the hearing aid and, without changing the VCW position, measure the 2-cm³ coupler gain with the same input intensity as used in the REAR.
■ Subtract the REIR from the 2-cm³ coupler gain, thus providing the customized CORFIG.
■ Add the CORFIG to the prescribed target REIG values, yielding the desired 2-cm³ coupler gain at use VCW position.
■ Add 10 dB for reserve gain; the resulting values will be the desired full-on 2-cm³ coupler gain.

CLINICAL APPLICATION

■ Customizes the 2-cm³ coupler gain order to optimize the chances of obtaining the prescribed target REIG.

REFERENCE

■ Chapters 9 and 12.

References

American National Standards Institute. (1977). *Criteria for permissible ambient noise during audiometric testing. ANSI S3.1-1977.* New York: American National Standards Institute, Inc.

American National Standards Institute. (1986). *Occluded ear simulator. ANSI S3.25-1979.* New York: American National Standards Institute, Inc.

American National Standards Institute. (1987). *Specification of hearing aid characteristics. ANSI S3.22-1987.* New York: American National Standards Institute, Inc.

American National Standards Institute. (1989). *Specification for audiometers. ANSI S3.6-1989.* New York: American National Standards Institute, Inc.

Angeli, G., Seestedt-Stanford, L., & Nerbonne, M. (1990). Consistency among/within manufacturers regarding electroacoustic properties of ITE instruments. *Hearing Journal, 43,* 23–27.

Ayers, E. (1953). A discussion of some problems involved in deriving objective performance criteria for a wearable hearing aid from clinical measurements with laboratory apparatus. *Proceedings, First ICA Congress, 1,* 141–143.

Beck. L. (1983). Assessment of directional hearing aid characteristics. *Audiological Acoustics, 22,* 178–191.

Beck, L. (1991). Amplification needs: Where do we go from here? In G. Studebaker, F. Bess, & L. Beck (Eds.), *The Vanderbilt hearing-aid report II* (pp. 1–9). Parkton, MD: York Press.

Beck, L., & Nance, G. (1989). Hearing aids, assistive listening devices and telephones: Issues to consider. *Seminars in Hearing, 10,* 78–89.

Bentler, R. (1989). External ear resonance characteristics in children. *Journal of Speech and Hearing Disorders, 54,* 264–268.

Bentler, R. (1991). Programmable hearing aid review. *American Journal of Audiology, 1,* 25–29.

Bentler, R., & Pavlovic, C. (1989). Transfer functions and correction factors used in hearing aid evaluation and research. *Ear and Hearing, 10,* 58–63.

Berger, K., Hagberg, E., & Rane, R. (1977). Prescription of hearing aids: Rationale, procedures, and results. Kent, OH: Herald Publishing.

Berger, K., Hagberg, E., & Rane, R. (1980). A reexamination of the one-half gain rule. *Ear and Hearing, 1,* 223–225.

Berger, K., Hagberg, E., & Rane, R. (1988). *Prescription of hearing aids: Rationale, procedures, and results.* Kent, OH: Herald Publishing.

Bratt, G. (1980). *Hearing aid receiver output in occluded ear canals of children.* Unpublished doctoral dissertation, Vanderbilt University, Nashville, TN.

Bratt, G., & Sammeth, C. (1991). Clinical implications of prescriptive formulas for hearing aid selection. In G. Studebaker, F. Bess, & L. Beck (Eds.), *The Vanderbilt hearing-aid report II* (pp. 23–35). Parkton, MD: York Press.

Brooks, D. (1973). Gain requirements of hearing aid users. *Scandinavian Audiology, 2,* 199–205.

Brooks, W., & Grimes, A. (1989). *Real ear assessment of personal communication devices.* Paper presented at the Annual Convention of the American Speech-Language-Hearing Association, St. Louis, MO.

Bruel, P., Frederiksen, E., & Rasmussen, G. (1976). Investigation of a new insert earphone coupler. *Hearing Instruments, 34,* 22–25.

Bryant, M., Mueller, H., & Northern, J. (1991).

Minimal contact long canal ITE hearing instruments. *Hearing Instruments, 42,* 12–15.

Bryant, M., Mueller, H., & Reidel, C. (1990). Establishing real ear insertion gain pass/fail criteria for ITE fittings. *Audiology Today, 2,* 27.

Burkhard, M., & Sachs, R. (1975). Anthropometric manikin for acoustic research. *Journal of the Acoustical Society of America, 58,* 214–222.

Burkhard, M., & Sachs, R. (1977). Sound pressure in insert earphone couplers and real ears. *Journal of Speech and Hearing Research, 20,* 799–807.

Burnett, E. (1989). *Handbook of hearing aid measurement: 1989.* Washington, DC: VA Medical Center.

Burnett, E., & Beck, L. (1987). A correction for converting 2 cm^3 coupler responses to insertion responses for custom in-the-ear nondirectional hearing aids. *Ear and Hearing, 8*(Suppl. 5), 89S–94S.

Byrne, D. (1987). Hearing aid selection formulae: Same or different? *Hearing Instruments, 38,* 5–11.

Byrne, D. (1992). Key issues in hearing aid selection and evaluation. *Journal of the American Academy of Audiology, 3*(2), 67–80.

Byrne, D., & Cotton, S. (1988). Evaluation of the National Acoustics Laboratories' new hearing aid selection procedure. *Journal of Speech and Hearing Research, 31,* 178–186.

Byrne, D., & Dillon, H. (1986). The National Acoustic Laboratories' (NAL) new procedure for selecting the gain and frequency response of a hearing aid. *Ear and Hearing, 7,* 257–265.

Byrne, D., Parkinson, A., & Newall, P. (1990). Hearing aid gain and frequency response requirements for the severely/profoundly hearing impaired. *Ear and Hearing, 11,* 40–49.

Byrne, D., Parkinson, A., & Newall, P. (1991). Modified hearing aid selection procedures for severe/profound hearing losses. In G. Studebaker, F. Bess, & L. Beck (Eds.), *The Vanderbilt hearing-aid report II* (pp. 295–300). Parkton, MD: York Press.

Byrne, D., & Tonisson, W. (1976). Selecting the gain of hearing aids for persons with sensorineural hearing impairments. *Scandanavian Audiology, 5,* 51–59.

Byrne, D., & Upfold, G. (1991). Implications of ear canal resonance for hearing aid fitting. *Seminars in Hearing, 12*(1), 34–41.

Carhart, R. (1946). Tests for selection of hearing aids. *Laryngoscope, 56,* 780–794.

Civantos, F., & Meyer, D. (1990). Ear canal resonance in surgically modified external auditory canals. *ASHA, 10,* 62.

Compton, C. (1989). Assistive listening devices. *Seminars in Hearing, 10*(1), 1–122.

Compton, C. (1991). Clinical management of assistive technology users. In G. Studebaker, F. Bess, & L. Beck (Eds.), *The Vanderbilt hearing-aid report II* (pp. 301–318). Parkton, MD: York Press.

Cox, R. (1979). Acoustic aspects of hearing aid-ear canal coupling systems. *Monographs in Contemporary Audiology, 1,* 1–44.

Cox, R. (1983). Using ULCL measures to find frequency-gain and SSPL90. *Hearing Instruments, 34,* 17–21, 39.

Cox, R. (1985). A structured approach to hearing aid selection. *Ear and Hearing, 6,* 226–239.

Cox, R. (1986). NBS-9A coupler-to-eardrum transformation: TDH-39 and TDH-49 earphones. *Journal of Acoustical Society of America, 79,* 120–123.

Cox, R. (1988). The MSU hearing instrument prescription procedure. *Hearing Instruments, 39,* 6–10.

Cox, R. (1989). Comfortable loudness level: Stimulus effects, long-term reliability, and predictability. *Journal of Speech and Hearing Research, 32,* 816–828.

Cox, R., & Alexander, G. (1990). Evaluation of an in-situ output probe-microphone method for hearing verification. *Ear and Hearing, 11,* 31–39.

Cox, R., & Alexander, G. (1991a). Preferred hearing aid gain in everyday environments. *Ear and Hearing, 12,* 123–127.

Cox, R., & Alexander, G. (1991b). Hearing aid benefit in everyday environments. *Ear and Hearing, 12,* 127–140.

Cox, R., & Moore, J. (1988). Composite speech spectrum for hearing aid gain prescriptions. *Journal of Speech and Hearing Research, 31,* 102–107.

Cox, R., & Risberg, D. (1986). Comparison of in-the-ear and over-the-ear hearing aid fittings. *Journal of Speech and Hearing Disorders, 51,* 362–369.

Cranmer, K. (1991). Hearing aid dispensing. *Hearing Instruments, 42*(6), 6–13.

Curran, J. (1988). Hearing aids. In N. Lass, L. McReynolds, J. Northern, & D. Yoder (Eds.), *Handbook of speech-language pathology and audiology* (pp. 1293–1314). Toronto, Canada: B.C. Decker.

Dalsgaard, S., & Dyrlund-Jensen, O. (1976). Measurements of the insertion gain of hearing aids. *Journal Audiologic Technique, 15,* 170.

Davies, J., & Mueller H. (1987). Hearing aid selection. In H. Mueller & V. Geoffrey (Eds.), *Communication disorders in aging* (pp. 408–436). Washington, DC: Gallaudet Press.

Davis, A., & Haggard, M. (1982). Some implications of audiological measures in the population for binaural aiding strategies. In O. Pederson & T. Paulson (Eds.), *Binaural effects in normal and impaired hearing (pp.167–179). Scandinavian Audiology* (Suppl. 15).

Davis, H., Hudgins, C., Marquis, R., Nichols, R., Peterson, G., Ross, D., & Stevens, S. (1946). The selection of hearing aids. *Laryngoscope, 56,* 85–163.

Dempster, J., & Mackenzie, K. (1990). The resonance frequency of the external auditory canal in children. *Ear and Hearing, 11,* 296–298.

Dillon, H. (1985). Earmolds and high frequency response modification. *Hearing Instruments, 36,* 8–12.

Dillon, H., & Murray, N. (1987). Accuracy of twelve methods for estimating the real ear gain of hearing aids. *Ear and Hearing, 8,* 2–11.

Dillon, H., & Walker, G. (1983). Compression: Input or output control. *Hearing Instruments, 34,* 20–22, 42.

Dirks, D., & Kincaid, G. (1987). Basic acoustic considerations of ear canal probe measurements. *Ear and Hearing, 8*(Suppl. 5), 60S–67S.

Dolan, T. (1991). High frequency biasing in measuring AGC responses. *Hearing Instruments, 42,* 3, 28, 46.

Ely, W., Curran, J., & Becker, A. (1978). *An investigation of blooming in AGC and peak-clipping hearing aids.* Paper presented at American Auditory Society Convention, San Francisco.

Erber, N. (1968). Variables that influence sound pressures generated in the ear canal by an audiometric earphone. *Journal of the Acoustical Society of America, 44,* 555–562.

Ewertsen, H., Ipsen, J., & Nielsen, S. (1956). On acoustical characteristics of the earmold. *Acta Otolaryngologica, 47,* 312–317.

Fabry, D. (1991a). Programmable and automatic noise reduction in existing hearing aids. In G. Studebaker, F. Bess, & L. Beck (Eds.), *The Vanderbilt hearing-aid report II* (pp. 65–75). Parkton, MD: York Press.

Fabry, D. (1991b). Hearing aid compression. *American Journal of Audiology, 1,* 11–13.

Feigin, J., Kopun, J., Stelmachowicz, P., & Gorga, M. (1989). Probe-tube microphone measures of ear-canal sound pressure levels in infants and children. *Ear and Hearing, 10,* 254–258.

Feigin, J., Nelson Barlow, N., & Stelmachowicz, P. (1990). The effect of reference microphone placement on sound-pressure levels at an ear-level hearing aid microphone. *Ear and Hearing, 11,* 321–326.

Fikret-Pasa, S., & Revit, L. (1992). Individualized correction factors in the pre-selection of hearing aids. *Journal of Speech and Hearing Research, 35*(2), 384–400.

Frye, G. (1986). High-speed real-time hearing aid analysis. *Hearing Journal, 39,* 21–26.

Frye, G. (1987). Crest factor and composite signals for hearing aid testing. *Hearing Journal, 40,* 15–18.

Gabbard, S., & Northern, J. (1987). Real ear hearing instrument measurements in children. *Hearing Instruments, 38,* 11–13, 67.

Gagne, J-P., Seewald, R., Zelisko, D., & Hudson, S. (1991). Procedure for defining the auditory area of hearing impaired adolescents with severe/profound hearing loss I: Detection thresholds. *Journal of Speech-Language Pathology and Audiology, 15,*13–20.

Gallagher, G. (1989). Real-ear measurement: Adding more science to the artful science of fitting. *Hearing Journal, 42,* 11–17.

Gilman, S., & Dirks, D. (1986). Acoustics of ear canal measurement of eardrum SPL in simulators. *Journal of the Acoustical Society of America, 80,* 783–792.

Gilmore, R., & Lederman, N. (1989). Inductive loop assistive listening systems: Back to the future? *Hearing Instruments, 40,* 14–20.

Gordon-Salant, S. (1991). Special amplification considerations for elderly individuals. In G. Studebaker, F. Bess, & L. Beck (Eds.), *The Vanderbilt hearing-aid report II* (pp. 245–261). Parkton, MD: York Press.

Grimes, A., & Mueller, H. (1988). Hearing aid distortion in the real ear. *ASHA, 30,* 150.

Grimes, A., & Mueller, H. (1991a). Using probe-microphone measures to assess telecoils and ALD's. Part I: Assessment of telecoil performance. *Hearing Journal, 44,* 16–21.

Grimes, A., & Mueller, H. (1991b). Using probe-microphone measures to assess telecoils and ALD's. Part II: Assessment of ALD's telephones, and telephone amplifiers. *Hearing Journal, 44,* 21–29.

Hagen, L., & Preves, D. (1982). Beyond the NBS-9A coupler: The probe microphone as an SPL determinant. *Hearing Aid Journal, 35,* 7–12.

Harford, E. (1981). Amplification for sensorineural hearing loss. In M. Paparella & W. Meyerhoff (Eds.), *Sensorineural hearing loss, vertigo and tinnitus* (pp. 121–127). Baltimore, MD: Williams & Wilkins.

Harford, E. (1982). Real ear measurements for prescribing a hearing aid. In M. Paparella & M. Goycoolea (Eds.), *Ear clinics international* (pp. 171–181). Baltimore, MD: Williams & Wilkins.

Harris, J. (1971). Summary of the symposium on amplification for sensorineural hearing loss. In *Harris on audiology.* Groton, CT: W. Shilling Co.

Hawkins, D. (1982). Overamplification: A well-documented case study. *Journal of Speech and Hearing Disorders, 47,* 382–384.

Hawkins, D. (1984). Selection of a critical electroacoustic characteristic: SSPL90. *Hearing Instruments, 35,* 28–32.

Hawkins, D. (1986). Selection of hearing aid characteristics. In W. Hodgson (Ed.), *Hearing aid assessment and use in audiologic habilitation* (3rd ed., pp. 128–151). Baltimore, MD: Williams & Wilkins.

Hawkins, D. (1987a). Assessment of FM systems with an ear canal probe tube microphone system. *Ear and Hearing, 8,* 301–303.

Hawkins, D. (1987b). Clinical ear canal probe tube measurements. *Ear and Hearing, 8*(Suppl. 5), 74S–81S.

Hawkins, D. (1987c). Variability in clinical ear canal probe microphone measurements. *Hearing Instruments, 38,* 30–32.

Hawkins, D. (1991). Acoustic measures of hearing aid performance. In G. Studebaker, F. Bess, & L. Beck (Eds.), *The Vanderbilt hearing-aid report II* (pp. 123–139). Parkton, MD: York Press.

Hawkins, D., Alvarez, E., & Houlihan, J. (1991). Reliability of three types of probe tube microphone measurements. *Hearing Instruments, 42,* 14–16.

Hawkins, D., Ball, T., Beasley, H., & Cooper, W. (1992). A comparison of SSPL90 selection procedures. *Journal of American Academy of Audiology, 3,* 46–50.

Hawkins, D., Beck, L., Bratt, G., Fabry, D., Mueller, H., & Stelmachowicz, P. (1991). *The Vanderbilt/Department of Veterans Affairs 1990 Conference Consensus Statement: Recommended components of a hearing aid selection procedure for adults. Audiology Today, 3,* 16–18.

Hawkins, D., Cooper, W., & Thompson, D. (1990). Comparisons among SPLs in real ears, 2 cm^3 and 6 cm^3 couplers. *Journal of American Academy of Audiology, 1,* 154–161.

Hawkins, D., Foley, J., Stelmachowicz, P., & New, T. (1992). Desired frequency response characteristics of CROS hearing aids. Study in progress.

Hawkins, D., Montgomery, A., Prosek, R., & Walden, B. (1987a). Examination of two issues concerning functional gain measurements. *Journal of Speech and Hearing Disorders, 52,* 56–63.

Hawkins, D., Morrison, T., Halligan, P., & Cooper, W. (1989). Use of probe tube measurements in hearing aid selection for children: Some initial clinical experiences. *Ear and Hearing, 10,* 281–287.

Hawkins, D., & Mueller, H. (1986). Some variables affecting the accuracy of probe tube microphone measurements. *Hearing Instruments, 37,* 8–12, 49.

Hawkins, D., & Naidoo, S. (1992). *The effect of peak clipping and compression limiting upon perceived sound clarity and quality.* Paper presented at annual convention of American Academy of Audiology, Nashville, TN.

Hawkins, D., & Schum, D. (1984). Relationships among various measures of hearing aid gain. *Journal of Speech and Hearing Disorders, 49,* 94–97.

Hawkins, D., & Schum, D. (1992). LDL measures: An efficient use of clinic time? *American Journal of Audiology, 1,* 8–10.

Hawkins, D., Walden, B., Montgomery, A., & Prosek, R. (1987b). Description and validation of an LDL procedure designed to select SSPL90. *Ear and Hearing, 8,* 162–169.

Hawkins, D., & Yacullo, W. (1984). Signal-to-noise advantage of binaural hearing aids and directional microphones under different levels of reverberation. *Journal of Speech and Hearing Disorders, 49,* 278–286.

Heide, V. (1991). Variables in real ear measurement. *Hearing Instruments, 42,* 24–25.

Hodson, W., & Tillman, T. (1966). Reliability of bone conduction occlusion effects in normals. *Journal of Auditory Research, 6,* 141–153.

Holmes, A., & Frank, T. (1984). Telephone listening ability for hearing-impaired individuals. *Ear and Hearing, 5,* 96–100.

Humes, L. (1986). An evaluation of several rationales for selecting hearing aid gain. *Journal of Speech and Hearing Disorders, 51,* 272–281.

Humes, L. (1991a). Understanding the speech understanding problems of the hearing impaired. *Journal of American Academy of Audiology, 2,* 59–69.

Humes, L. (1991b). Prescribing gain characteristics of linear hearing aids. In G. Studebaker, F. Bess, & Beck, L. (Eds.), *The Vanderbilt hearing-aid report II* (pp. 13–23). Parkton, MD: York Press.

Humes, L., & Hackett, T. (1990). Comparison of frequency response and aided speech-recognition performance for hearing aids selected by three different prescriptive methods. *Journal of American Academy of Audiology, 1,* 101–108.

Humes, L., & Houghton, R. (1992). Beyond insertion gain. *Hearing Instruments, 43*(3), 32–35.

Humes, L., & Kirn, E. (1990). The reliability of functional gain. *Journal of Speech and Hearing Disorders, 55,* 193–197.

Humes, L., Hipskind, N., & Block, M. (1988). Insertion gain measured with three probe tube systems. *Ear and Hearing, 9,* 108–112.

Ickes, M., Hawkins, D., & Cooper, W. (1991). Effect

of loudspeaker azimuth and reference microphone location on ear canal probe tube microphone measurements. *Journal of American Academy of Audiology, 2,* 156–163.

Jerger, J. (1987). On the evaluation of hearing aid performance. *ASHA, 29,* 49–51.

Jerger, J., Johnson, K., & Smith-Farach, S. (1989). Signal processing. *Hearing Instruments, 40,* 12–18.

Jerger, J., Malmquist, C., & Speaks, C. (1966). Comparison of some speech intelligibility tests in the evaluation of hearing aid performance. *Journal of Speech and Hearing Research, 9,* 253–258.

Johansen, P. (1975). Magnitude of the acoustical feedback as a function of leakage in earmold. *Scandinavian Audiology,* (Suppl. 5), 271–279.

Kawell, M., Kopun, J., & Stelmachowicz, P. (1988). Loudness discomfort levels in children. *Ear and Hearing, 9,* 133–136.

Killion, M. (1978). Revised estimate of minimum audible pressure: Where is the "missing" 6 dB. *Journal of Acoustical Society of America, 63,* 1501–1508.

Killion, M. (1988a). An "acoustically invisible" hearing aid. *Hearing Instruments, 39*(10), 39–44.

Killion, M. (1988b). The "hollow voice" occlusion effect. In J. Jensen (Ed.), *Hearing aid fitting: Theoretical and practical views* (pp. 231–241). Copenhagen, Denmark: Stougaard.

Killion, M., & Monser, E. (1980). CORFIG: Coupler response for flat insertion gain. In G. Studebaker & I. Hochberg (Eds.), *Acoustical factors affecting hearing aid performance* (pp. 149–168). Baltimore, MD: University Park Press.

Killion, M., & Revit, L. (1987). Insertion gain repeatability versus loudspeaker location: You want me to put my loudspeaker W H E R E? *Ear and Hearing, 8*(Suppl. 5), 68S–73S.

Killion, M., Staab, W., & Preves, D. (1990). Classifying automatic signal processors. *Hearing Instruments, 41, 8,* 24–26.

Kirkwood, D. (1990). 1990 U.S. hearing aid sales summary. *Hearing Journal, 43*(12), 7–13.

Kirkwood, D. (1991). 1991 U.S. hearing aid sales summary. *Hearing Journal, 44*(12), 9–15.

Klar, I., & Trede, K. (1986). Real ear measurements: A second generation instrument. *Hearing Instruments, 37,* 15–16.

Kopun, J., Stelmachowicz, P., Carney, E., & Schulte, L. (1992). Coupling of FM systems to individuals with unilateral hearing loss. *Journal of Speech and Hearing Research, 35*(1), 201–208.

Koschmann, D., & Garstecki, D. (1987, November). *Probe tube microphone measures in assistive listening*

device evaluation. Paper presented at the ASHA Convention, New Orleans.

Kruger, B. (1987). An update on the external ear resonance in infants and young children. *Ear and Hearing, 8,* 333–336.

Kruger, B., & Ruben, R. (1987). The acoustic properties of the infant ear. *Acta Otolaryngologica, 103,* 578–585.

Kuhn, G. (1979). The pressure transformation from a diffuse sound field to the external ear and to the body and head surface. *Journal of Acoustical Society of America, 65,* 991–1000.

Larson, V., Egolf, D., & Cooper, W. (1991). Application of acoustic impedance measures to hearing aid fitting. In G. Studebaker, F. Bess, & L. Beck (Eds.), *The Vanderbilt hearing-aid report II* (pp. 165–175). Parkton, MD: York Press.

Larson, V., Studebaker, G., & Cox, R. (1977). Sound levels in a 2-cc cavity, a Zwislocki coupler, and occluded ear canals. *Journal of American Auditory Society, 3,* 63–70.

Leijon, A., Eriksson-Mangold, M., & Bech-Karlsen, A. (1984). Preferred hearing aid gain and bass-cut in relation to prescriptive fitting. *Scandinavian Audiology, 13,* 157–161.

Leijon, A., Harford, E., Liden, G., Ringdahl, A., & Dahlberg, A. (1983). Audiometric earphone discomfort level and hearing aid saturation sound pressure level for a 90 decibel input signal (SSPL90) as measured in the ear canal. *Ear and Hearing, 4,* 185–189.

Leijon, A., Lindkvist, A., Ringdahl, A., & Israelsson, B. (1990). Preferred hearing aid gain in everyday use after prescriptive fitting. *Ear and Hearing, 11,* 299–305.

Libby, E. (1985). State-of-the-art hearing aid selection procedures. *Hearing Instruments, 36,* 30–38, 62.

Libby, E. (1986). The 1/3-2/3 insertion gain hearing aid selection guide. *Hearing Instruments, 37,* 27–28.

Libby, E., & Westermann, S. (1988). Principles of acoustic measurement and ear canal resonances. In R. Sandlin (Ed.), *Handbook of hearing aid amplification: Theoretical and technical considerations* (pp. 165–220). Boston: College-Hill Press.

Lybarger, S. (1955). *Basic manual for fitting Radioear hearing aids.* Pittsburgh: Radioear Corporation.

Lybarger, S. (1985). Earmolds. In J. Katz (Ed.), *Handbook of clinical audiology* (3rd ed., pp. 885–910). Baltimore: Williams & Wilkins.

Lybarger, S., & Teder, H. (1986). 2 cc coupler curves to insertion gain curves: Calculated and experimental results. *Hearing Instruments, 37,* 36–40.

Macrae, J. (1982). Invalid aided thresholds. *Hearing Instruments, 33,* 21–22.

Macrae, J., & Frazer, G. (1980). An investigation of variables affecting aided thresholds. *Australian Journal of Audiology, 2,* 56–62.

Madsen, P. (1986). Insertion gain optimization. *Hearing Instruments, 37*(1), 28–32.

Mahon, W. (1986). Real-ear probe measurements: A procedure comes of age. *Hearing Journal, 39,* 7–10.

Martin, D. (1989). Probe microphones, prescriptions and children. *Hearing Instruments, 40,* 28–29.

Martin, F., & Morris, L. (1989). Current audiologic practices in the United States. *Hearing Journal, 4,* 25–44.

Mason, D., & Popelka, G. (1986). Comparison of hearing-aid gain using functional coupler, and probe-tube measurements. *Journal of Speech and Hearing Research, 29,* 218–226.

Mauldin, L., & Trede, K. (1991). Real-ear measurements: Considerations on instrumentation and applications. *Hearing Instruments, 37*(1), 4–14.

McCandless, G. (1982). In the ear canal acoustic measurements. In G. Studebaker & F. Bess (Eds.), *Vanderbilt hearing aid report* (pp. 170–174). Upper Darby, PA: Associated Hearing Instruments.

McCandless, G., & Lyregaard, P. (1983). Prescription of gain/output (POGO) for hearing aids. *Hearing Instruments, 34,* 16–21.

McDonald, F., & Studebaker, G. (1970). Earmold alteration as measured in the human auditory meatus. *Journal of Acoustical Society of America, 48,* 1366–1372.

Morgan, D., Dirks, D., & Bower, D. (1979). Suggested threshold sound pressure levels for frequency modulated warble tones in the sound field. *Journal of Speech and Hearing Disorders, 44,* 37–54.

Moryl, C., Danhauer, J., & DiBartolomeo, J. (1992). Real ear unaided responses in ears with tympanic membrane perforations. *Journal American Academy of Audiology, 3,* 60–65.

Mueller, H. (1981). Directional hearing aids: A 10 year report. *Hearing Instruments, 32,* 16–19.

Mueller, H. (1989). Individualizing the ordering of custom hearing instruments. *Hearing Instruments, 40,* 18–22.

Mueller, H. (1990). Probe tube microphone measures: Some opinions on terminology and procedures. *Hearing Journal, 42*(1), 1–5.

Mueller, H., & Bright, K. (1992, April). *Study of the occlusion effect using probe microphone measurements.* Paper presented at American Academy of Audiology Convention, Nashville, TN.

Mueller, H., & Bryant, M. (1991). Some commonly overlooked uses of probe microphone measurements. *Seminars in Hearing, 12,* 73–91.

Mueller, H., Bryant, M., Brown, W., & Budinger, A. (1991). Hearing aid selection for high-frequency hearing loss. In G. Studebaker, F. Bess, & L. Beck (Eds.), *The Vanderbilt hearing-aid report II* (pp. 269–287). Parkton, MD: York Press.

Mueller, H., & Budinger, A. (1990). Selection of hearing aid style. *Reports in Hearing Instrumentation and Technology, 2,* 5–10.

Mueller, H., Budinger, A., & Grimes, A. (1990). Insertion gain comparisons of ITE telecoils. *Reports in Hearing Instrumentation and Technology, 2,* 11–15.

Mueller, H., Cuttie, V., & Shaw, T. (1990). Surgical and prosthetic restoration of binaural hearing in an 88-year-old man. *Ear and Hearing, 11*(6), 460–462.

Mueller, H., & Grimes, A. (1983). Speech audiometry for hearing aid selection. *Seminars in Hearing, 4*(3), 255–272.

Mueller, H., & Grimes, A. (1986). Amplification systems for the hearing impaired. In J. Alpiner & P. McCarthy (Eds.), *Handbook of aural rehabilitation* (3rd ed., pp. 115–160). Baltimore: Williams & Wilkins.

Mueller, H., & Hawkins, D. (1990). Considerations in hearing aid selection. In R. Sandlin (Ed.), *Handbook of hearing aid amplification, volume II: Clinical considerations and fitting practices* (pp. 31–60). San Diego: College-Hill Press.

Mueller, H., Hawkins, D., & Sedge, R. (1984). Three important options in hearing aid selection. *Hearing Instruments, 35,* 14–17.

Mueller, H., & Jons, C. (1989). Some clinical guidelines for the fitting of custom hearing aids. *ASHA, 10,* 57.

Mueller, H., & Killion, M. (1990). An easy method for calculating the articulation index. *Hearing Journal, 43,* 14–17.

Mueller, H., & Sweetow, R. (1987). A clinical comparison of probe microphone systems. *Hearing Instruments, 38,* 20–21, 57.

Nielsen, H., & Rasmussen, S. (1984). New aspects in hearing aid fittings. *Hearing Instruments, 35,* 18–21.

Northern, J., & Downs, M. (1991). *Hearing in children* (4th ed.). Baltimore: Williams & Wilkins.

Northern, J., & Hattler, K. (1970). Earmold influence on aided speech identification tasks. *Journal of Speech and Hearing Research, 13,* 162–172.

Orchik, D., Cowgill, S., & Parmely, J. (1990). Peritympanic soft hearing instrument fitting in high frequency hearing loss. *Hearing Instruments, 41*(11), 28–32.

Palmer, C. (1991). *The influence of individual ear canal and eardrum characteristics on speech intelligibility and sound quality judgments.* Unpublished doctoral dissertation. Northwestern University, Evanston, IL.

Pascoe, D. (1978). An approach to hearing aid selection. *Hearing Instruments, 34,* 12–16, 36.

Pascoe, D. (1980). Clinical implications of nonverbal methods of hearing aid selection and fitting. *Seminars in Hearing, 1,* 217–229.

Pavlovic, C. (1991). Speech recognition and five articulation indexes. *Hearing Instruments, 42,* 20–24.

Preves, D. (1977). Effects of earmold venting on coupler, manikin and real ears. *Hearing Aid Journal, 30,* 43–46.

Preves, D. (1982). Coupler and in situ measurements. In G. Studebaker & F. Bess (Eds.), *Vanderbilt hearing aid report* (pp. 74–77). Upper Darby, PA: Associated Hearing Instruments.

Preves, D. (1984). Levels of realism in hearing aid measurement techniques. *Hearing Journal, 37,* 13–19.

Preves, D. (1987). Some issues in utilizing probe tube microphone systems. *Ear and Hearing, 8*(Suppl. 5), 82S–88S.

Preves, D., Beck, L., Burnett, E., & Teder, H. (1989). Input stimuli for obtaining frequency responses of automatic gain control hearing aids. *Journal of Speech and Hearing Research, 32,* 189–194.

Preves, D., & Sullivan, R. (1987). Sound field equalization for real ear measurements with probe microphones. *Hearing Instruments, 38,* 20–26, 64.

Punch, J., Chi, C., & Patterson, J. (1990). A recommended protocol for prescriptive use of target gain rules. *Hearing Instruments, 41,* 12–19.

Rankovic, C. (1991). An application of the articulation index to hearing aid fitting. *Journal of Speech and Hearing Research, 34,* 391–403.

Rasmussen, S. (1984). How insertion gain measurements can take the guess work out of hearing aid fittings. *Hearing Instruments, 34,* 20, 48.

Revit, L. (1987). *New loudspeaker locations for improved reliability in clinical measure of the insertion gain of hearing aids.* Unpublished master's thesis, Northwestern University, Evanston, IL.

Revit, L. (1990). A software program for calculating 2cc full-on gain and SSPL90 targets. *Hearing Instruments, 41,* 34–35.

Revit, L. (1991a). New tests for signal-processing and multichannel hearing instruments. *Hearing Journal, 44,* 20–23.

Revit, L. (1991b). The articulation index and hearing aid fitting. *Larry's Corner,* Summer.

Revit, L. (1991c). My voice sounds like it's in a barrel. *Larry's Corner,* Autumn.

Revit, L. (1991d). An open letter: New thinking on the proper application of real-ear unaided response measurements to prescriptions and fittings. *New Zealand Audiological Society Bulletin, 1,* 1–17.

Ringdahl, A., & Leijon, A. (1984). The reliability of insertion gain measurements using probe microphones in the ear canal. *Scandinavian Audiology, 13,* 173–178.

Rintlemann, W., & Bess, F. (1988). High-level amplification and potential hearing loss in children. In F. Bess (Ed.), *Hearing impairment in children* (pp. 278–309). Parkton, MD: York Press.

Romanow, F. (1942). Methods for measuring the performance of hearing aids. *Journal of Acoustical Society of America, 13,* 294–304.

Roeser, R., & Crandell, C. (1991a). More on "The responsibility of audiologists in cerumen management." *Audiology Today, 3,* 20–21.

Roeser, R., & Crandell, C. (1991b). The audiologist's role in cerumen management. *ASHA, 33,* 51–53.

Ryals, B., & Auther, L. (1990). Difference in hearing instrument gain as a function of age. *Hearing Instruments, 41,* 26–28.

Sachs, R., & Burkhard, M. (1972a). Earphone pressure response in ear and couplers. *Journal Acoustical Society of America, 52,* 183(A).

Sachs, R., & Burkhard, M. (1972b). Making pressure measurements in insert earphones, couplers, and real ears. *Journal Acoustical Society of America, 51,* 140(A).

Sanders, J. (1964). Masking in audiometry. *Archives of Otolaryngology, 80,* 541–556.

Schum, D. (1990). Noise reduction strategies for elderly, hearing-impaired listeners. *Journal of American Academy of Audiology, 1,* 31–36.

Schwartz, D. (1982). Hearing aid selection methods: An enigma. In G. Studebaker & F. Bess (Eds.), *Vanderbilt hearing aid report* (pp. 180–187). Upper Darby, PA: Associated Hearing Instruments.

Schwartz, D., Lyregaard, P., & Lundh, P. (1988). Hearing aid selection for severe-to-profound hearing loss. *Hearing Journal, 41,* 13–17.

Schwietzer, H. (1986). Time: The third dimension of hearing aid performance. *Hearing Instruments, 37,* 17–19.

Schwietzer, H., Sullivan, R., Beck, L., & Cole, W. (1990). Developing a consensus for real-ear hearing instrument terms. *Hearing Instruments, 41,* 28, 46.

Seewald, R. (1988). The desired sensation level approach for children: Selection and verification. *Hearing Instruments, 39,* 18–22.

Seewald, R. (1990). *Probe-tube microphone measurements with children.* Paper presented at the Fourth Hearing Aid Conference, Washington University School of Medicine.

Seewald, R. (1992). The desired sensation level method for fitting children. Version 3.0. *Hearing Journal, 45,* 36–46.

Seewald, R., & Ross, M. (1988). Amplification for young hearing-impaired children. In M. Pollack (Ed.), *Amplification for the hearing-impaired* (pp. 213–271). Orlando, FL: Grune & Stratton.

Seewald, R., Ross, M., & Spiro, M. (1985). Selecting amplification characteristics for young hearing-impaired children. *Ear and Hearing, 6,* 48–53.

Seewald, R., Ross, M., & Stelmachowicz, P. (1987). Selecting and verifying hearing aid performance characteristics for children. *Journal of the Academy of Rehabilitative Audiology, 20,* 25–37.

Seewald, R., Zelisko, D., Ramji, K., & Jamieson, D. (1991). *DSL 3.0 user's manual.* London, Ontario, Canada: University of Western Ontario.

Shaw, E. (1974). Transformation of sound pressure from the free field to the eardrum in the horizontal plane. *Journal of the Acoustical Society of America, 56,* 1848–1861.

Shore, I., Bilger, R., & Hirsch, I. (1960). Hearing aid evaluation: Reliability of repeated measurements. *Journal of Speech and Hearing Disorders, 25,* 152–170.

Sigelman, J., & Preves. D. (1987). Field trials of a new adaptive signal processor hearing aid circuit. *Hearing Journal, 40,* 4, 24–27.

Simon, C., & Harlow, B. (1987). Real ear measurement — A practical perspective. *Hearing Instruments, 38,* 12–14, 57.

Skadegard, H. (1987). Real ear measurements — A professional tool. *Hearing Instruments, 38,* 13.

Skinner, M. (1988). *Hearing aid evaluation.* Englewood Cliffs, NJ: Prentice-Hall.

Skinner, M., Pascoe, D., Miller, J., & Popelka, G. (1982). Measurements to determine the optimal placement of speech energy within the listener's auditory area: A basis for selecting amplification characteristics. In G. Studebaker & F. Bess (Eds.), *The Vanderbilt hearing aid report* (pp. 161–169). Upper Darby, PA: Associated Hearing Instruments.

Smaldino, J., & Hoene, D. (1981). A view of state of

hearing aid fitting practices: Part I. *Hearing Instruments, 32,* 14–15, 38.

Staab, W., & Finlay, B. (1991). A fitting rationale for deep fitting canal hearing instruments. *Hearing Instruments, 42,* 6–10, 48.

Stach, B., Speerschneider, J., & Jerger, J. (1987). Evaluating the efficacy of automatic signal processing hearing aids. *Hearing Journal, 40,* 15–19.

Stelmachowicz, P. (1991). Clinical issues related to hearing aid maximum output. In G. Studebaker, F. Bess, & L. Beck (Eds.), *The Vanderbilt hearing-aid report II* (pp. 141–148). Parkton, MD: York Press.

Stelmachowicz, P., & Lewis, D. (1988). Some theoretical considerations concerning the relation between functional gain and insertion gain. *Journal of Speech and Hearing Research, 31,* 491–496.

Stelmachowicz, P., & Seewald, R. (1991). Probe-tube microphone measures in children. *Seminars in Hearing, 12,* 62–72.

Stelmachowicz, P., Lewis, D., Seewald, R., & Hawkins, D. (1990). Complex and pure-tone signals in the evaluation of hearing-aid characteristics. *Journal of Speech and Hearing Research, 33,* 380–385.

Stuart, A., Durieux-Smith, A., & Stenstrom, R. (1990). Critical differences in aided sound field thresholds in children. *Journal of Speech and Hearing Research, 33,* 612–615.

Stuart, A., Durieux-Smith, A., & Stenstrom, R. (1991). Probe tube microphone measures of loudness discomfort levels in children. *Ear and Hearing, 12,* 140–143.

Stuart, A., Stenstrom, R., MacDonald, O., Schmidt, M., & MacLean, G. (1992). Probe-tube microphone measures of vent effects with in-the-canal hearing aid shells. *American Journal of Audiology, 1*(2), 58–62.

Studebaker, G. (1991). Measures of intelligibility and quality. In G. Studebaker, F. Bess, & L. Beck (Eds.), *The Vanderbilt hearing-aid report II* (pp. 185–195). Parkton, MD: York Press.

Studebaker, G. (1992). The effect of equating loudness on audibility-based hearing aid selection procedures. *Journal of the American Academy of Audiology, 3*(2), 113–118.

Studebaker, G., Cox, R., & Wark, D. (1982). Earmold modification effect measured by coupler, threshold, and probe techniques. *Audiology, 17,* 173–186.

Studebaker, G., & Zachman, T. (1970). Investigation of the acoustics of earmold vents. *Journal of Acoustical Society of America, 47,* 110–115.

Sullivan, J., Levitt, H., Hwang, J., & Hennessey, A. (1988). An experimental comparison of four hearing aid prescription methods. *Ear and Hearing,* 9, 22–32.

Sullivan, R. (1985). An acoustic coupling-based classification system for hearing aid fittings. *Hearing Instruments,* 9 (Part I), 25–28; 12, (Part II & III), 16–22.

Sullivan, R. (1987). Aided SSPL 90 response in the real ear: A safe estimate. *Hearing Instruments, 38,* 36.

Sullivan, R. (1988). Probe tube microphone placement near the tympanic membrane. *Hearing Instruments, 39,* 43–44, 60.

Sullivan, R. (1989a). Custom canal and concha hearing instruments: A real ear comparison. *Hearing Instruments, 40,* 23–29.

Sullivan, R. (1989b). Custom canal and concha hearing instruments: A real ear comparison. *Hearing Instruments, 40,* 30–36, 58.

Sullivan, R. (1990). Acoustic coupling classification system and custom hearing aids. *Reports on Hearing Instrumentation and Technology, 2,* 15–22.

Surr, R., & Hawkins, D. (1988). New hearing aid users' perception of the "hearing aid effect." *Ear and Hearing, 9,* 113–118.

Sweetow, R. (1991). The truth behind "non-occluding" earmolds. *Hearing Instruments, 42,* 25.

Sweetow, R., & Mueller, H. (1991a). The interfacing of hearing aids and probe microphone measures. *Audecibel, 40,* 2, 19–22.

Sweetow, R., & Mueller, H. (1991b). The interfacing of programmable hearing aids and probe microphone measures (Part 2). *Audecibel, 40,* 3, 17–20.

Talbott, C., & Matsumoto, J. (1990). Effects of ventilating tubes on external ear resonance in infants. *ASHA, 32*(10), 62.

Tecca, J. (1990). Clinical application of real-ear probe tube measurement. In R. Sandlin (Ed.), *Handbook of hearing aid amplification, volume II: Clinical considerations and fitting practices* (pp. 225–255). Boston, MA: College-Hill Press.

Tecca, J. (1991a). Reliability of insertion gain measures. *Seminars in Hearing, 12*(1), 15–25.

Tecca, J. (1991b). Real ear vent effects in ITE hearing instrument fittings. *Hearing Instruments, 42,* 10–12.

Upfold, G., & Byrne, D. (1988). Variability of ear canal resonance and its implications for the design of hearing aids and earplugs. *Australian Journal of Audiology, 10,* 97–102.

Valente, M. (1990). Intratester and test-retest reliability of insertion gain measures. *Ear and Hearing, 11,* 181–184.

Valente, M. (1991). Reliability and intersubject variability of the real ear unaided response. *Ear and Hearing, 12,* 216–220.

Valente, M., Valente, M., & Vass, W. (1990). Selecting an appropriate matrix for ITE/ITC hearing instruments. *Hearing Instruments, 41,* 20–24.

Valente, M., Valente, M., & Vass, W. (1991). Use of real-ear measures to select the gain and output of hearing aids. *Seminars in Hearing, 12,* 53–61.

Walker, G., Dillon, H., & Byrne, D. (1984). Sound field audiometry: Recommended stimuli and procedures. *Ear and Hearing, 5,* 13–21.

Walker, G., Dillon, H., Byrne, D., & Christen, R. (1984). The use of loudness discomfort levels for selecting the maximum output of hearing aids. *Australian Journal of Audiology, 6,* 23–32.

Wallber, M., MacKenzie, D., & Clyme, E. (1987). *Telecoil evaluation procedure.* National Technical Institute for the Deaf, Rochester Institute of Technology. St. Louis: Auditec of St. Louis.

Watson, N., & Knudsen, V. (1940). Selective amplification in hearing aids. *Journal of Acoustical Society of America, 11,* 406–419.

Weiner, F., & Ross, D. (1946). The pressure distribution in the auditory canal in a progressive sound field. *Journal of Acoustical Society of America, 18,* 401–408.

Wetzell, C., & Harford, E. (1983). Predictability of real ear hearing aid performance from coupler measurements. *Ear and Hearing, 4,* 237–242.

Wimmer, V. (1986). The occlusion effect from earmolds. *Hearing Instruments, 37,* 19, 57–58.

Zelisko, D., Seewald, R., & Gagne, J-P. (1990). Reliability of a procedure for measuring loudness discomfort in children. *Journal of Speech-Language Pathology and Audiology, 14,* 56.

Zemplenyi, J., Dirks, D., & Gilman, S. (1985). Probe-determined hearing-aid gain compared to functional and coupler gains. *Journal of Speech and Hearing Research, 28,* 394–404.

Zemplenyi, J., Gilman, S., & Dirks, D. (1985). Optical method for measurement of ear canal length. *Journal of Acoustical Society of America, 78,* 2146–2148.

Zwislocki, J. (1970). *An acoustic coupler for earphone calibration.* Report LSC-S-7, Lab Sensory Communication, Syracuse University, NY.

Zwislocki, J. (1971). *An ear-like coupler for earphone calibration.* Report LSC-S-9, Lab Sensory Communication, Syracuse University, NY.

■ INDEX ■